TEACHING EMS:
An Educator's Guide to Improved EMS Instruction

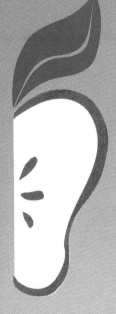

TEACHING EMS:
An Educator's Guide to
Improved EMS Instruction

Catherine A. Parvensky, MEd, RN, EMT

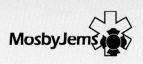

An Affiliate of Elsevier Science

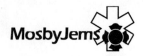

An Affiliate of Elsevier Science

Publisher: David Dusthimer
Executive Editor: Claire Merrick
Editor: Rina Steinhauer
Developmental Editor: Melissa Blair
Project Manager: Chris Baumle
Production Editor: Stacy M. Guarracino
Design Manager: Nancy J. McDonald
Cover Illustrator: Margie Caldwell-Gill

Printed in the United States of America

Mosby, Inc.
11830 Westline Industrial Drive
St. Louis, Missouri 63146

Library of Congress Cataloging–in–Publication Data
Parvensky, Catherine A.
    Teaching EMS: an educator's guide to improved EMS instruction/
  Catherine A. Parvensky.
        p. cm.
    Includes bibliographical references and index.
    ISBN (invalid) 0-8151-6611-7 (alk. paper)
    1. Emergency medical services—Study and teaching. I. Title.
RA645.5P37 1995   95-4793
616.02'5'071—dc20
03 04 05 / 9 8 7 6 5 4

AUTHOR'S ACKNOWLEDGMENTS

One of the most difficult parts of writing a book is recognizing all those individuals who have influenced, or assisted in some form, with the completion of the text. While I am certain to inadvertently omit someone, I will attempt to acknowledge those individuals that have contributed in some manner.

First and foremost, I would like to thank my family. To Mom (Irene), Mary, John, Andi, Paula, Emil, Anna, Margaret, and David, thank you for all your love and support.

To Philip Barwell, my soon to be husband, thank you for your love, support, encouragement, and strength. Without it, this past year would have been a nightmare.

To Jerry Peters, thank you for your continued encouragement. Were it not for you, this project would probably never been initiated. Thanks for being so pushy.

To Gail Dubs, Everitt Binns, and John Lewis, a special thanks for taking me under your wing. Your knowledge and experience have been a valuable learning tool for me. You have certainly helped me to achieve all I have, and for that I thank you. A special thanks to you Gail, for providing so much of the information and examples outlined in the games section of this text.

To Bill Milheim, Marilyn Lake-DelAngelo and the rest of the Penn State gang, I told you I could get a Masters Degree in nine months. The professors of the Instructional Systems Masters Program taught me more than I thought possible and significantly added to the contents of this text. Thank you for your imparted knowledge and wisdom.

To John Haynes, Carol Hammond, Latta White, John Weer, and Grace Manuel, I include you because you threatened me if I did not. From the early years of EMS to the current days of 911 and training, thanks for your continued support and assistance. You are great co-workers and staff.

To the staff of JEMS and Mosby Lifeline, my wholehearted thanks. To Nancy Peterson, thank you for initiating this project. To Melissa Blair, Rina Steinhauer, and Stacy Guarracino, thanks for keeping me on track and imparting your publishing expertise on me. And, especially to Claire Merrick, thank you for having enough faith in my ability to complete a project of this size.

Finally, to all the individuals I forgot to mention who either knowingly or incidently imparted some of the wisdom contained in this text, I thank you.

PUBLISHER'S ACKNOWLEDGEMENTS

The editors wish to acknowledge and thank the reviewers of this book. Their comments were invaluable in the development of this manuscript.

Chip Boehm, RN, EMT-P
Training Coordinator
Maine Emergency Medical Services
Augusta, Maine

Everitt F. Binns, PhD
Executive Director
Eastern Pennsylvania EMS Council
Allentown, Pennsylvania

Robert Elling, MPA, NREMT-P
Senior EMS Representative
New York State EMS Program
Albany, New York

Note on Gender Terminology

Throughout this text, reference to the gender of students, providers, and instructors is in the masculine. This usage stems from the generally accepted standards of grammar and is not in any way indicative of any desire on the part of the author or editors to deny the very real role played by members of both sexes in providing prehospital emergency care and EMS education.

FOREWORD

The road to finally having an EMS Instructor text has been a long and arduous one. It began in the early 1980s. When the National Highway Traffic Safety Administration (NHTSA) assumed responsibility for the development of Emergency Medical Services training programs, their intent was to develop programs of the highest quality with current and up-to-date status in both technical content and instructional strategy. While NHTSA developed numerous training programs for EMS personnel, the instructional delivery of those standardized programs varied markedly. The fact was that in the majority of programs nationwide, instructors had little or no formal education or training in how to teach. To that end, NHTSA contracted to develop a training program specifically for EMS Instructors.

In 1983, pilot courses for the EMS Instructor Training Program began. As a participant in one of those early pilot courses, I closely observed the actions of Nels Sandahl, Mike French, Janet Head and Rocco Morando. I found myself wishing that I could fix some of those memorable classroom exchanges in my mind for instant recall when needed. There was, of course, nothing more than a notebook of outlines for us to jot our notes. In 1986, the first edition of *Emergency Medical Services Instructor Training Program: A National Standard Curriculum* was published. Since that time, the EMS Instructor Training Program has become a mandatory course in many states for those who wish to teach in EMS. There still, however, is only a curriculum with lesson plans and a Student Study Guide; there is no textbook that satisfactorily meets the intent and objectives of the course as well as the needs of the participants.

Catherine's book is such a text. I was delighted to be asked to review it and even more excited to discover in its contents the essence of what EMS Instructors need to know. This text is the perfect compliment to the EMS Instructor Training Program and a handy source for those of us who have taken the course and need a ready reference.

While the content of this text meets the intent and objectives of the EMS Instructor Training Program, it also surpasses those basic guidelines. There are additional sections on cross cultural communications, current technological advances such as computer aided instruction, remediation of learning deficiencies, behavior modification and preparing students for certification exams.

With the advent of this text and the continuing work of educators, such as Janet Head and Catherine Parvensky and others, we are also seeing the advent of a move toward professionalism of the EMS Instructor. The days of selecting someone to be an instructor just because they are a good practitioner are coming to a close. EMT courses that are worth college credit and paramedic courses that are worth an Associate Degree are becoming more frequent. The effort toward enhancing critical thinking skills and strengthening a student's ability to make sound field judgements is requiring more skills of the instructor than just how to recognize the compensated shock patient. This move toward teaching higher levels of cognitive processing is, in turn, requiring more education of its instructors. Thus, the critical need for a text for EMS Instructors.

The very element that makes the good practitioner the one chosen to be the instructor is their functioning knowledge of the context within which the material is taught. While the value of field experience can never be overestimated, neither should the education of the practitioner into an instructor. If that field knowledge can not be translated into an understandable form that helps students make the transition from the classroom to the field, it is for nothing. The ability to make that transition not only calls for a functioning knowledge of the field, but also a knowledge of teaching techniques and a knowledge of the characteristics of the adult learner. Together, these three factors, when correctly applied to any classroom situation, have the potential to positively effect the lives of many hundreds of patients as well as the EMTs who care for them...and isn't that what we are about? Now we have Catherine's book to help us.

Twink Dalton
April, 1995

PREFACE

My father passed away many years ago. At the age of only forty-five, he suffered a massive heart attack while on a business trip. He left behind nine children of which I am the youngest. At only eleven years of age, I could not comprehend why he had died, I only knew he wasn't coming home.

In an effort to decrease the instances in which other small children lose a parent, I entered the health care field. I started as a hospital nurse but soon contracted that "EMS bug" and entered into the pre-hospital medical arena. My first call–cardiac arrest; my partner–my instructor. Then it hit me... the only thing I knew was what he had taught me... It must have worked, the patient survived. Then I got the "EMS Teaching Bug."

Several years later, in the middle of the night, my brother-in-law phoned and told me my sister had fallen on the driveway and was bleeding severely. I hurried to her house and arrived with the rest of the ensemble: the QRS unit, the Ambulance and the Medic Unit. I hurried to her side and looked around, only to notice that most of the EMS providers were once students of mine, and I thought... "Oh my God, they only know what I taught them"; what a scary thought.

From that day forward, I set out to ensure that anyone within our County, in need of emergency medical treatment, would receive it from the most qualified and competently trained individuals. Where to start? With the instructors.

EMS education is in part a skill of its own, but so much of the basic art of teaching stems from sound principles of learning. This text is a compilation of the most current educational concepts, strategies and techniques. It is designed to help you, the new or seasoned EMS instructor, understand learning principles and adapt teaching strategies to increase the effectiveness of the classes you teach.

Learning is a never-ending process. In fact, the day we stop learning is the day we die. As such, no single text can contain all the solutions to all the problems you will encounter, nor can it provide all the ideas for improved instruction. *Teaching EMS* will, however, provide a solid foundation from which you can evolve as an effective instructor. Once you have the basic knowledge, add a little experience and you're on your way to never worrying "Oh my God, they only know what I've taught them."

I have attempted to lace this text with helpful strategies to improve EMS instruction. Throughout your teaching journeys, I welcome any ideas you have for new teaching methods, solutions to common problems encountered in classes, new games or techniques for increasing learning retention or student motivation, or even problems or concerns which you would like addressed. Please send your ideas or questions to the address below, and I will try to incorporate them into future editions of this text.

Mosby Lifeline
Re: Parvensky / Teaching EMS
7250 Parkway Drive, Suite 510
Hanover, MD 21076

Good luck and happy teaching.

CONTENTS

1 The Learning Process

OBJECTIVES

Upon completion of this chapter, the reader will have sufficient information to:

1. Identify the three domains of learning.
2. List the six levels of the cognitive domain, the five levels of the psychomotor domain, and the five levels of the affective domain.
3. Define hemisphericity.
4. Describe various characteristics of right-brain and left-brain students.
5. List five characteristics for students with each perceptual modality (visual, auditory, and kinesthetic).
6. Describe six social styles that may affect how students learn and participate in classroom activities.
7. Describe the process of Witkin's testing for field dependence and identify seven characteristics for both field-dependent and field-independent students.
8. Identify five methods to increase student motivation, based on field dominance.
9. Define conceptual tempo and describe the differences between impulsive and reflective individuals.
10. List the characteristics for each of the four types of students identified in the 4MAT system.
11. Describe four methods to determine learning style preferences.
12. Identify eight potential barriers to the learning process.
13. List eight factors that affect student learning rates.
14. Describe five methods to increase learning rates.
15. Describe the importance of knowing the individual characteristics of learning styles.

KEY TERMS

Affective domain One of three domains of learning, pertaining to student attitudes, values, and emotional growth; includes five categories: receiving, responding, valuing, organization and characterization

Affective strategies Learning strategies directed toward improving the successful attainment of objectives targeted toward the affective domain; strategies include focusing student attention, maintaining motivation, and managing time in an attempt to improve student involvement

Automaticity The result of overlearning a behavior to the point where it can be performed without conscious thought

Baseline A natural occurrence of behavior before any intervention

Behavioral objectives Statements regarding a desired outcome or specific change instructors intend to produce in student behavior

Cognitive domain One of the three domains of learning pertaining to intellectual abilities, comprising six levels: knowledge, comprehension, application, analysis, synthesis, and evaluation

Cognitive style The way in which a student consistently responds to perceptual tasks; also referred to as *learning style*

Conceptual tempo A cognitive style referring to the speed at which individuals respond to a task and the number of errors they make in such responses, usually referred to as *impulsive* or *reflective*

Education The general acquisition of information in order to better oneself; education is the process by which one learns study habits, problem-solving, and general principles that govern the learning process throughout one's life; education alone, however, will not prepare someone for a specific vocation

Field-dependent A cognitive style in which a student operates in a global manner and is distracted by background elements

Field-independent A cognitive style in which a student is capable of overcoming the effects of distracting elements within a field or background when attempting to differentiate important aspects of a particular situation

Hemisphericity The identification of two halves of the human brain, each controlling different functions; the right hemisphere appears to be primarily responsible for spatial relationships and imagination, while the left side is primarily responsible for verbal abilities and sequencing

Impulsive A dimension of conceptual tempo in which students respond quickly, thereby making a moderate number of errors

Intelligence The capacity that allows a student to learn, solve problems, or successfully interact with the environment

Learned helplessness A situation in which students learn, over time and through constant failure, that they cannot control the outcome of events affecting their lives

Learning An active process of communication between students and instructors, resulting in the gaining of knowledge and mastering of information; learning results in a relatively permanent change or modification in behavior as a result of experience or training

Learning style Similar to cognitive styles, these are individual differences that influence the way in which a student learns and processes information

Locus of control An individual's perception of whom or what is responsible for the outcome of events and behaviors in their lives

Mastery learning An instructional strategy that allows students to study material until they master it

Perceptual modalities Any one of the sensory channels through which a student receives information

Programmed instruction An instructional process in which material is developed in a particular sequence and in small steps, requiring students to respond and providing immediate feedback

Psychomotor domain One of three domains of learning, primarily affecting the physical ability to perform skills or other type movement

Reflective Dimension of conceptual tempo in which students are slow to respond and tend to make fewer errors

Self-concept The total organization of perception that an individual has of himself; often used interchangeably with *self-esteem*

Self-efficacy The belief that one can successfully execute the behavior required to produce a particular outcome

Self-esteem The value or judgement a student places on his behavior; often used interchangeably with *self-concept*

Teaching A system of actions intended to induce learning

Training The process of acquiring specific knowledge and skills necessary to perform a skill or task; training is common in the industry in order to prepare workers for specific tasks and is designed to affect performance by teaching skills

INTRODUCTION

Teaching is a system of actions intended to induce learning. Learning is a process by which behavior is either modified or changed through experience or training. Although teaching and learning are related, they are independent processes. Sometimes teaching leads to learning, but not always. Although an instructor may facilitate it, each student must take responsibility for his or her own learning.

Training is the process of acquiring the specific knowledge and skills necessary to perform a skill or task, whereas educating is the general acquisition of information in order to better oneself. An effective EMS training program incorporates learning, education, and training. In addition to teaching students *how* to perform a specific skill, it is also important to inform them of *when* and *why* the skill is performed. While some EMS educators will argue that the responsibility of an instructor is to train and not educate, the two go hand in hand.

An effective EMS training program incorporates learning, education, and training.

In order for training to be effective, the following criteria must be met:

- Students must be taught how, when, and why to perform a specific task.
- Students must have the psychomotor ability to perform the task.
- Students must have the desire or motivation to perform the task.

It is common for instructors to encounter students who memorize an entire text and can recite every indication and contraindication for performing a skill, yet have absolutely no coordination and cannot pass a practical examination. It is important for instructors to understand that it is impossible to teach students to be coordinated; they either are or they are not. All that can be done in an attempt to help sharpen a student's coordination, is to offer assistance and perhaps extra time for practice.

How students process information does not make them stupid, slow, or difficult—only unique. Kiersey and Bates' book *Please Understand Me* identifies such differences and stresses the importance of empathy— walking in the shoes of another before casting blame that they are not trying to learn or are too stupid[1]. These students may simply process information differently than the instructor is presenting it. This difference may cause a conflict resulting in the inability of the student to learn.

While it may not be practical to modify presentations to meet all of the needs of every student, it is important for instructors to identify the majority of styles and to provide information in a fashion students can understand.

Identifying a student's style proves invaluable for remedial training. If a student has been unable to comprehend certain information, instructors should not simply cast them aside as being unable to learn, but rather should find out the student's style and present the information according to the way the student processes it. Chances are they will learn just fine.

DOMAINS OF LEARNING

The learning process involves three steps: obtaining information, processing it, and attaching value to it. In emergency medical service (EMS), the value attached through training results in judgement. This judgement allows EMS providers to take classroom knowledge and, in a given situation, act appropriately. More specifically, the value a student attaches to the training he receives will result in the ability to recognize a problem and intervene with the proper treatment in an appropriate amount of time, in order to affect patient outcome positively.

Theorists have identified three primary domains involved with the learning process: the cognitive, psychomotor, and affective domains, as shown in Figure 1.1. The cognitive domain deals with the intellect, the knowledge of information and facts. The psychomotor domain deals with the learning of skills requiring motion or muscle coordination of some sort. The affective domain is the most difficult to understand and teach, as it focuses on attaching attitudes, values, and feelings to information learned.

Cognitive Domain
The cognitive domain[2] is described based on a continuum of intellectual learning, from most simple to most complex. It is in the cognitive

> The learning process involves three steps: obtaining information, processing it, and attaching value to it.

> It is in the cognitive domain that students deal with facts, knowledge, and information.

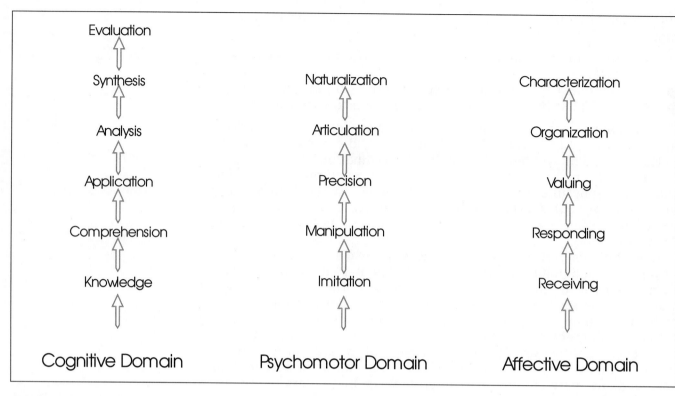

FIGURE 1.1   The Three Domains of Learning

domain that students deal with facts, knowledge, and information. There are six levels in this domain.

Knowledge

This category of the cognitive domain generally requires memorization of information for immediate recall. In EMS education, it is at this level that students can recall facts, *eg*, the ability to recite signs and symptoms, or components of the respiratory system. Such memorization and recall of facts is considered the lowest level in this domain.

> Behavioral terms indicating that objects within this category have been met include the following: identify, define, list, name, and recognize.

Comprehension

At this level the student interprets the information he or she receives. Comprehension includes the ability to understand the meaning behind information. For example, the ability to evaluate the effectiveness of the cardiovascular system based on a patient's blood pressure, pulse, respiratory rate, level of consciousness, and capillary refill requires the student to comprehend the symptoms of cardiovascular compromise.

> Behavioral terms indicating that objectives within this category have been met include the following: evaluate, describe, explain, estimate, interpret, and summarize.

Application

It is at this level that students apply the knowledge they gained to what they are doing. This category is very important in EMS education, since students must be able to take classroom information and apply it in real-life situations.

The application phase of the cognitive domain requires students to take information they have learned and apply it in a new situation. An example of this level is a student knowing from the signs and symptoms a person exhibits that he is about to go into shock, and taking measures to prevent it from happening.

Behavioral terms indicating that objectives within this category have been met include the following: demonstrate, explain, calculate, identify, and apply.

Analysis

This level requires students to separate information into pieces in order to analyze and thoroughly understand its structure. In EMS, an example of this is responding to the aid of an unconscious victim; the student must take all available data and determine the cause of such unconsciousness. Such data might include witnesses, medical alert tags, physical surroundings, medications, and a physical assessment.

Behavioral terms indicating that objectives within this category have been met include the following: distinguish, outline, identify, and discriminate.

Synthesis

This component of the cognitive domain requires students to combine pieces of information into a new structure. It is at this level that students put information analyzed at the previous level together differently.

An example of this level is the student with the same unconscious patient mentioned above, evaluating all available data, and realizing that the patient is taking insulin and, therefore, has a past medical history of diabetes. Family members state that the patient has not eaten all day, thus the student concludes that the patient is suffering from a diabetic emergency and requires the administration of glucose.

Behavioral terms indicating that objectives within this category have been met include the following: design, organize, formulate, determine, create, and compose.

Evaluation

The final level in this domain deals with putting a worth on knowledge by making judgements against specific criteria. In EMS education, an example would include determining whether a patient requires the use of an aeromedical evacuation unit based on information gathered.

Behavioral terms indicating that objectives within this category have been met include the following: examine, evaluate, judge, compare, contrast, and critique.

The psychomotor domain is a skills domain.

Psychomotor Domain

The second domain, the psychomotor domain, is a skills domain consisting of five levels.

Imitation

At this level students simply imitate what is done by instructors. An example of this is watching the instructor insert an airway, then inserting one the same way.

Manipulation

It is at this level that students change what they are doing and start performing the skill their own way. Students may make mistakes, but should keep practicing to work out their own "style" for performing a skill. For example, when applying a spinal immobilization device, students must practice the application of this device and develop their own way of doing it quickly and accurately.

Precision

At this stage students practice and perform skills more easily and accurately. An example of this is taking a blood pressure measurement. After performing this task repeatedly, it becomes second nature.

Articulation

At this level everything that has been learned fits together nicely. The student knows how to perform a skill, does it proficiently, and fits it into all surrounding skills. An example of this is the application and use of an automated external defibrillator (AED) device. The student may be proficient at individual skills such as the primary survey, airway obstruction, performing cardiopulmonary resuscitation (CPR), maintaining airway control, and the actual AED application and discharge of electric current. Here all the components fit together so the student flows easily through the entire process.

Naturalization

It is at this, the final level of the psychomotor domain, that everything comes naturally. The student arrives at a situation, knows what to do, and does it without a hitch. An example of this is a cardiac arrest scenario. From arriving to find the patient, assessing the patient, initiating CPR, assembling and administering oxygen through a bag-valve-mask device, and transporting the patient to the hospital—proficiently, quickly, and without incident—the process has become automatic.

Affective Domain

The third and final domain is the affective domain. The affective domain involves attaching emotions, attitudes, and values to information and learning[3]. A student cannot achieve the highest level of the cognitive or psychomotor domain without achieving the affective domain. There are five levels of attitudes, interests, or personal involvement within this domain, each dealing with the students' degree of positive feelings about what they are learning.

The affective domain involves attaching emotions, attitudes, and values to information and learning[3].

Receiving

This component of the affective domain is the most basic and involves an awareness of the importance of learning and the willingness to concentrate on the information being presented. An example of this component in EMS includes the attentiveness of students in the classroom.

Behavioral terms indicating that objectives within this category have been met include the following: observe, attend, demonstrate, listen, ask, and concentrate.

Responding

This area involves the willingness of the student to participate actively in learning and deriving some amount of satisfaction from doing so. In EMS education, an example of this component might include volunteering with an ambulance service to help those in need and to practice the knowledge they have learned.

Behavioral terms indicating that objectives within this category have been met include the following: volunteer, perform, participate, assist, help, and answer.

> **"If a man does not keep pace with his companions, perhaps it is because he hears a different drummer. Let him step to the music which he hears, however measured or far away."**
> **Henry David Thoreau**

Valuing

This involves the perception that a behavior or object has worth. It also includes commitment to the task at hand. In EMS, an example of valuing is volunteering to take an ambulance call rather that attending a party because of the belief that the ambulance call is more important.

Behavioral terms indicating that objectives within this category have been met include the following: appreciate, differentiate, justify, select, and value.

Organization

This next component of the affective domain is more complex and involves integrating differing values and beliefs, reconciling such differences, and formulating a consistent value system within oneself. An example of use of this component within the EMS system is an ambulance call in which two emergency medical technicians (EMTs) disagree as to the proper treatment. Comparing strategies to determine the appropriate action to take might involve explaining, defending, or compromising in order to best serve the patient, and may result in the development of a new value system.

Behavioral terms indicating that objectives within this category have been met include the following: explain, defend, compare, combine, organize, synthesize, recognize, and integrate.

Characterization

This is the value system that governs a student's behavior. It is because of this characterization that students act and react in a certain fashion, one that is consistent with one's own value system.

Behavioral terms indicating that objectives within this category have been met include the following: act, perform, practice, demonstrate, and influence.

LEARNING STYLES

Students process information in different ways and usually have a preference in the way they receive information. Because of this it is important that instructors understand these differences and modify their presentation styles to recognize and adapt to the various learning styles of their students.

Students process information in different ways and usually have a preference in the way they receive information.

Hemisphericity

Students usually have a dominant way in which information is organized within the cerebral hemisphere[4]. Each side of the brain, although connected and working together, functions differently. If a student is "right-brained," the processing of information is done primarily in the right side of the brain, leading to a more global or intuitive student. In contrast, if a student is "left-brained," the processing of information is done primarily in the left side of the brain, leading to a more analytical or logical student. Each of these types of students exhibits various characteristics, as identified in Figure 1.2.

Right-Brain Students

Students who think predominantly with the right side of the brain tend to be more global, visual, emotional, creative, innovative, and intuitive. They tend to use intuition, beliefs, and opinions when forming conclusions and selecting strategies. Right-brain students tend to focus on spacial relationships.

These students tend to be artistic and are less rigid with structure. Although their desks may be cluttered with piles of papers, and they are often referred to as "messy," they know exactly where something is located.

In EMS, these students are good at recognizing the global picture and, thus are good at incident command responsibilities since they are able to develop an overall plan for handling an emergency situation.

> *Students who think predominantly with the right side of the brain tend to be more global, visual, emotional, creative, innovative, and intuitive.*

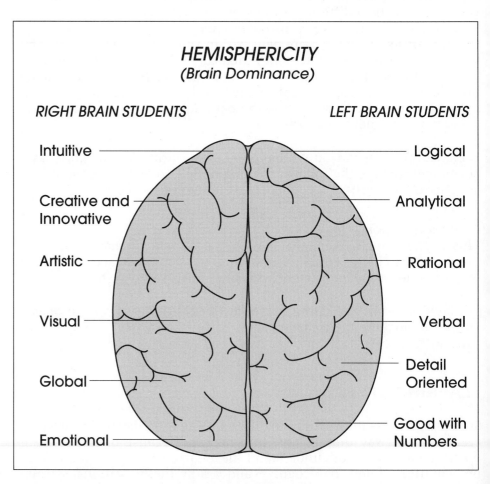

FIGURE 1.2 Characteristics of Students Based on Hemisphericity

In education, however, it is necessary for instructors to take measures to increase the use of the left hemisphere of right-brain students so these students can become more analytical when necessary.

Left-Brain Students

Students who think predominantly with the left side of the brain tend to be analytical, rational, verbal, abstract, and logical. They are generally good at speech, reading, and mathematics. These students are generally very analytical and detail-oriented. They tend to be good spellers and can remember peoples names easily. Extreme left-brain students know exactly how much money they have in their wallets and usually have the presidents facing the same direction.

Sequence is important to left-brain students. As such, they may not see the "big picture." While they generally remember learned information, they tend to have difficulty applying some of that knowledge.

Although students are predominantly right- or left-brain learners, it is essential for instructors to challenge all students to use the "weaker" side of the brain whenever possible. This can be accomplished through the selection of audiovisual materials or by planned activities that focus on skills using both sides of the brain.

For example, visual media such as a slide that presents a picture of a properly applied short board on one side of the slide, and the specific sequence in words for applying the board on the other side, will meet the needs of both the right-brain (visual and global) and left-brain (verbal and detail-oriented) students while forcing them to use the nondominant side as well. Activities such as brain teasers or scenarios requiring both creative and analytical or logical reasoning can also help increase the use of a nondominant brain hemisphere.

> Students who think predominantly with the left side of the brain tend to be analytical, rational, verbal, abstract, and logical.

Perceptual Modalities

As with hemisphericity, students tend to have a preference in how they process information. *Perceptual modalities* are the ways in which students receive information, and include all five senses. While most students receive information in a variety of ways, there is usually a preference for receiving the information, *eg,* seeing, hearing, or feeling material.

Students exhibit certain characteristics depending on their preferred modality, as identified in Box 1.1.

> While most students receive information in a variety of ways, there is usually a preference for receiving the information, *eg,* seeing, hearing, or feeling material.

Visual Learners

Students who prefer to see the information being presented are referred to as "visual learners." They tend to paint a visual picture of the information presented and respond best when instructors use visual aids such as slides, handouts, or overhead transparencies so they do not miss important information transmitted verbally or kinesthetically. Videotapes are very beneficial to this type of student.

Auditory Learners

Students who prefer to hear the information being presented are referred to as "auditory learners." These students learn best through verbal instructions from themselves or others. They listen attentively during classroom lectures and tend to disregard information they see on slides, handouts, or overhead transparencies. Audiocassettes of a lesson are very beneficial to this type of student.

BOX 1.1 Perceptual Modalities

VISUAL LEARNER	AUDITORY LEARNER	KINESTHETIC LEARNER
Expresses feelings by facial expressions (staring, smiling, pouting, *etc*)	Expresses feelings through tone, pitch, and volume of voice	Cannot sit still; fidgets or plays with things
Learns by looking at visual materials	Likes to talk about what to do	Points when reading
Likes to examine things	Would rather listen to a story than read it	Gestures when talking
Exhibits a greater immediate recall when information is presented visually	Often talks or counts to oneself	Responds physically when listening to stories
Likes the written word	Learns best through oral presentation of directions	Likes action words
Is quieter, more organized, and more deliberate	Subvocalizes to remember things	Expresses feelings physically (push, tug, stomp, *etc*)
Is first to notice changes in the classroom	Is easily distracted by sounds	Is often a poor speller; needs to write words down to see if they "feel" right
Would rather read a story than listen to it being read	Responds well to lecture and discussion sessions	Understands more when able to handle and examine things
Has trouble remembering verbal directions.		
Has a vivid imagination and thinks in pictures		
Is impatient with extensive listening activities		

Characteristics of learners based on modalities (adapted from Barbe et. al, 1979).

Kinesthetic Learners

Students who prefer to receive information through tactile stimulation are referred to as "kinesthetic learners". These students learn by doing or touching. For example, rather than hearing a lecture on how to perform CPR, kinesthetic learners prefer to jump right in and play with the manikins. Unfortunately, only a portion of EMS education cater to kinesthetic learners. As a result, these students are often forced to strengthen their auditory or visual tendencies for learning or they will most likely do poorly on written examinations.

Social Styles
How students react in various learning environments may affect how they learn[6].

How students react in various learning environments may affect how they learn[6].

Large Group Participators
These students are most comfortable when surrounded by many others, thereby making them feel somewhat anonymous. While they feel free to speak out, participate and ask questions in a large group, they sometimes feel uncomfortable participating in small groups.

Small Group Participators
These students are most comfortable in small group discussions in which they feel free to speak out. They prefer to work in groups and tend not to participate or ask questions in large group sessions where they feel somewhat intimidated or overwhelmed.

Soloists
These students prefer to learn information on their own. While they may take part in listening to a larger group session, they rarely participate because they feel uncomfortable and intimidated. Programmed learning programs are beneficial to this type of student.

"Oral" Students
These students have a certain oral fixation that does not disappear when they enter the classroom. They learn best when chewing, drinking, or eating. Consequently, it is important for instructors to understand that this behavior helps students learn and should not be forbidden in the classroom environment or it may impede the learning process.

"Noise" Students
These students learn best when surrounded by some degree of background noise. They may need the noise from a radio or television to focus their attention toward learning. While this is most likely not practical in the classroom environment, it is important for instructors to understand that some students have an inherent need to watch television or listen to music while studying.

"Pacing" Students
These students are very active and find it difficult to sit still during classroom presentations. This may be due to a physical problem (eg, cramping, low back injuries) making sitting still uncomfortable. These students may find it difficult to learn in an environment in which they are forced to stay still.

Field Dependence
The theory of field dependence focuses on the student's ability to overcome the effects of distracting background elements in order to differentiate more relevant aspects of a particular situation or object, such as that identified in Figure 1.3[7]. While some students who are labeled highly field–independent can quickly identify an object that is surrounded by other objects, highly field-dependent students find it difficult to locate the object and need to have it identified for them. Most students fall somewhere between these two extremes[8]. There are many

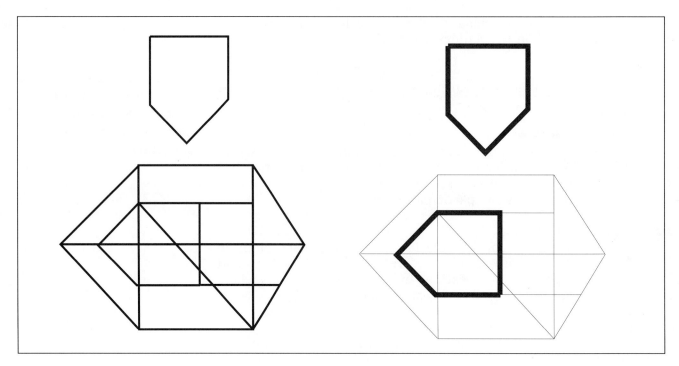

FIGURE 1.3   Field Dependence/Independence Testing

> Whether a student is field-dependent or field-independent affects how he learns, teaches, and generally interacts with others.

tests available to identify whether a student is field-dependent or field-independent.

Whether a student is field-dependent or field-independent affects how he learns, teaches, and generally interacts with others. Box 1.2 provides a list of learning characteristics for both styles. Box 1.3 identifies characteristics of instructors based on field-dependent or field-independent teaching styles. Finally, Box 1.4 identifies ways in which instructors should interact with students based on their learning styles in order to motivate them in the classroom setting.

BOX 1.2   Field Dependence Learning Styles

FIELD-DEPENDENT	FIELD-INDEPENDENT
Look at information globally	Analyze information
Adhere to structure provided	Self-impose structure or restrictions
Identify generalizations ("gray area")	Identify specific tendencies ("black/white")
Socially oriented to the world	Impersonal orientation to the world
Seek externally defined goals	Have self-defined goals
Need organization to be provided	Can self-structure situations and information
Greatly affected by criticism	Less affected by criticism

Learning styles (adapted from Guild and Garger, 1985).

BOX 1.3 Field Dependence Teaching Styles

FIELD-DEPENDENT	FIELD-INDEPENDENT
Is strong in developing a warm learning climate, emphasizing personal aspects of instruction	Is strong in organizing and guiding students in learning, emphasizing intellectual aspects of instruction
Prefers using interactive, discussion-type teaching methods to allow for interaction	Prefers impersonal teaching methods such as lecture or problem solving activities, emphasizing cognitive aspects of learning
Uses student centered activities	Uses teacher-organized activities
Provides minimal feedback	Provides specific corrective feedback
Uses questions to check on student achievement following instruction	Uses questions to introduce topics and throughout instruction
Is viewed by students as "teaching the facts"	Is viewed by students as "encouraging them to apply principles"

Teaching styles (adapted from Garger and Guild, 1984).

Field-Dependent Students

A student who is incapable of ignoring distracting elements is generally more global, and is referred to as field-dependent. For example, a student who has a difficult time following skill sheets to properly apply a short board would most likely be field-dependent.

Field-dependent students are generally very social and people-oriented, looking to others for help in defining their own attitudes and beliefs. They are often drawn to people and favor occupations that require active involvement with others, such as teaching, social work and nursing.

Field-dependent students are generally very social and people-oriented, looking to others for help in defining their own attitudes and beliefs.

BOX 1.4 Instructor Motivation Styles

FIELD-DEPENDENT	FIELD-INDEPENDENT
Uses verbal praise	Uses grades
Asks students for help	Uses games for competition
Uses external rewards (eg, prizes, points)	Uses a personal goal chart to track progress
Identifies goal value to others	Identifies goal value to the student
Provides outlines and structure to students	Allows freedom for students to design their own structure

Instructor motivation styles (modified from Garger and Guild, 1984).

These students find it more difficult to internalize necessary structure in order to organize material and learn information. They need a structured learning environment in order to benefit fully from classroom learning. When material is organized adequately, the learning ability of a field-dependent student equals that of a field-independent one.

Field-Independent Students

A student is generally referred to as field-independent when he is not distracted by background elements. This type of student is usually more analytical and logical. Field-independent students usually show greater interest in impersonal, abstract aspects of information.

A field-independent student is more likely to favor occupations in which there is less emphasis on interpersonal interaction, such as engineering, astronomy or accounting. They tend to favor subjects such as mathematics and physical sciences that stress the impersonal and abstract.

These students are able to internalize and structure instructional material in order to learn. They work well in minimally supervised activities such as independent study or programmed learning activities.

Conceptual Tempo

Individual students vary in the speed at which they learn and respond to information, questions, or problems. While some students take a long time to think before they respond, others respond almost immediately. Kagan et al.[10] coined the term *conceptual tempo*, which refers to the speed at which individuals respond and to the number of errors made in association with such responses.

Impulsive

Impulsive students are those who tend to respond rapidly, thereby making a fair amount of errors. They are often the first to turn in tests and papers due to their quick response to questions without adequate time for thinking. This behavior can result in poorer test scores because the student did not take enough time to read a question accurately, thereby leading to an incorrect response.

Reflective

Reflective students tend to take more time prior to responding, and consequently make fewer errors. They usually spend extra time reviewing answers to test questions and pondering over their answers prior to turning the test in. This type of student may waste time mulling over answers that really do not require much attention.

The 4MAT System

The 4MAT system, researched by Bernice McCarthy[11-13] was an adaptation of the learning style dimensions developed by David Kolb in the early 1970s. Kolb identified two major dimensions of learning, perception and processing[8]. The 4MAT system contains eight elements of instruction based on the individual learning styles identified by Kolb, as well as brain hemisphere dominance.

All students feel, reflect, think, and do; the time one takes performing each task, however, is what develops learning style differences. Some students are watchers while others are doers. Watchers tend to step back and analyze a situation in order to create meaning while doers immediately act on new information.

A field-independent student is more likely to favor occupations in which there is less emphasis on interpersonal interaction, such as engineering, astronomy or accounting.

Conceptual tempo refers to the speed at which individuals respond and to the number of errors made in association with such responses.

"Instruction begins when you the teacher, learn from the learner, put yourself in his place so that you may understand what he learns and the way he understands it."

Kierkegaard

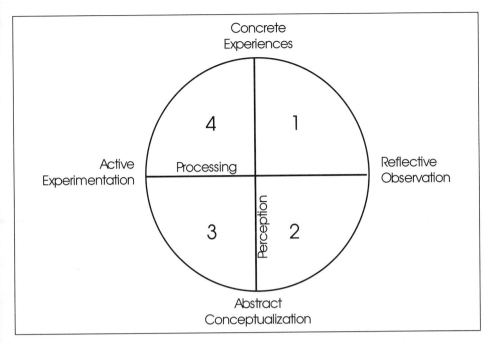

FIGURE 1.4 Kolb's Learning Style Dimensions *(adapted from Guild and Garger, 1985).*

Kolb's Learning Style Dimensions

Perception
There are two extremes in the way in which students perceive information. At one end of the continuum, students perceive through abstract conceptualization. At the other end, they receive information through concrete experiences.

Processing
There are also two extremes at which students process the information they perceive. At one end of the continuum, they process through active experimentation and at the other end through reflective observation.

The result of this research led to Kolb's formation of a four-quadrant model of learning styles, as shown in Figure 1.4. McCarthy[11-13] then incorporated research of hemisphericity into Kolb's learning dimensions to develop the 4MAT system identified in Figures 1.5 and 1.6.

McCarthy's 4MAT System

Type One: Imaginative Learners
The upper right quadrant of the 4MAT system identifies what Mc-Carthy refers to as "Type 1" learners. These students perceive information through sensing and feeling (concrete experiences) and process it through watching (reflective observation). They have a great need to grow and understand, and require personal involvement to learn.

The right hemisphere of the brain then tries to incorporate information into the student's own personal experiences; the left hemisphere tries to analyze the experience to find understanding. The student asks "Why?" and searches for the meaning behind how learning affects them personally based on their beliefs and values. Because these students tend to see all sides to a situation, and reflect upon it, they generally take more time making decisions.

All students feel, reflect, think, and do; the time one takes performing each task, however, is what develops learning style differences.

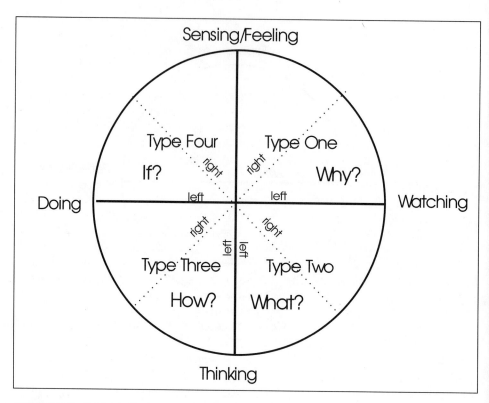

FIGURE 1.5 McCarthy's 4Mat System *(adapted from Guild and Garger, 1985).*

Type Two: Analytical Learners

The second quadrant identifies "Type 2" learners who perceive information by thinking (abstract conceptualization) and process it by watching (reflective observation). These students are concerned with

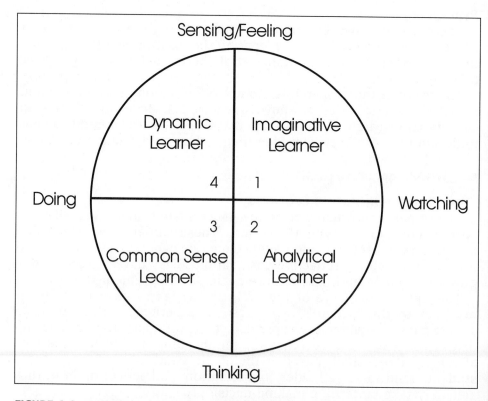

FIGURE 1.6 McCarthy's 4Mat System Learning Styles *(adapted from McCarthy, 1990).*

"What?" they know. They are very thorough and pay keen attention to detail. They devise their own theories by incorporating observations into what is known and need facts to deepen their understanding.

The right hemisphere of the brain is concerned with integrating information with past experiences; the left hemisphere is concerned with acquiring new information. Type 2 learners pay attention to detail, respect authority and expertise, and require accurate information. They are often fascinated by ideas and knowledge, tend to read large amounts of information, and speak fluently.

Type Three: Common Sense Learners

The third quadrant identifies "Type 3" learners. These students perceive information through thinking (abstract conceptualization) and process it through doing (active experimentation). They are concerned with "How?" something works.

These students tend to integrate theory into practice, and learn by testing theories and applying common sense. They are skills-oriented with a keen need to know "how" something works. These students enjoy problem-solving and trying to figure things out for themselves; they resent being given answers. They prefer to use and apply the knowledge they have gained immediately, often feeling frustrated in classroom situations.

The right hemisphere of the brain is concerned with how to apply information learned; the left hemisphere looks at more global general applications for information. These students are very practical and desire information that has a concrete purpose. They prefer to participate actively in the learning process by *doing* something.

Type Four: Dynamic Learners

The fourth quadrant identifies "Type 4" learners. These students perceive information through sensing and feeling (concrete experience) and process it by doing (active experimentation) and self-discovery. They are concerned with "If?" and have been called innovators because of their ability to apply learning in new and different ways.

These students are extremely flexible and enjoy change and new ideas. They tend to learn by trial and error. While they do not need logical justification for action, they are often risk takers and are sometimes viewed as "pushy" because of their need to influence others.

Figure 1.7 provides a list of skills at which each type of student excels. Because students learn and process information differently, it is important for instructors to use an assortment of methods when teaching. While students tend to have a strong preference for certain teaching styles, instructors should challenge their students by designing training programs that use diverse strategies within the 4MAT System.

IDENTIFYING LEARNING STYLE PREFERENCES

Instructors can usually identify learning preferences by listening to their students. Visual learners tend to make statements such as "I **see** what you mean," "I **saw** a presentation at a conference," or "I never **noticed** that before." Auditory learners tend to make statements such as "I **hear** what you're saying," "I **heard** a speaker at a conference," or "I never **heard** it stated that way." Kinesthetic learners, on the other hand, may make statements such as "I **feel** there is a problem" or "Could you **touch** on the differences between . . ."

In addition, instructors should look at other individual characteristics such as those listed in Box 1.5. For example, how do students in-

Instructors can usually identify learning preferences by listening to their students.

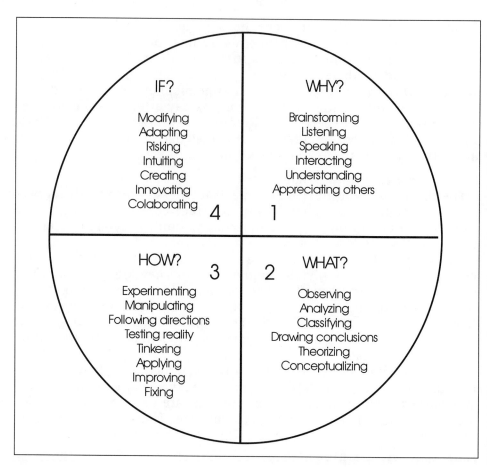

FIGURE 1.7 Skills Associated with Individual Learning Styles *(adapted from McCarthy, 1985).*

teract within the classroom environment; do they take part in large or small group activities or do they sit off on their own? Are they constantly placing something in their mouths, chewing on gum or on a pen or pencil, fidgeting in their chairs or tapping their fingers?

Finally, instructors should ask their students how they learn best. Do they learn best with the use of visual resources such as slides, by hands-on practice, or by listening to step-by-step instructions? Students often know how they learn best and can offer suggestions for instructors to improve their learning experience.

BARRIERS TO LEARNING

Various circumstances may interfere with a student's ability to attend training programs or adequately learn information. There are three primary categories of learning barriers: dispositional, situational, and environmental.

Dispositional Factors

Adult learners bring with them certain personal characteristics that may interfere with their willingness to attend training programs. Some have been out of the classroom setting for many years and feel they are too old to learn. Others simply lack the self-confidence needed to succeed in learning. Still others, especially "doers," are easily bored when attending training programs.

Adult learners bring with them certain personal characteristics that may interfere with their willingness to attend training programs.

BOX 1.5 Learning Style Diagnosis

FACTORS	DIAGNOSIS
Time	When is the student most alert: early morning, afternoon, evening, or late at night?
Schedule	What is the student's attention span: continuous or short bursts of concentrated effort?
Noise	What type of sounds produce a positive behavior: music, talking, or laughter? How much noise can a student tolerate: none, minimal, or high-level conversation?
Type of work group	How does the student work best: alone, in small study groups, or in large work groups?
Amount of pressure	How much pressure does a student need to perform optimally: a relaxed environment, light, moderate, or extreme pressure? (Some students do best by waiting until the last minute to study for a test.)
Motivation	What helps to motivate a student: expectations (self or outside influence), deadlines, rewards, recognition of achievement?
Place	Where does a student learn best: home, school, library, at a desk, on the couch, on the floor?
Type of assignments	With what type assignments does a student perform best: contracts, self-directed projects, or instructor-directed activities?
Perceptual strengths and styles	How does a student learn best: visual material, printed media, tactile experiences, multimedia packages, audiotapes, or a combination of the above?
Structure and evaluation	Under what degree of structure does a student perform best: strict, flexible, self-determined, jointly arranged, continual, or terminal assessment?

Learning style diagnosis (adapted from Dunn and Dunn, 1972[14]).

It is important for instructors to understand these characteristics and take steps to minimize the negative effects on learning should a barrier be identified within a student. If a student is bored, instructors should use various motivational strategies to maintain interest, such as improving presentation methods, making class sessions as interactive as possible, and using alternative teaching methods.

In addition, it is important that instructors are very careful when handling students with low self-confidence or with the perception that they are too old. These students may be looking for an excuse to withdraw from training. It is important that these problems be identified early in a training program and that steps be taken to offer praise and encouragement to these students.

Situational Factors

Situational barriers to learning include certain circumstances preventing a student from attending training program. One such barrier is time; the EMT-Basic curriculum is a minimum of 110 hours, plus extra time for remedial training, exams, and continuing education. Paramedic and nursing programs require significantly more time. For some students, it is quite difficult to commit such a large number of hours to attending training programs. When these students do agree to participate in such a program, they expect a quality education that does not waste any of their time.

In addition to time, some students have transportation constraints that interfere with their ability to participate in training programs. If a student does not have a car, or if training programs are often offered in areas without access to public transportation, it may not be feasible for him or her to attend such training. Instructors must be aware that this barrier exists.

While it is the students responsibility to get to and from class, changes in location midstream, requirements for field trips, or scheduling certain classes away from the original class location can be unfair to students with transportation difficulties.

Child care may also present a barrier for students with children. These students expect class to start and end on time so they can relieve their children's caretakers. In addition, when children are sick, students may miss or be late for a class. While child care problems do not provide an excuse for students to miss classes, instructors should be aware of these possible constraints and be accommodating whenever possible.

"Excess baggage" refers to outside issues a student brings into the classroom that may interfere with the learning process. Such issues might include financial worries, work issues, family problems, sick loved ones, or any other situation that causes a student's mind to wander from the learning tasks at hand. The student caught "day-dreaming" is most likely thinking about excess baggage.

Environmental Factors

Environmental factors that prevent students from attending training programs or cause negative feelings include inconvenient schedules or restricting locations. For example, if an EMT course is only offered during the evening, and a potential student works the evening shift, it becomes impossible for him to participate in training without the stress of changing schedules. Sometimes it is even impossible for students to change schedules. Likewise, if a Saturday class is required, such as for vehicle extrication practices, and a student works on Saturdays, a barrier has been placed on learning for that individual.

The location of training becomes an issue when travel time is significant. If programs are offered only at a location 2 hours away, chances are participants will be quite hesitant about attending. Such a commute could also cause students to be anxious about their return trip during the class session. Inclement weather increases the detrimental effect of a long commute.

Excessive fees may also prevent students from attending training programs. Some institutions may provide financial assistance. If not, a student may be unable to participate in training, or may be required to travel to a different area where tuition is cheaper. There is a wide range of costs for all levels of EMS training programs, and while some organizations send members free of charge, others do not.

As is discussed in Chapter 4, the classroom environment itself can be an environmental barrier to learning. If a room is too hot or cold, poorly lit, inappropriately arranged, or too noisy, learning will be affected.

FACTORS AFFECTING INDIVIDUAL LEARNING RATES

Students learn at different rates. There are both intrinsic and external factors that are responsible for such differences.

Intrinsic Factors

Past learning experiences can affect the speed at which a student learns new information. If a student has attended training programs consistently, and has been successful in doing so, he is most likely comfortable with the learning process and is able to learn relatively quickly. If, however, this is the first time back to the classroom setting for a student, learning may be more difficult, requiring additional time and energy for success.

Past learning experiences can affect the speed at which a student learns new information.

In addition, past experiences may result in certain expectations on the part of students. If a student last attended a superior interactive multimedia training program, he may be expecting a similar class. If the next program is dramatically different, learning may take more time.

Likewise, if a student attended a program in which the instructor taught directly toward a test, additional time may be required to retrain the student to take appropriate notes and identify key information on his own.

Training programs previously attended on the same or similar course content can also affect learning rates as well. If a student has background in first aid or CPR, or has completed a first responder training program, he may already have advanced knowledge in certain areas. This student is able to build on past knowledge more easily and at a faster rate than a student who has had no exposure to the content presented in a particular course.

Learning rates are also affected by sensory abilities. If a student is visual, and information is presented in an auditory or kinesthetic modality, learning may take more time. Likewise, if a student is kinesthetic and is not given the opportunity to examine or use equipment, learning may be delayed.

If a student is sensory-challenged *eg*, visually-impaired without corrective lenses, learning will be more difficult in a visual environment. Likewise, hearing-impaired students may have a difficult time in an auditory learning environment.

Obviously, motivation has a great effect on learning rates. If a student is highly motivated, learning will take place quickly. Even if the student is intellectually challenged, motivation will help him or her practice, study, and review until the information is learned.

Conversely, if a student is not motivated, either intrinsically or externally, learning will be more difficult and will take more time. Motivation is discussed in more detail in Chapter 2.

External Factors

External factors associated with learning rates are often controllable factors. One such factor is the learning environment. The learning climate an instructor develops and maintains will greatly affect learning

External factors associated with learning rates are often controllable factors.

rates. The classroom environment is discussed in detail in Chapter 4.

The instructor also effects learning rates. A poorly prepared or organized instructor will create a barrier to learning, thereby increasing the time needed to learn information accurately. Likewise, the attitude of instruction influences learning rates. A negative attitude hinders motivation and increases learning rates. A positive attitude and well-designed and -presented training session on the part of an instructor should decrease the time necessary for learning to take place. Characteristics of an effective instructor are discussed in detail in Chapter 4.

Support and encouragement from outside persons also affects learning rates. If family members and friends of students encourage them to do well in training, they will usually try harder to succeed. If that support and encouragement are not present, however, the student must overcome extra obstacles to learn.

METHODS OF INCREASING LEARNING RATES

There are various techniques instructors can use to increase learning rates. The first is to individualize instruction by identifying entry knowledge and skill requirements, ensuring that the students meet these requirements, and continually monitoring student progress throughout the course. In addition, instructors need to make themselves available to students for remedial training and extra practice if at all possible. If a student seeks out additional help, it should be easily available.

Instructors must also advise students of the intended outcomes, goals, and objectives at the beginning of a training program. Without knowledge of what is expected of them, students cannot gauge how they are progressing. Once they know what is expected, instructors should evaluate progress continually and intervene early with students who fail to meet course objectives.

In order to identify learning deficiencies early in a program, instructors must:

- Identify the tasks to be accomplished (expected knowledge and skills).
- Identify student abilities (current knowledge and skills).
- Identify deficiencies (tasks – abilities = deficiency).

Once a deficiency is identified, instructional strategies need to be designed and implemented in order to overcome the deficiency. Throughout this process, instructors should involve students in selecting instructional delivery methods, course design, evaluation strategies and feedback, and the learning environment itself, in order to determine methods that meet the individual needs of the students.

KEY POINTS

1. Theorists have identified three domains of learning. The cognitive domain is responsible for knowledge of information and facts; the psychomotor domain is responsible for the learning of skills requiring motion or coordination; and the affective domain focuses on attaching attitudes, values, and feelings to information learned.

2. The six levels of the cognitive domain, from simplest to most complex, are knowledge, comprehension, application, analysis, synthesis, and evaluation.

3. The five levels of the psychomotor domain include imitation, manipulation, precision, articulation, and naturalization.

4. The five levels of the affective domain include

KEY POINTS continued

receiving, responding, valuing, organization, and characterization.

5. Students process information differently and usually have a preference in they way they receive and process information. *Hemisphericity* refers to the way in which information is organized within the cerebral hemisphere. Students who think predominantly with the right side of the brain tend to be more global, artistic, and emotional, whereas students who think predominantly with the left side of the brain tend to be more organized, rational, and analytical.

6. *Perceptual modalities* are the ways in which students receive information through the senses. While students can receive information with the use of all five senses, they usually prefer to receive information by seeing, hearing, or touching.

7. Visual learners prefer to see information and learn best when visual aids are used. Auditory learners prefer to hear the information presented and respond best when information is presented in oral form, generally through lectures or audiotapes. Kinesthetic learners prefer to receive information through tactile stimulation and respond best when they are given "hands-on" instruction.

8. There are various social styles by which students act in classroom situations. Some are more comfortable in large classes, others in small classes, and still others prefer independent learning.

9. Whether a student is capable of ignoring distracting background elements in order to differentiate more relevant aspects of a particular situation or object is referred to as field dependence. A field-dependent learner is incapable of ignoring such distractions and views information and situations more globally. These students generally need more

structure in training programs and usually look to others to determine their own attitudes and beliefs. A field-independent learner is not easily distracted by background elements. These students are usually more logical, analytical, and show greater interest in impersonal and abstract aspects of information.

10. Conceptual tempo refers to the speed at which individuals respond to information, questions, or problems, and the number of errors made in association with their responses. Impulsive students respond quickly, making a fair amount of errors. Reflective students tend to take more time thinking prior to responding, and consequently make fewer errors.

11. The 4MAT system identifies four types of students based on the way they perceive and process information. Imaginative students perceive information by sensing or feeling and process it by watching others. Their favorite question is "Why?" Analytical students perceive information by thinking and process it by watching. Their favorite question is "What?". Common sense students perceive information by thinking and process it by doing. Their favorite question is "How?". Dynamic students perceive information by sensing and feeling and process it by doing. Their favorite question is "If?".

12. Adult learners bring with them certain characteristics that may interfere with their willingness to attend training programs. Whether a student feels he is too old to learn, lacks self-confidence, is easily bored, or has time or transportation constraints or other outside interference can prevent learning from taking place. It is that important that instructors understand these barriers to learning and try to assist students in overcoming such to improve their chances of success in training programs.

FOLLOW-UP ACTIVITIES

1. Analyze a slow learner within the classroom setting. Determine his learning style and identify instructional methods that can improve the learning process based on these styles.
2. Identify an objective for each level of the following three domains of learning:
    Cognitive
    Knowledge
    Comprehension
    Application
    Analysis
    Synthesis
    Evaluation
    Psychomotor
    Imitation

FOLLOW-UP ACTIVITIES continued

    Manipulation
    Precision
    Articulation
    Naturalization
  Affective
    Receiving
    Responding
    Valuing
    Organization
    Characterization

3. Identify your own learning/teaching styles. Are you:
_____ Field-dependent or _____ Field-independent
_____ Visual Learner or _____ Auditory Learner or _____ Kinesthetic Learner
_____ Type 1 Learner or _____ Type 2 Learner or _____ Type 3 Learner or
_____ Type 4 Learner

REFERENCES

1. Keirsey D, Bates M. *Please Understand Me.* Del Mar, CA: Prometheus Nemesis Book Company; 1984.
2. Bloom B, Englehart N, Furst E, Hill W, Krathwohl D. *Taxonomy of Educational Objectives: Handbook I. Cognitive Domain.* New York: McKay; 1956.
3. Krathwohl D, Bloom B, Masia B. *Taxonomy of Educational Objectives; Handbook II. Affective Domain.* New York: McKay; 1964.
4. Bjorklund D. *Children's Thinking: Developmental Function and Individual Differences.* Pacific Grove, CA: Brooks/Cole; 1989.
5. Barbe W, Swassing H, Milone M. *Teaching Through Modality Strengths.* Columbus, OH: Zaner-Bloser, Inc.; 1979.
6. Bourn S. *Building Blocks for the Adult Learner.* Paper presented at the EMS Today Conference, Albuquerque, NM; 1990.
7. Witkin H, Goodenough D. *Cognitive Styles: Essence and Origins.* New York: International Universities Press, Inc.; 1981.
8. Guild P, Garger S. *Marching to Different Drummers.* Alexandria, VA; Association for Supervision and Curriculum Development; 1985.
9. Garger S, Guild P. Learning styles: the crucial differences. *Curriculum Review.* 1984; 23:9-12.
10. Kagan J, Rosman B, Day D, Albert J, Phillips W. Information processing in the child: significance of analytic and reflective attitudes. *Psychological Monographs,* 1964; 78 (1, Whole No. 578).
11. McCarthy B. Using the 4MAT system to bring learning styles to schools. *Educational Leadership.* 1990;48(2):31-37.
12. McCarthy B. What 4MAT training teaches us about staff development. *Educational Leadership.* 1985;61-68.
13. McCarthy B. *The 4MAT System: Teaching to Learning Styles with Right/Left Mode Techniques.* Barrington, IL: Excel, Inc.; 1980.
14. Dunn R, Dunn K. *Practical Approaches to Individualizing Instruction.* West Nyack, NY: Parker; 1972.

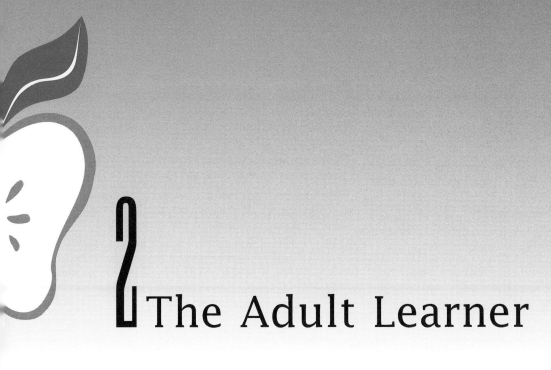

2 The Adult Learner

Upon completion of this chapter, the reader will have sufficient information to:

1. List five assumptions of adult learners.
2. Define andragogy and pedagogy.
3. Describe 10 differences between andragogy and pedagogy.
4. Identify seven strategies for teaching adult learners.
5. Describe the seven steps of Maslow's Hierarchy of Needs.
6. Describe the differences between intrinsic and extrinsic motivation.
7. List 15 factors leading to negative motivation and strategies instructors should use to combat each.
8. Identify three types of goal structures.
9. List interaction and motivation strategies for each type of goal structure.
10. Describe four methods for motivating students.
11. List nine behaviors exhibited by highly anxious students.
12. Identify five strategies instructors can use to assist low-level students to perform better.

KEY TERMS

Andragogy The methodology of life-long education for adults

Creativity The capacity of students to produce a novel or original answer, product, or method of doing something

Evaluation The process of obtaining information to form judgements so that educational decisions can be made

External locus of control A feeling that one has little control over one's fate and the failure to perceive a cause-and-effect relationship between actions and consequences

Extrinsic motivation Motivation influenced by external events such as grades, points, or money

Goal structure The way in which students relate to one another and to the instructor while working toward the attainment of instructional goals; includes cooperative, competitive, and individualistic goal structures

Hierarchy of Needs Maslow's classification of human needs

Internal locus of control A feeling of control over one's fate and the belief that effort and reward are connected

Intrinsic motivation Motivation influenced by personal factors such as satisfaction or enjoyment

Learned helplessness A situation in which students learn, over time and through constant failure, that they cannot control the outcome of events affecting their lives

Locus of control An individual's perception of who is responsible for the outcome of events and behavior in their lives

Long-term memory The part of the information processing system that retains encoded information for long periods

Negative reinforcement The termination of an unpleasant condition following a desired response; the termination serves to reinforce the desired response

Pedagogy The methodology of formalized education of children

KEY TERMS continued

Positive reinforcement A procedure that maintains or increases the rate of a response by presenting a positive reinforcer following a response

Prompting The presentation of additional stimuli to increase the probability that an appropriate response will be given

Punishment A procedure in which an adverse stimulus is presented immediately following a response, resulting in a reduction in the rate of response

Reward An object, stimulus, or outcome that is perceived as being pleasant

Self-actualization Maslow's term for the psychological need to develop one's capabilities and potential in order to enhance personal growth

Self-concept The total organization of the perceptions individuals have of themselves

Self-esteem The value or judgement individuals place on their behavior; self-esteem and self-concept are often used interchangeably

Short-term memory The part of information processing in which conscious mental activity is carried out; information is held in short-term memory for only a few seconds

INTRODUCTION

> A majority of the students encountered in EMS training programs are adults. Many have not been in the classroom setting in many years.

A majority of the students encountered in EMS training programs are adults. Many have not been in the classroom setting in many years. Adult students are anxious about learning, and especially about being tested. In general, adult students are very different from elementary, and even secondary students. This chapter is designed to assist the instructor in identifying the differences that exist among adult students, and finding a practical approach to modifying their presentations to address the needs of these students.

MALCOLM KNOWLES' MODEL OF HUMAN LEARNING

In 1978, Boston University professor Malcolm Knowles, sparked a revolution in adult education and training by introducing his theory of andragogy[1]. Although Knowles was not the first to discover the differences between educating adults and children, his principles and theories governing andragogy have been publicized widely over the past two decades. His theory had been referred to as the "theory of andragogy," but Knowles no longer refers to it as such and prefers to call it a "model of human learning"[2].

Andragogy vs. Pedagogy

> Andragogy is defined as "the art and science of helping adults learn." It is the student's responsibility to learn the material, and the instructor's responsibility to facilitate the learning process.

Andragogy is defined as "the art and science of *helping* adults learn." Conversely, *pedagogy* is defined as "the art and science of *teaching* children"[3]. Andragogic methods of teaching involve assisting the adult learner reach his academic potential. It is the student's responsibility to learn the material, and the instructor's responsibility to facilitate the learning process. In pedagogic methods, the instructor assumes the dominant role as "teacher" and controls all the learning taking place. With this method, it is the instructor's responsibility to provide all required information.

The traditional pedagogic approach views students as passive recipients of knowledge. Based on this theory, students rarely take the initiative to learn; rather they are merely sponges that absorb information as it is presented. Students are viewed as having blank slates with no prior experience to influence or hinder learning. According to this model, pedagogic students are subject-oriented, primarily interested in the content to be learned, and motivated by extrinsic rewards[4].

The traditional andragogic approach, on the other hand, is based on certain assumptions and characteristics of the adult learner. One basic characteristic of adult learners is that they cannot be forced to learn; although they can be directed to attend a training session, they cannot be forced to learn the information presented[5]. Box 2.1 identifies differences between the andragogic and pedagogic approaches to learning.

Assumptions of Adult Learners

Knowles' model of human learning is based on five fundamental assumptions that distinguish adult learners from children[1]:

1) **Adults have a need to be self-directing and in control of the learning process.** They learn because they want to, not because someone says they should.

2) **Adults have a resource base for learning that consists of past experiences**; they build learning on what they know. They tend to bring a greater quantity and quality of experiences to the classroom, and are able to share these experiences to make new information more meaningful and relevant to "real-life" practical applications.

3) **Adults learn based on need**; that is, they will learn only what they need to know. They have a practical approach to learning and want to know how the training is going to help them now. They tend to learn more quickly when they see immediate benefit. Therefore, adults accept practical applications better than theory-based lecture.

4) **Adults are task-oriented** and seek knowledge and skills that apply to the real-life problems they face. Adults are generally motivated to learn because of some immediate need in their lives (*eg*, a career change, modification of habits, financial in-

---

BOX 2.1 Characteristics of adult and child learners

ADULTS	CHILDREN
Experienced	Inexperienced
Oriented by need/problem	Oriented by subject/content
Learners decide content	Instructors determine content
Concerned with learning for immediate needs	Concerned with learning for the future
Prefer active learning	Prefer passive learning
Skills-oriented	Grade-oriented
Learn best in informal settings	Usually learn best in structured environment
Prefer self-directed learning	Prefer guided learning
On more of an "equal" level with instructor	View instructors as being "superior"
Motivated by intrinsic rewards	Motivated by external rewards

Characteristics of adult and child learners (adapted from Zemke and Zemke, 1988).

vestments). They want to know that the information they receive from training is relevant, with immediate reward.

5) **Adults are more motivated by intrinsic factors**, such as self-esteem and achievement, than by external rewards such as pay raises.

Children learn in a structured environment. Remember when you were in elementary school and you had to raise your hand to go to the bathroom? Children learn best in that type of environment; they feel they cannot do something unless they are told to. Adults on the other hand, tend to think they can do something unless they are told they cannot. In general, adults learn best in an a flexible environment that promotes participation. Adults try to relate new knowledge to past experiences and apply that knowledge to problems they encounter in life.

In general, adults learn best in an a flexible environment that promotes participation.

Strategies for Adult Learners

In order to increase the effectiveness of adult training, it is important to accommodate adult learner characteristics by incorporating the above assumptions into the design process. Tailoring specific strategies for adult learners, to meet their inherent needs will result in efficient and more meaningful learning for this population. The following strategies can help achieve this result.

Maintain an atmosphere that promotes learning

Instructors must prepare an environment that is conducive to learning, both physically and psychologically. Physically, the classroom should provide ample room for a lecture and individual spaces for small group practice. In addition, traditional "school-like" seating arrangements should be avoided by arranging chairs in a circle or U-shape, thereby eliminating an inhibiting classroom atmosphere.

Instructors must prepare an environment that is conducive to learning, both physically and psychologically.

Adults learn best in an informal environment. Psychologically, the classroom environment should promote mutual respect and trust between students and instructors. Finally, the environment should be pleasant, interesting, and nonthreatening[2]. Learning does not have to be dull or emotionally draining, but should be stimulating and thought-provoking.

Involve students in the planning process

Adult learners prefer to have input in what they are doing. Although the curriculum is outlined for students, they should have some input into the type of learning activities in which they will participate. Would they prefer lecture or group discussions, oral or written presentations, weekly or monthly quizzes? Do they learn better with one night of lecture followed by one night of practice, or one night of combined lecture and then practice on that topic?

While the final authority rests with the instructor or coordinator, students should have some input into flexible subjects. Participation in areas of planning will result in more involvement and commitment on the part of the student[2].

Involve students in determining their learning needs

Again, although the curriculum may be defined already, certain items can be altered to incorporate specific needs of students. For example, practice time can be geared toward a specific skill, scenarios, role playing, or "putting it all together" after the basics are mastered. Asking students what they feel are key areas to focus on promotes an environment that is competency-based, thereby placing some responsibility on the class.

Involve students when formulating learning objectives and designing lesson plans

Again, in EMS training, this principle may not appear practical, since the curriculum and lesson plans are standardized by the Department of Transportation. Nonetheless, to whatever extent possible, allowing students to have a say in what they want to get from a class will ensure that their needs are being met.

Adult learners have expectations of what they will learn from a course, and it is extremely important that the goals and objectives of the program be identified by both the students and instructor. Any differences should be negotiated and resolved from the onset[5].

Practice using information immediately after it is presented

Research has shown that retention of information is significantly higher when immediate practice is provided. Practice can take many forms, including skills demonstration, role playing, games, or simulations. With adult learners, practice definitely makes perfect, and perfect practice leads to retention of information.

Adults learn by doing. In fact, research has shown that if adults do not have the opportunity either to be involved actively in the learning process or to practice, they will forget, within 24 hours, approximately 50% of the information presented, and will forget an additional 25% within 2 weeks[6]. Adults must have the opportunity to use the information they learn before they forget it.

Adults learn by doing.

Incorporate student past experience

Adult learners bring with them a different quality of experience, including:

- A broader base of experience to which they attach new ideas and skills for more meaning
- A wider range of backgrounds, interests, abilities, and learning styles
- Developed habits and biases

Adult learners need to integrate new material with previously learned concepts and knowledge in order to increase the retention and usability of new information. If this new information does not "fit" with previous knowledge, the student will probably reject it. Conversely, if the new information is related to, and built on, past knowledge and experiences, learning will be augmented and will hold more meaning.

Adult learners need to integrate new material with previously learned concepts and knowledge.

Involve students in evaluating learning

Giving students the opportunity to evaluate the learning process serves multiple functions. First, exams test only a portion of the students' knowledge. Students know how competent they feel and should be able to provide input as to how the course was run and ways to improve it.

In addition, adults want guidance, not grades. They are often frightened by exams and fear being humiliated by low scores, especially when they may have been away from school for a prolonged period of time. Reassurance of satisfactory progress and sincere praise and guidance throughout the course should help prevent students from becoming anxious about tests or discouraged after poor test scores.

Finally, the evaluation process should analyze whether students have met their learning objectives, as well as the quality of the program. Obtaining 90% on a written exam does not hold any meaning if the student cannot transfer the information into real-life situations. Therefore, instructors should evaluate learning with case studies, presentations, or other practical methods to verify adequate knowledge of information and the transfer of this knowledge in relevant situations. This will ensure that students have met both their and your objectives.

Knowles' theory of andragogy identifies the adult need to be self-directing[1]. Unfortunately, most adults have been through a pedagogic school system and automatically take the submissive role in the learning environment. Because the role of the student traditionally has been a dependent one, adults often give up their need to be self-directing in return for education.

Over the past two decades, theorists have scrutinized Knowles and his theories. Although adult educators still view these andragogic methods as superior to pedagogic methods, Knowles himself now concedes that many of his theories apply to children as well as adults. The one factor that clearly distinguishes adult learners from children, however, is the experiences that adults bring to the classroom. Because of these life experiences, instructors must restructure their teaching style to accommodate these adult learners.

Adult education generally consists of participants from a wide range of ages, attitudes, goals, and learning styles. It is a challenge for adult educators to find commonalities among participants in the classroom setting. Therefore, it is important to identify patterns relating to developmental stages, ages, and life experiences in order to make use of these as resources for learning.

It is imperative that adult educators understand differences that exist between andragogy and pedagogy and develop a blend of instructional techniques that meet the needs of all students in the adult learning environment. It is equally important that instructors evaluate students in order to determine their characteristics and developmental stages. Only then can instruction that meets everyone's learning styles and needs be developed.

> It is important that instructors evaluate students in order to determine their characteristics and developmental stages.

MASLOW'S HIERARCHY OF NEEDS

Abraham Maslow has been influential in understanding the basic human motivations of students. His theory is based on the assumption that within all of us there are forces that both seek and resist. Maslow's hierarchy of needs (Figure 2.1) helps in understanding the basic need gratification of individuals[7].

According to Maslow, physiologic needs such as food, sleep, clothing, and shelter are basic and must be met before one can be concerned with higher needs. If a student is placed in a cold, dark room or has not eaten all day, he or she may not be focused on learning but may be thinking of warmth or food instead. Likewise, if the student is having financial difficulties and is wondering how to support a family, his or her mind may be on issues other than the class session. In circumstances in which physiologic needs are not satisfied, learning may not take place.

Once the physiologic needs have been met, needs at the next level emerge—those of safety. Safety needs include the need to be free from

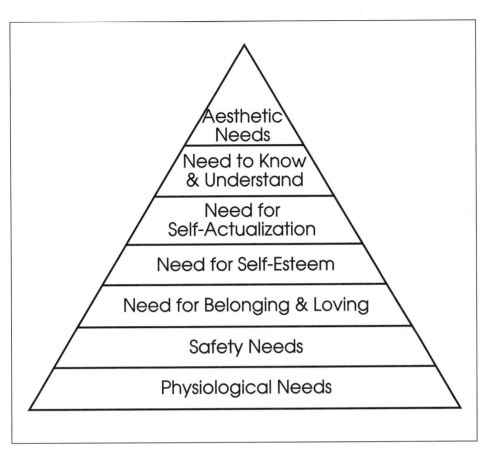

FIGURE 2.1 Maslow's Hierarchy of Needs *(adapted from Dembo, 1991).*

harm and danger, and the need for good health. Again, if someone is sick or being harassed or in some other danger, learning may be difficult.

After the need for safety has been satisfied, the need for belonging and loving becomes important. It is at this level one has the need for family and friends, or the need to belong to a group. In the event this need cannot be satisfied, the student may be motivated to behave in different ways to gain acceptance. Some may substitute achievement for love; this achievement may come in the form of intelligence or athletics.

Satisfaction of the need for belonging and love is followed by the need for self-esteem. This level includes the need to gain the respect and admiration of others, and the need for self-confidence. Such needs are often portrayed during training sessions. Students inherently need to succeed in order to build their self-confidence. When they do well in a class session, they practice more and become proficient with their skills.

Students inherently need to succeed in order to build their self-confidence.

Likewise, when students do poorly, their self-confidence is diminished and they are embarrassed by lack of coordination and, therefore, are scared to practice. This fear causes them not to learn the skill and possibly fail the course, thereby leading to the lack of self-confidence that began the cycle. This cyclic response is called the self-fulfilling prophecy. The cycle needs to be broken early in the program in order to minimize the negative and build confidence so students strive for excellence.

The next level on the hierarchy is self-actualization. Once all lower-level needs have been satisfied, motivation is directed toward the need to develop one's potential to be the best he can be. Self-actualization is

It is at this level that we hope our students are—with the need to seek knowledge and understanding.

very personal: it is not important what the student does, but rather how he feels about doing it. The inherent need is to do more—be more productive, earn higher scores, or take more calls.

Once the need for self-actualization has been satisfied, motivation is directed toward the need to know and understand. It is at this level that we hope our students are—with the need to seek knowledge and understanding. Learning is a never-ending phenomenon; this basic need results in the satisfaction of curiosity.

The final need of Maslow's hierarchy is that of esthetics. Some students possess a need for order and closure. Those at this level seek a conclusion to one aspect of life (a project, skill, or exam) before they can move on to the next aspect.

It is essential that instructors understand the concept of Maslow's hierarchy of needs in order to look beyond a troubled student to identify why he is having difficulty. Is the student falling asleep in class because he works two jobs? Is the student not paying attention because he is thinking of family problems, or needs to use the rest room? All these needs result in a lack of attention, which instructors may misread as a lack of interest or motivation. This is not to suggest that instructors become help counselors, but there are some strategies that can be used to assist students with these basic needs to help meet the goals and objectives of training programs.

MOTIVATION

Remember, adults learn what they want to learn.

Regardless of how prepared an instructor is, or how exciting the course material is, if a student is not receptive to the information presented, little or no learning will take place. Remember, adults learn what they want to learn. The key then is to convince them to want to learn what they need to know. It is important that instructors instill in students the desire to participate in the learning process.

There are two categories of motivation: intrinsic and extrinsic. Intrinsic motivation is influenced by personal factors such as satisfac-

Motivating Students

CURIOSITY

Provoke curiosity in students before stating the topic for a lesson by identifying a problem or conflict or giving a pretest to make them realize how much they do not know about a given topic. Arouse surprise and feelings of contradiction by presenting a dilemma that violates their expectations or past knowledge and experiences. Arouse doubt, uncertainty, and even bafflement by presenting a problem with no indication for its solution, such as how to remove a victim from the top of an oil tower.

ATTENTION

Arouse students' attention by beginning a class session with something unique, different, or unusual. Maintain their attention and interest through variety throughout the class session. Refrain from starting and ending classes the same way day after day.

tion, enjoyment, power, personal growth, and self-esteem. Extrinsic motivation is influenced by external events such as grades, points, raises, promotions, money and better working conditions. The WIIFM (What's In It For Me?) phenomena may incorporate factors of both types.

Primarily, students want to know what they will get out of a training session. If there is nothing "in it for them," they will most likely not be motivated to learn. As such, instructors need to find some element that relates to students in order to make the training have some meaning for them.

Motivation is usually high when students are introduced to a new topic. However, as the course continues, learning, enthusiasm, and motivation level off. During this plateau, instructors should introduce some change such as a new activity or instructional technique.

When examining what motivates students to learn, there seem to be two factors that must be addressed: the need to achieve and the need to avoid failure. As identified in Figure 2.2, the degree to which each factor is important to students determines how they attack tasks.

Research has shown that students with a stronger need to achieve than to avoid failure set goals of intermediate difficulty, in which their efforts are neither doomed for failure nor guaranteed success. Students with a stronger need to avoid failure tend to prefer very easy tasks in which they are certain to succeed or difficult tasks in which they can rationalize failing; either way they cannot lose.

As identified in Box 2.2, there are many factors that lead to negative motivation. It is essential that instructors understand these negative influences in order to take steps to minimize them and create a positive learning experience. Box 2.3 lists ways to minimize negative influences.

Negative motivation results from various components, including the student, instructor, instructional techniques, and evaluation methods. Any one component or a combination of all four can promote or prevent learning from taking place.

> *Research has shown that students with a stronger need to achieve than to avoid failure set goals of intermediate difficulty, in which their efforts are neither doomed for failure nor guaranteed success.*

REINFORCEMENT

Use positive reinforcement appropriately. Praise and encouragement should be used especially for those students suffering from a lack of self-confidence. Provide encouraging comments on assignments and examinations rather than just a grade. Provide continual feedback to students regarding how they are doing in a course.

REDUCE STUDENT ANXIETY

Provide information regarding what is expected of students early in a program. Students need sufficient time to complete assignments and study for tests so that classwork does not become overwhelming, or lead to feelings of inadequacy and failure. Allow students to "pass" on a question rather than defeat their self-esteem when they do not know the answer. Refrain from posting grades and scores with names on them; use social security numbers instead. Finally, use relaxation training as well as test-taking skills to decrease students' anxieties.

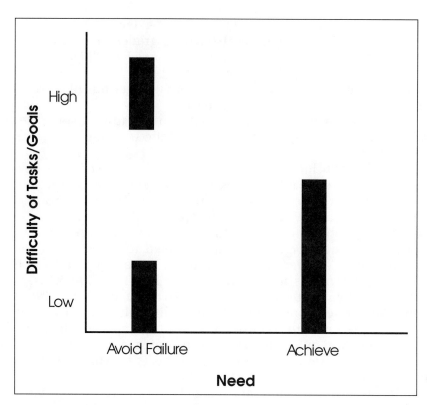

FIGURE 2.2 Needs vs. Risks Analysis

Negative Motivation Related to the Student

Poor self-concept

If students are not confident in their ability to learn and perform necessary skills, they will be apprehensive from the outset. It is essential that instructors put students at ease by promoting a positive attitude toward learner abilities and convincing them that they **can** succeed.

When students have confidence in their ability to master tasks, they are usually more eager to learn and to work harder at a task until it is successfully completed, thereby instilling further self-confidence. Students with a high level of self-confidence tend to choose more difficult tasks, expend more efforts, persist longer at trying to achieve goals, and have less fear and anxiety relative to the task.

Learned helplessness

Severely failure-oriented students may become convinced that they have no control over the outcome of events and that there is no relationship between effort and the attainment of goals. These students tend to not try to their full potential because they feel that whether or not they achieve is beyond their control.

These students need considerable attention to convince them that hard work and practice do make a difference. It is not that they are unmotivated; they may in fact be extremely motivated. Unfortunately, they are usually motivated to avoid failure rather than to succeed. Instructors need to identify these students and establish classroom conditions in which students learn that effort leads to success and through practice and study they can achieve their educational goals. Providing these students with short-term attainable goals and the strategies necessary to meet such goals will assist them to succeed academically.

It is essential that instructors put students at ease by promoting a positive attitude toward learner abilities and convincing them that they can succeed.

Establish classroom conditions in which students learn that effort leads to success and through practice and study they can achieve their educational goals.

BOX 2.2 Contributing Factors of Negative Motivation

STUDENT	INSTRUCTOR	INSTRUCTION	EVALUATION
Poor self-concept	Communicating low expectations	Emphasis on performance rather than mastery of goals	Emphasis on grades rather than retention of skills and knowledge
Learned helplessness			
Anxiety of learning	Poor self-confidence in the ability to teach	Emphasis on extrinsic rather than intrinsic goals	Emphasis on ability rather than effort
Past failure			
		Poor presentation methods	Public evaluation leading to evaluation (test) anxiety
		Lack of student involvement with task selection	
		Lack of interactivity	
		Uni-dimensional classroom presentation style	
		Focusing on one type of goal structure	

Factors contributing to negative motivation.

BOX 2.3 Minimizing Contributing Factors of Negative Motivation

STUDENT	INSTRUCTOR	INSTRUCTION	EVALUATION
Promote a positive attitude toward student abilities	Communicate **high** expectations	Place emphasis on mastery of goals and objectives	Place emphasis on retention of knowledge and ability to perform skills rather than on grades
Let the student know he **can** succeed	Increase own self-confidence with ability to teach	Place emphasis on intrinsic rather than extrinsic goals; make students **want** to learn	Place emphasis on effort as well as ability to perform
Make learning fun, not anxiety-provoking	Practice teaching methods to gain confidence		
Let students know they can not succeed if they do not at least **try**	Complete an honest self-evaluation after every class session	Improve presentation methods	Reduce test anxiety with games; never put down a student's ability in public; council in private
		Increase student involvement with task selection	
		Make class session as interactive as possible	
		Use multi-dimensional classroom presentation styles and techniques	

Factors to reduce negative motivation.

The Highly Anxious Student

Students who are highly anxious in learning situations often behave in ways that account for low levels of performance. For example:

- They attempt to avoid evaluation situations.
- They choose, and are more successful at, easy tasks in which success is more certain.
- They do not attend to tasks in sufficient detail because they are preoccupied with failure.
- As instructors are presenting information, they are thinking of inadequacies that will make it difficult for them to learn the material.
- They have difficulty with instructional methods that require them to rely on short-term memory or to perform quickly.
- They exhibit difficulty in learning material that is not well organized and perform better with highly structured material.
- They are not as successful with independent study or programmed learning instructional strategies.
- They exhibit lower self-concepts, blame themselves for failure, and daydream extensively.
- They may exhibit headaches, a stomach disorder not relating to a physical illness, nail-biting, sweating, restlessness, irregular motor coordination, or other general distractions.

Anxiety of learning

As previously discussed, adult learners are often anxious about returning to the classroom setting. By making learning an enjoyable process and assuring students that goals and objectives are attainable, instructors can help decrease the anxiety associated with learning.

Past failure

Failure comes in many shapes and sizes. Students set different goals for themselves. Obtaining a score of 70% on an exam may be a goal to one student and failure to the student who set a goal of 85%. Regardless of the individual goals, if a student consistently fails to meet goals, he will become less motivated to try and will begin to set lower goals that can be met.

It is important that instructors instill a sense of need in students to try to achieve goals that may seem out of their reach. Students need to know that they cannot succeed if they do not at least *try*.

Negative Motivation Related to the Instructor

Communicating low expectations

It is essential that instructors consistently push their students to achieve higher goals to get progressively better every time they perform a skill or score higher on a quiz. Challenge students to meet their full potential. If an instructor exhibits low expectations for students, such as scoring 70% on an examination, students may only study hard enough to meet that goal even though their potential could result in a score of 90% if they were motivated to study harder. This is not to say that instructors should set outrageous goals. Goals must be realistic in order to be effective.

Success comes in cans; failure comes in cannots. You will always miss 100% of the shots that you never take.

It is important that instructors instill a sense of need in students to try to achieve goals that may seem out of their reach.

Challenge students to meet their full potential.

There are ways in which instructors can assist low-level students perform better.

- Reassure them they are capable of succeeding and that they will be accepted and liked regardless of their academic performance, as long as they do their best.
- Be careful not to compare low-level students with higher-level students or publicly question the nature of their difficulties.
- Because anxious students are more dependent and have a greater need to be liked, it is important the instructor not ignore the student's performance. Neglecting these students reinforces their feeling of inadequacy.
- Since anxious students have difficulty memorizing and retrieving information, and perform better in a more structured learning environment, use instructional methods such as outlines, diagrams, and other methods for organizing information.
- Refrain from using self-directed learning activities such as independent study or discussion groups since low-level learners need to know exactly what is expected of them in order to control their anxiety.

Poor self-confidence

If an instructor is not confident with his teaching abilities, it will be reflected in the way he presents material and in the general undertone of the classroom environment. Without demonstrated competence in teaching methods, students will begin to doubt the instructor and all of the information presented. It is essential, therefore, that the instructor be confident and project this confidence in the classroom setting.

In order to gain self-confidence, instructors should practice various teaching methods to find the one that is the most comfortable. In addition, instructors should complete an honest self-evaluation after every class session to determine which methods work, which do not, and ways to modify presentation skills to meet the objectives most effectively.

Practice various teaching methods to find the one that is the most comfortable.

Negative Motivation Related to Instructional Strategies

Emphasis on performance rather than mastery

Goals and objectives are outcomes students are expected to obtain prior to the end of a training program and students reach these goals in various ways. Instructors should evaluate whether or not students meet objectives rather than how they meet them. Perhaps a student is not the most methodical in his way to assess and treat a patient, but if he completes the assessment and identifies and treats all the patient's injuries in an appropriate manner, does it matter in what order tasks were completed?

Instructors teach skills in a certain sequence, usually the most logical. Remember, students process information in different ways, and information relayed to the student may be processed in the brain in a

Instructors should evaluate whether or not students meet objectives rather than how they meet them.

different order, an order that is more easily retrieved by that student. If instructors demand that students only remember something one specific way, or perform a skill in one specific order (when it is not medically necessary to do so), the student will focus on learning that one task and may become frustrated and not have enough time to learn the remaining skills.

Emphasis on extrinsic rather than intrinsic goals
While some students are motivated by extrinsic factors, others are motivated by intrinsic factors. Intrinsic motivation can be used to guide much of classroom learning, but students may need some external incentives to learn material in which they are less interested.

Research has shown that instructors can undermine intrinsic motivation and learning by placing too much emphasis on external rewards or incentives. This is not to say that instructors should not reinforce student behavior, but that they should reduce the use of extrinsic rewards when the activity is interesting or enjoyable.

One theory suggests that when extrinsic rewards are used as an incentive to make students engage in a task, instructors should try to shift student attention away from the reward and toward the importance of the task and feelings of competence that performing the skill to mastery will instill, thereby focusing on intrinsic rewards.

Shift student attention away from the reward and toward the importance of the task.

Poor presentation methods
How information is presented influences how a student perceives a class session and whether or not participation is worth the time. If students view a class as boring or a waste of time, motivation will be minimal and little learning will take place. If presentation methods such as discussion, role playing or simulations are used, students will be more motivated to participate in class sessions.

Lack of student involvement with task selection
As discussed earlier, students are more motivated when they have input in what they learn and how they learn it.

Lack of interactivity
If the instructor chooses a straight lecture, with no interactivity with the audience, students will be less motivated than if a more interactive approach is taken. Using games such as Jeopardy or Trivial Pursuit customized for the course will enlist enthusiasm from students and increase their motivation toward learning.

Uni-dimensional presentation style
Using various presentation methods will increase student motivation, while maintaining a uni-dimensional style will prove boring and ineffective after the first few class sessions. Using a mix of lecture, demonstrations, small group discussions and other methods proves most beneficial in keeping students motivated. Incorporating audiovisual aids such as videos and even computer-based training programs also increases motivation.

Using various presentation methods will increase student motivation.

Negative Motivation Related to Evaluation Methods

Emphasis on grades rather than retention
Some instructors place too much emphasis on evaluation, and grade every activity and performance. They believe that unless an activity is

graded, students will not complete the task. Unfortunately, placing so much emphasis on the extrinsic motivation of grades may result in lost intrinsic motivation. Instructors need to encourage an increase in student knowledge and motivation to learn, not necessarily the completion of a task.

Emphasis on ability rather than effort

While the ability to perform tasks is a necessary part of EMS training programs, students must be rewarded for effort as well. Instructors are often more patient with a student who cannot pass an exam after spending hours studying and highlighting every chapter in the text. When it is obvious that the student is trying and giving an honest effort, it is the instructor's responsibility to alter teaching methods to find one that works for each student.

Students who need to avoid failure often do not try to succeed since expending effort and still failing poses a serious threat to their self-esteem. If the student fails after not trying, he can rationalize that he would have been successful if he had studied. This type of student always has an excuse at hand to save his pride in the event of failure. One such example is the student who announces he does not plan to study much for an exam. If this student does well on the exam, he is praised for success with little apparent effort. If the student does poorly, he can fall back on his previously announced excuse that he had not studied.

While instructors should value achievement, they must make an effort to reward more and punish less those students who have at least made an effort, regardless of their ability. Punishment should be saved for those who do not try.

Public evaluation leading to test anxiety

Research has shown that small amounts of anxiety can facilitate learning. If a student is well prepared and confident about an exam, a little anxiety can serve as motivation to excel. However, high levels of anxiety can prove detrimental to achievement. In fact, test anxiety is one of the most important factors of negative motivation, having debilitating effects on learning.

Remember the instructor who moves through a row of students asking a list of questions? The typical student is not paying attention to the questions but is instead counting down the row to find the question that will be asked of him. During this time, students miss all previous questions and learn little from the exercise. While learning the information presented during the exercise is important, some students are more motivated to avoid failure than to learn the lesson content.

When a student is severely afraid of failure, he is likely to fail to show up for class when unprepared, especially on exam days. Watch for this type of student and try to intervene early in the program while there is still time for remediation.

GOAL STRUCTURES

Goal structure refers to the way in which students relate to one another and to the instructor while working toward the attainment of instructional goals. As identified in Box 2.4, there are three types of goal structures—cooperative, competitive, and individualistic[7].

> Encourage an increase in student knowledge and motivation to learn.

> High levels of anxiety can prove detrimental to achievement.

BOX 2.4 Goal Structures

TYPE	MOTIVATION	USES/EXAMPLES
Cooperative	Positive interpersonal relations, including trust, acceptance, sharing, and helping	Preparing students to work in teams as they will in the field, eg, working together to extricate an entrapped patient in a motor vehicle accident
		Matching a low-level student with a high-level student since a cooperative setting is more likely to produce an increased level of motivation to learn because the interaction patterns encourage and support one's efforts to achieve
Competitive	Promotes little trust and acceptance and generates more attempts to mislead and obstruct others; competitive nature leads to an instinctive drive to succeed	Persons participating in an Emergency Vehicle Operations Course (EVOC) where students are awarded points based on selected criteria and the student with the highest score wins the competition
		Preparing for exams when individual skills are necessary
Individualistic	Promotes interaction with the instructor rather than with peers and minimizes positive affective (emotional) outcomes	Students working individually to prepare for and successfully complete an exam in which grades are based on their own progress
		Remedial learning to increase individual knowledge and skills

Goal structures

Cooperative Structure
Students work together in order to accomplish shared goals. There are no losers associated with a cooperative goal structure.

Competitive Structure
Students work against each other in order to achieve goals that only a few students can attain. Competitive environments produce both "winners" and "losers."

Individualistic Structure
Here, one student's achievement of the goal is unrelated to other student's achievement of the goal.

Different patterns of interaction and motivation are elicited by each type of goal structure. All three types are effective under certain conditions relating to specific goals and objectives of a lesson. Knowing when to use each type of learning strategy is an important decision instructors must make.

KEY POINTS

1. Adult students are different from traditional school-age students. Consequently, it is necessary for instructors to understand such differences and use instructional strategies to incorporate these differences to improve learning.
2. Malcom Knowles was the leader in defining what makes adult students different from children. While some of his original theories have been modified, others have been the cornerstone for building effective learning strategies.
3. Abraham Maslow's Hierarchy of Needs identifies various needs students must satisfy in order for learning to take place.
4. The most basic of these needs are the physiologic needs of food, sleep, clothing, and shelter. The second most basic need is that of safety in which students have a need to be in good health and free from harm and danger.
5. Both physiologic and safety needs must be met in the classroom environment. It is essential that instructors provide an atmosphere that promotes learning. Students need an environment that is warm, free from outside noise, and appropriately lighted.
6. It is important that instructors provide adequate breaks so students can meet other physiologic needs.
7. In addition to providing an appropriate learning environment and using instructional strategies with which adult students learn best, it is important that instructors motivate students to learn. There are two types of motivation factors; intrinsic and extrinsic.
8. Intrinsic motivation is influenced by personal factors such as satisfaction or an internal drive to succeed.
9. External motivation is influenced by external factors such as grades, title, points, or money.
10. Whichever type of motivation is most important to the individual student should be emphasized to make a connection and identify what is "in it for them."
11. Students learn what they want to learn. It is important that instructors make students want to learn what they need to know.
12. There are many factors that lead to negative motivation including those relating to the student, instructor, instructional techniques, and evaluation methods.
13. Any one component or a combination of all four can promote or prevent learning from taking place. The key is for instructors to recognize why students are exhibiting poor behavior or low performance, and use strategies to modify their behavior and increase performance and learning.
14. How individual students relate to one another and to the instructor is referred to as *goal structure.*
15. With a cooperative goal structure, students work together to accomplish shared goals.
16. With a competitive goal structure, students work against each other in order to achieve goals that only a few students can attain.
17. With an individualistic goal structure, one student's achievement of a goal is unrelated to another student's achievement of that goal.
18. Each type of goal structure elicits different patterns of interaction and should be used under certain conditions to improve understanding and retention of information.

FOLLOW-UP ACTIVITIES

1. Observe a classroom session and identify characteristics of the students. Note the differences between students in secondary school versus those returning to the classroom setting after many years.
2. Remember instructors who have had significant positive and negative impacts on you. What behavior did they exhibit that motivated you? What did not?
3. Think of factors that would have positive and negative influences on student motivation within each of the following categories:
   a. The student
   b. The instructor
   c. The course content
   d. The methods of instruction
   e. The evaluation process

FOLLOW-UP ACTIVITIES continued

4. Remember how you felt and how motivated you were in the following situations:
   a. Attended class without eating
   b. Had to use the bathroom but were uncertain when the next break would be
   c. Were in a room that was extremely cold or hot
   d. Were new in a class and did not know any other student
   e. Were scared
5. Think of how you felt as an EMT or paramedic students in the middle or three-quarters of the way through a class. How was the motivation level of the group? What can you do as an instructor to increase motivation levels?
6. Observe a few students in one of your class sessions:
   a. How often do low, middle, and high achievers interact in activities (*eg,* ask questions, engage in discussion)?
   b. How often do low, middle, and high achievers ask for assistance?
   c. Which students work independently at their work stations?

REFERENCE LIST

1. Knowles MS. *The Adult Learner: A Neglected Species.* Houston: Gulf Publishing Company; 1978.
2. Feuer D, Geber B. Uh-Oh... Second thoughts about adult learning theory. *Training.* 1988; December:31-39.
3. Davenport J III, Davenport JA. Andragogical-pedagogical orientations of adult learners. *Lifelong Learning.* 1986; September:58–59.
4. Newstrom JW, Lengnick-Hall ML. One size does not fit all. *Training & Development.* 1991; June:43-48.
5. Zemke R, Zemke S. 30 things we know for sure about adult learning. *Training.* 1988; July:57–61.
6. *Effective Training: A guide for the company instructor.* Intext, Inc.; 1979.
7. Dembo M. *Applying Educational Psychology in the Classroom.* White Plains, NY: Longman Publishing Group; 1991.

3 Principles of Learning

OBJECTIVES

Upon completion of this chapter, the reader will have sufficient information to:

1. Describe the three principle "laws" of learning and state their importance in EMS education.
2. State six factors to consider when selecting an instructional strategy.
3. List the three categories of informational material presented during instructional programs.
4. Identify the purpose of ice-breakers during an EMS program and list four ice-breaker exercises.
5. Identify techniques for improving the effectiveness of a lecture.
6. Describe techniques for improving the effectiveness of group discussions.
7. Determine appropriate methods for handling difficult groups during a group discussion session.
8. Identify techniques for improving the effectiveness of demonstrations and practice.
9. Describe the purpose of small group interaction, role playing, simulations, brainstorming, consultation triads, and case studies as instructional strategies.
10. Describe the purpose of team teaching during a training session.
11. List three different basic responses elicited by questions.
12. Describe the techniques involved with asking questions.
13. List the five steps involved in processing an answer.
14. Identify three possible effects of causing questions to increase learning.
15. Describe four actions to refrain from in order to increase the effectiveness of questioning.

KEY TERMS

Consultation triad An instructional strategy in which teams of three students participate in practice exercises

Demonstration An instructional strategy in which instructors show students the steps involved with a particular skill for training purposes

Group discussion An "open forum" of group interaction to talk about problem-solving issues

Longevity A learning principle stating that reinforcement and practice lead to retention of information and skills

Primacy A learning principle stating that the way one learns something the first time is the way one learns it best

Probing A strategy of trying to get a student to reach a correct answer; may involve restating the question or asking related questions to help the student

Programmed learning An instructional strategy that guides a student independently through a training session

Prompting Giving a student hints in an attempt to extract the correct response to a question

Recitation A series of questions teachers ask to elicit student responses

Recency A learning principle stating that what a student learns last is what he or she will most likely remember

Simulation A well-defined exercise designed to make a practice session as realistic as possible

Vivacy A learning principle stating that the more vivid the experience, the more likely the student is to learn and remember it

LAWS OF LEARNING

There are certain principles associated with learning that instructors should follow when teaching. These principles are referred to as the "laws" of learning and include primacy, vivacy, and longevity.

The law of primacy is extremely important when teaching students new information. This principle states that what students learn first is what they will remember. The law of primacy can be likened to having a clean chalkboard and writing information on it. If the information in wrong, and the instructor tries to erase it, there is still an imprint on the board of the original information.

Primacy occurs when teaching standards change. Prior to 1986, the American Heart Association taught students to open a victim's airway by using the head-tilt/neck-lift maneuver. In 1986, this standard was replaced by the head-tilt/chin-lift method. However, since students were taught the neck-lift first, and had practiced it for many years, the procedure was imbedded in memory and became a habit. Changing a habit is extremely difficult; even years after the change in this standard, students continue to perform the neck-lift.

Primacy also occurs when inaccurate information is presented. If an instructor must correct erroneous information, students may become confused since they are more likely to remember the information initially presented.

Along with the law of primacy is the law of recency. Recency simply means that what a student learns last is what he is most likely to remember. Therefore, it is important for the instructor to reinforce key points at the end of a lecture so that these items are discussed last.

The second law, the law of vivacy, refers to the way in which information is presented. Making information more vivid in the student's mind increases the likelihood the student will remember it. The more vividly something is presented, the more real and memorable it becomes. For example, using moulage during a practice scenario embeds a picture in the student's mind of what a particular injury looks like.

Vivacy also refers to audiovisual aids used during a presentation. Videos, slides, and transparencies all increase the likelihood that a student will remember information. Vivacy is increased by providing information in more than one way and by using more than one of the senses. By seeing, hearing, reading, and doing, students are more likely to understand and remember information, and be better able to perform skills adequately.

The third law of learning is longevity. Longevity is the principle belief that practice makes perfect, and that repetition breeds reinforcement, resulting in greater retention. This principle is somewhat obvious in that the longer and more often a student performs a skill, the more proficient he will become at that skill.

ENHANCING RECALL

Instructional strategies are various methods for organizing and presenting material during a course. Although variety in instructional methods is good, it is most important that you be effective as an instructor. The purpose of EMS instruction is to provide students with key information, teach them practical skills, provide the opportunity for practice and facilitate the learning process so they are able to understand what is presented and rapidly recall and process the infor-

> The more vividly something is presented, the more real and memorable it becomes.

> The purpose of EMS instruction is to provide students with key information, teach them practical skills, provide the opportunity for practice and facilitate the learning process so they are able to understand what is presented and rapidly recall and process the information during an emergency.

mation during an emergency. Therefore, when choosing an appropriate strategy, it is important to choose the one that will accomplish these goals most effectively[2].

The selection of a strategy depends primarily on the material being presented. There are multiple instructional strategies that can be effective in EMS programs. When choosing a method, it is important to keep the following in mind.

- **Instructor self-confidence.** Use techniques with which you are comfortable. As the instructor you must be comfortable, relaxed, and confident with the strategy you choose in order for it to be effective.
- **Time and materials needed for preparation.** Obviously some instructional strategies require many hours of preparation to be effective. Do not skimp on preparation. If you are not adequately prepared, the session will be a waste; go with a second choice.
- **Availability of materials, equipment and instructional adjuncts.** If available, ready-made instructional packages are easy and effective. Know in advance what instructional adjuncts are available in your area and how to obtain them.
- **Classroom size and environment**. If space is limited it may be difficult to break into small groups. In addition, if lighting is inadequate or the classroom is extremely warm, the class may fall asleep during a lecture. The addition of another instructional strategy may be required to maintain class interest and keep the students awake.
- **The size and makeup of the group.** If the group is large, make certain there are enough assistant instructors for small group discussions. Otherwise, a lecture format may be more appropriate. If the students are quick students and all that is necessary is a review of key points, alternative instructional strategies can be used. Games, such as Jeopardy or crossword puzzles, are more effective with a refresher program than a straight lecture since these students possess background information. In addition, the use of certain audiovisual equipment may not be effective with large groups.
- **The type of information being presented.** Informational material presented during a program falls into three categories:

1) **Factual information**—Facts, such as the definitions of dyspnea, anatomy and physiology, or the number of bones in the body. Factual information is more effectively presented in a lecture format. Puzzles and games can be very effective when used to reinforce or review factual information for refresher students.
2) **Subjective information**—Material that requires input of feelings, attitudes, and beliefs. Subjective information is best communicated by lectures, group discussion, simulation, and role playing.
3) **Physical skills**—The knowledge of and ability to perform specific physical tasks such as applying a traction splint or immobilizing the spine. Teaching physical skills is best done by demonstration, simulation, and guided practice.

TYPES OF INSTRUCTIONAL STRATEGIES

The following are various types of instructional strategies[2]. Each method can be used on its own or in combination.

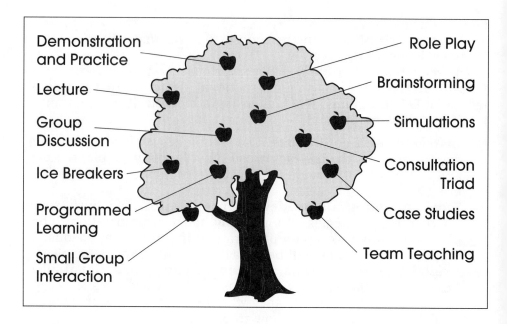

Ice breakers are short exercises designed to get a class "warmed-up."

Ice Breakers

Ice breakers are short exercises designed to get a class "warmed-up." They are generally used on the first day of class to familiarize students with each other and to serve as an introduction. If the class is relatively short, icebreakers may not be necessary; however, they are highly recommended for the first night of first responder, EMT, and paramedic training programs.

Besides providing a means for students to introduce themselves to each other, ice breakers provide the opportunity for instructors to meet students and for students to become familiar with persons other than those with whom they came. Since most EMS courses require students to find partners, many students choose the classmates they know—a relationship that often proves detrimental. Just because a student is a friend does not make him or her a good choice for partner. Often the opposite is true and students are better off finding a different partner early. Ice breakers provide the opportunity for all students to mingle with each other and find new partners before "cliques" begin. The following ice breakers have proven beneficial for the first night of class.

The Name Game

Students and instructors form a circle. The person to the left of the instructor begins by stating his name and one bit of personal information such as a hobby. The person to the left then states the first student's name and hobby and then introduces himself and states his hobby. The next student will state the first student's name and hobby, the second student's name and hobby, and add his own information. This process continues until the instructor has to repeat everyone's name and hobby, and then introduce himself. Class members should help out if a participant gets stuck on one particular person. If time permits, when one student forgets the previous information on his turn, the preceding student should repeat his turn, providing the opportunity for review. This exercise lasts between 20 and 30 minutes depending on the size of the class. Besides providing an opportunity for introductions, the name game lets students know that through repetition anything can be learned.

Paired Introductions

Students pair off with a classmate, introduce themselves, and discuss personal background with each other. When the group gets back together, students introduce their partners to the rest of the group.

Written Exercises

Students are given index cards on which they are asked to write one or two items, such as what outcome they expect from the course, fears, expectations, concerns, or problems they would like addressed. Cards are then given to the instructor for review or kept by the student for future reference. At the conclusion of the course, students are again given index cards and asked to complete the same task. The cards can then be compared to identify whether goals were achieved, problems solved, and fears conquered.

The Scavenger Name Hunt

Students are given a worksheet with multiple questions pertaining to class makeup. Students are then asked to circulate and mingle with other classmates to determine which student each question identifies, and write that person's name next to the question. Each student's name can be used only once. Like the name game, this process provides the opportunity for participants to meet each other, make new friends, and find new partners. This exercise is very effective and works well on the first day of a long course such as the EMT or paramedic programs. Questions can be either serious or fun.

Scavenger Name Hunt

- Who is from the southern part of the county? _____
- Who is wearing mismatched socks? _____
- Who has ever wrecked an ambulance? _____
- Who has the initials C.P.? _____
- Who has ever flown in a hot air balloon? _____
- Who has ever done CPR in the field? _____
- Who wears three or more patches on their jacket? _____
- Who has their scanner on 24 hours a day? _____

Lecture

A *lecture* is a prepared, organized speech on a specific topic. Lectures are given to provide information, analyze issues and ideas, or describe personal experiences. During a lecture, there is little or no student participation or feedback, depending on the size of the class. Since lecture involves solely listening to the instructor, the students tend to remember little of what is presented.

Although lecture is very useful in certain circumstances, all information does not need to come from the instructor. Lecture is primarily a pedagogical method of instruction and works best in a traditional classroom setting. Historically, students expect to walk into the classroom and have the instructor "spoon feed" all the information they need to know. While lecturing is still the predominant instructional strategy in EMS education, the addition of other strategies will ultimately increase the amount of learning actually taking place in the classroom.

Lectures allow the instructor to present pertinent information in a relatively short period of time with little effort. If the instructor is ill

Lectures are given to provide information, analyze issues and ideas, or describe personal experiences.

prepared, however, a straight lecture can be ineffective. Students do not generally come to class with a "clean slate," and can often add to a lecture with case scenarios, past experiences, and questions. Therefore, try to involve students as often as possible to make the information relative to their needs as well as keep them awake.

When presenting a lecture, try to keep it short and to the point. Provide enough information to cover key areas and then move on to a different instructional strategy. Remember, when dealing with adult students, it is not the instructor's responsibility to provide all of the necessary information. It should be emphasized often to the class that students are expected and required to read all appropriate materials. Instructors simply point out key issues, facilitate the learning process, and provide the opportunity for evaluation and remedial training. Instructors are not present to spoon feed information to the students.

The following suggestions may increase the effectiveness of a lecture:

- **When presenting information in lecture format, try to use instructional media** to augment the lecture and provide a visual impression of what is being presented. The addition of audiovisual materials will increase the retention of the information provided.

- **Prepare an outline of the material to be covered, and provide it along with any additional handouts** that may be helpful to the students. An outline helps students follow the instructor and allows them to listen to the lecture rather than taking copious notes.

- **Make certain everyone can see you;** if they cannot, it may be necessary to stand on a podium. Students tend to block out the speaker they cannot see.

- **Use examples to reinforce the information you are providing** whenever possible. Examples and relevant real-life experiences increase the effectiveness of a lecture. Students need to be able to relate information to situations in order to make it meaningful, so it can be remembered and used as needed. Be careful, however, not to overuse "war stories."

- **Allow ample time for questions and answers.** If you do not know an answer, do not try to con the student or you will lose credibility. Simply say you do not know the answer but that you will research the question and have an answer for the next class. Make certain to follow-up with the answer.

- **When speaking to a large group, make certain everyone can hear you**. It may be necessary to use a microphone or have the group move closer to you.

Group Discussion

Group discussion provides the opportunity for instructors to ascertain the knowledge level of students.

Group discussion provides the opportunity for instructors to ascertain the knowledge level of students. By encouraging group discussion as an instructional strategy, the instructor can draw from students' past experiences and knowledge base. In addition, the open dialogue promotes the feeling of respect between the instructor and students, since they are adults and often have something important to add to a lecture. Group discussions provide a very simple, effective training strategy that promotes student interaction.

Group discussion is primarily an exchange of ideas. It is an active process that allows the instructor to monitor learning by listening to the students' interpretation or regurgitation of information. Discussion also stimulates thinking and modification of attitudes, provides for a pooling of ideas, maintains class interest, and facilitates the retention of key issues.

Group discussion can take place in large groups, but it is recommended that groups be kept small to provide all students the opportunity to participate. More interaction takes place and students view the experience as more valuable, when groups are small.

During a discussion, it is important to maintain control of the group while providing the opportunity for student participation. The instructor should guide and facilitate the group's discussion but not dominate the process. The idea of a discussion is for the students, not the instructor, to discuss information. Obviously, the instructor needs to participate in the process during controversial issues or lulls, but try not to impose your own ideas on the students if the information they are providing is adequate. Offer information as "food for thought," but don't hinder their thought process. If during a situational review, for example, the group decides on a method for immobilizing and extricating a victim of a car accident that is technically accurate, but perhaps not the method of choice, the instructor can provide an alternative without telling the students their idea is wrong. In emergency care procedures there are many correct methods for performing treatments; let students experiment, when possible, for what works for them.

It is important to provide feedback to students during a discussion. React to what students are saying. If a student provides incorrect information, ask the rest of the class what they think about this idea. Allow the opportunity for the group to correct the information without your direct interference. If the group is way "off base" you will need to bring them back on line. Likewise, react in a positive way if student comments are accurate. Comments such as "That's a good point" or "What does the rest of the group think?" will assist in the facilitation of the discussion.

> It is important to provide feedback to students during a discussion. React to what students are saying.

When leading the discussion process, remember to look at those who are providing input. Eye contact lets students know you are interested in what they have to say and that you are listening. Remember, this is neither a "free for all" session nor the opportunity for the instructor to take a break. The instructor is an integral part of the discussion process. Try to get the entire group involved in the discussion and keep the pace moving. Then, at the conclusion of a group discussion, bring the group together to summarize what learning has taken place.

> At the conclusion of a group discussion, bring the group together to summarize what learning has taken place.

All groups are different so there will be times when the instructor encounters problems during the discussion process. The following practical tips may be helpful when handling these difficulties in order to keep the discussion on track.

The quiet group
In this group nobody has anything to add to the discussion. Some students do not interact well with others, while others may not understand what is expected from them. Try to motivate students to participate, but if the discussion does not get started, step back, regroup, and try a different instructional strategy.

The fighting group
In this group students disagree among each other. If the disagreement is on subject matter, try to resolve the issue. If the problem is personal, try to resolve it or break up the group. Solve problems quickly to prevent wasting valuable time.

The "know-it-all" in the group

This person may complete all the tasks or answer all the questions within the first 10 minutes. Historically, if one student in the group offers all of the answers, other group members tend not to offer input. It is easier to not have to participate in the discussion and just let the know-it-all answer for them. Try to encourage all students to participate and offer opposing views to the discussion. It may become necessary to tell the know-it-all to let others participate; do so in a non-threatening manner.

The lingering group

Students in this group refrain from answering and cannot come to a consensus on an issue, and consequently tend to spend the entire time on the first issue. If the discussion is productive, revolving around key issues, let it continue. If the discussion is not productive, stop it and try to get the students back on the track of the discussion and move on to the next issue.

The straying group

In this group, students cannot keep their attention on the task at hand, but rather tend to stray from the intent of the discussion. When circulating around different groups, if you hear a group that seems to be "off the track" of the topic they should be discussing, stop and look at the group. This is usually enough to get them back on track. If not, you may need to interrupt and tell them they seem to have wandered off the subject. If the group continues to stray, it may be necessary to reorganize the groups.

Demonstration and Practice

Demonstrations arouse students' interest and motivate them to learn.

Demonstration as an instructional strategy is based on the premise that you must see something being done in order to do it yourself, and you must do it in order to know it. Demonstrations arouse students' interest and motivate them to learn. In EMS education, demonstration is necessary for students to effectively learn practical skills. Demonstrations serve multiple purposes in instruction: they arouse student interest in a topic, motivate student participation, direct attention to what is important, and put meaning behind what the instructor is presenting.

When performing a demonstration, it is important that you explain what you are doing and why you are doing it. Remember, the audience is passive during a demonstration. You must therefore make certain that students are attentive during the demonstration and understand what is taking place. To save time and embarrassment, be sure to check the equipment prior to the class session to make certain it is in working order.

In order to make the process more effective, the following factors are important to remember when offering a demonstration.

- **Make certain that all the students can see**. Ask anyone who cannot see what you are doing to move. Do not force them to move, but mention it.
- **Be accurate when performing the demonstration**. Remember the law of primacy. If you perform a skill incorrectly and then correct yourself, the way you did it first is the way students will remember and mimic it.
- **Repetition is a key factor in the learning process**. Demonstrations should be performed more than once and should be followed by guided practice. It is important to monitor the students' performance and provide feedback to correct or reinforce

performance. If a student performs a skill incorrectly, stop him at the point of the error and make him start the skill over from the beginning. This repetition forces the student to understand what he is doing wrong and provides the opportunity to imprint the correct way to perform the skill.

🍎 **When practicing skills, optimize the experience by providing the opportunity for all students to participate**. Have one student act as the victim and two others as rescuers. Make another student a bystander at the scene. The other two students can serve as "evaluators" for the station. When the scenario is completed, ask the students how they did and provide the opportunity for them to correct their mistakes. Then ask the evaluators how the students did and areas in need of improvement. This process allows all the students to participate during the entire session instead of only when they are acting as the rescuers.

Programmed Learning

Programmed learning is an instructional method using various training materials to guide a student through the learning process step by step. Programmed learning requires students to learn a small portion of material, practice it, and then repeat the information. Various programmed learning packages exist, including video packages, workbook self-study guides, and computer-assisted instructional packages.

Although programmed learning is extremely useful for remedial training or to make up a missed session, it is not very beneficial in a large group setting nor to learn a large amount of material. In small groups, however, programmed learning can be beneficial provided the student is interested in learning the material. Interaction is required to make this process work.

Programmed learning allows students to work through a curriculum at their own pace, paying more attention to those areas in which they need additional help. If the student feels comfortable with knowledge of the content of the material, he moves on to the next topic, thereby participating in the evaluation of his own progress. Programmed learning is not recommended for the learning of practical skills since instructor evaluation and feedback are necessary.

Small Group Interaction

Small group discussion sessions are extremely effective as an instructional strategy. Dividing large groups into smaller groups of no more than six students each provides the ultimate environment for providing information, demonstrations, and practice, and for allowing regurgitation and processing of knowledge. When planning a small group work session, it is best to have set goals, objectives, and tasks outlined. Having the session well planned will assist the group in understanding what is expected of them, the process to get there, and the time constraints placed on them.

In EMS training programs, small groups are useful for both discussion and practice sessions. They are useful for comparing viewpoints on how to perform a specific skill, how to deal with a particular situation, how to identify a specific illness or injury, and how to prioritize. During practice sessions, small groups provide the opportunity for accomplishing multiple tasks in a short period of time. Divide the class into groups of six students each. Have each group practice a specific skill with an instructor at each station. Allow ample time for students to practice a skill or run through a scenario and then send the

> Programmed learning requires students to learn a small portion of material, practice it, and then repeat the information.

> In EMS training programs, small groups are useful for both discussion and practice sessions.

group on to the next station. Rotate the groups until they have all completed each station and have accomplished the objectives for the session. By working in smaller groups, each student has the opportunity to practice every skill instead of only a select few.

Instructors can also use small groups for gathering information for discussion. For example, the instructor can divide the class into small groups and give each group one topic to research (*eg*, diabetes mellitus, myocardial infarction, or cerebrovascular accident). Each group can then identify the pathophysiology, signs and symptoms, and emergency care for each illness. Each group should take notes on their discussion and, when the class is brought together, a recorder from each group can present key points for their subject matter. One word of caution about this format is that groups are more likely to know their particular topic best and may not get the remainder of necessary information if other groups are not accurate or if the recorder is not a good presenter of information.

Although small group discussion is an extremely effective method of instruction, be careful not to overuse it. Students expect a certain amount of teaching to come from the instructor and do not like to do all the work involved with learning. Used in moderation, however, small groups are generally a well accepted and very useful instructional strategy.

Role Play

Role play is an instructional strategy used to act out roles involved in cases studies. One student plays the part of the victim, and two play the rescuers. Role play is designed to focus on the feelings of both victims and rescuers. EMS providers develop a new feeling for delivering patient care once they have acted as a victim, either through role play or under actual circumstances. There is no written script involved; each participant acts and reacts to one another as the scenario progresses.

> Role play is designed to focus on the feelings of both victims and rescuers.

In EMS education, role play is useful for practicing patient interviews, histories, and identification of illnesses and injuries. Pre-plan the scenario with the "victims," explaining what to expect and how to act for the exercise. Decide on the illness or injury, setting, and mechanism of injury. Then have the rescuers interview the patient and obtain information to determine the problem. At the end of the exercise, have a general discussion about it to ascertain how well the rescuers conducted the interview phase and identification of the illness or injury.

An alternative approach to role play is to stop the scenario periodically, analyze how the exercise is progressing, and elicit audience participation. Ask the students how they feel the scenario is progressing and whether the rescuers are performing their roles and responsibilities adequately. Then ask the students what steps should be taken next.

The key to success when using role play is student participation. Explain what is expected of the students and the anticipated outcome of the exercise. Evaluate the effectiveness of the exercise. If students are receptive to the process, continue with the next exercise; if not, decide on an alternative instructional strategy.

Simulations

A *simulation* is a well-defined exercise in which field situations are imitated and the students are expected to respond and perform in a manner consistent with their training. Simulations include programmed patient situations, role play, problem-solving situations, computer simulations, and the use of simulators, models, and manikins. Simulations are generally designed around case studies. In EMS training programs, simulation is an extremely effective instructional strategy. Next to real-life experience simulations are the best way to evaluate students' knowledge of a specific subject and their ability to perform practical skills. It is also the best and most realistic means for student practice.

Simulating experiences is the second most effective learning method. Since students simulate the actual field environment, allowing practice of frequently and infrequently encountered situations, they are better prepared to handle emergency situations at the conclusion of training. In addition, simulations allow the instructor to measure the total performance levels of students objectively, including their decision-making capabilities. By subjecting students to the stresses of the occupations, simulations provide them with realistic situations to allow them to determine objectively whether they actually want to pursue a career in EMS.

One disadvantage of simulations is the time needed for their preparation, presentation, and evaluation. In addition, these experiences often require additional equipment and personnel. Two ways around these constraints are to use a student as the victim, thereby decreasing the need for additional faculty to fill that role, and to break the skills into multiple scenarios requiring different skills in order to spread the equipment needs throughout the class.

Simulations should be scenario-based, and moulage should be used in order to add realism to the exercise. Similar to case studies and role play, simulations require student participation in order to be effective. To develop an effective situation, first decide what skills are to be included. Then decide on a simulation that would result in the illness or injury requiring the use of those skills. Next, choose one victim and two or three rescuers, and program the victim with appropriate information, such as the types of injuries involved, the appropriate answers to questions during the patient interview, and how to respond to different types of treatment.

Describe the scenario to the rest of the class beginning with dispatch information *eg*, "You are dispatched to an injury from a fall to find a 26-year-old woman lying on the sidewalk". Tell the rescuers what is expected of them, explain that there is equipment available for their use, and let them proceed. When they have completed the tasks of identifying injuries, performing a patient assessment and interview, and providing appropriate treatment, ask the students how they think they handled the situation. Then ask the rest of the class for input in evaluating the exercise.

When using simulations, try to involve as much of the class as possible. Smaller groups are most effective for this type of exercise, providing there is adequate equipment and supervision to correct mistakes.

The main difference between simulations and role play is the use of practical skills. In role play, emergency care is not performed but may be discussed. The objective of role play is patient assessment, interview, and discussion of actions in order to identify an illness or injury. Role play is a verbal exercise while a simulation is a hands-on practical skills exercise.

Brainstorming

Brainstorming is a creative thinking session designed to have students suggest ideas on a specific topic in order to bring about the information necessary to handle a problem. Brainstorming is a broad information-gathering session that will become more focused later. In EMS programs, brainstorming is useful to identify knowledge levels of stu-

Next to real-life experience, simulations are the best way to evaluate students' knowledge.

Brainstorming is a broad information-gathering session that will become more focused later.

dents, evaluate whether students have read necessary materials, and discover alternative methods for handling certain situations.

In order for brainstorming to be effective, groups should consist of no more than eight students. Each group should be provided with a pen and paper to keep track of their ideas. Start the class off by giving a scenario and ask students for input regarding appropriate actions. One such scenario could be, "Suppose you were dispatched to the scene of a multi-vehicle accident. There are four cars and one bus involved, with a total count of 16 patients. How would you handle this situation?" Then ask for student input on the logistics of what they would do in this incident.

A second approach would be to describe a specific situation and have students provide input into different ways to handle it. An example is, "You are dispatched to an injured person. You arrive at the scene of a domestic dispute involving a hostage situation. What should you be aware of during this situation and what actions would you take?" Or, "You arrive on location of an apparent suicide. What do you do?" Each of these situations requires specific actions, but the order and method by which the students perform them is their choice.

Another way to use brainstorming in the EMS classroom is to provide information and have students decipher what you are describing. For example, provide a listing of signs of symptoms of a specific illness and have the students identify the illness, or tell the students the illness and have them list the signs and symptoms or treatment.

Brainstorming is based on the premise that all students come to class with various backgrounds and ways to look at certain situations. Suggesting ideas for discussion allows students to discover different viewpoints on various topics.

Consultation Triad

A consultation triad is a group of three students working as a team in assigned roles.

A *consultation triad* is a group of three students working as a team in assigned roles. One student acts as the victim, one the rescuer, and the other as an observer. This exercise includes three phases in which students have the opportunity to function in each role. As a result, each student has a chance to practice performing skills, providing feedback, and getting a first-hand look at what the victim experiences at the scene of an incident.

Consultation triads are very effective because of the high level of student participation. Provide the groups with general guidelines about what is expected of them and set a time limit. Generally 15 to 20 minutes is ample time to complete the exercise. Then provide an additional 5 minutes to allow students to evaluate the exercise. Repeat the process until all class members have had the opportunity to function in each of the three roles. At the conclusion of the exercise, bring the group together to provide the opportunity for a wrap-up to evaluate the effectiveness of the exercise and discuss what the students have learned from it.

Case Studies

Case studies provide a method of discussion regarding how specific situations are handled.

Similar to role play and simulations, case studies provide a method of discussion regarding how specific situations are handled. The instructor should prepare handouts describing cases that are appropriate for a specific content area. For example, when teaching environmental emergencies, design some cases for a drowning victim, a heat stroke victim, and a hypothermic patient. For a handout, prepare a description of the scenario and the emergency treatment provided.

Give each student a copy of the cases to be studied. Then read the scenario, what was determined to be the illness, and what emergency care was provided. Next, have the class discuss whether the illness or injury was accurately determined and if the emergency care provided was appropriate. If it is decided that the illness or injuries were not accurately determined or that actions were not appropriate, it is important to ascertain why not and what changes should have been made. These case studies are invaluable in EMS training programs.

Team Teaching

In team teaching, two or more instructors share the responsibility of planning and coordinating a course, teaching the lessons, and evaluating student progress. Team members plan each session and assign roles. Responsibilities include planning the session, developing resource material, teaching the material, gathering and checking equipment, and assisting the lead instructor.

In team teaching, members learn from each other's instructional styles and abilities. Team members are then able to augment and complement each other by relating personal experience and expertise into each class session. Conflicts may arise if teaching styles are substantially different; be careful not to let these conflicts interfere with effective instruction. Remember that with team teaching the effectiveness of the program relies on the effectiveness and cohesiveness of the instructors. When planning team teaching, make certain to choose instructors who work well together.

In EMS programs, team teaching is extremely effective. Because programs are often taught by multiple instructors, cohesiveness of instruction is sometimes questioned. Through team teaching, however, cohesiveness is reinforced. Using the same group of people for an entire course allows instructors to know what information has been presented and what is yet to come. It also allows students to build a rapport with the instructors. Finally, team teaching allows for better control and evaluation of the program.

> In team teaching, two or more instructors share the responsibility of planning and coordinating a course, teaching the lessons, and evaluating student progress.

THE ART OF QUESTIONING

Recitation refers to a series of questions an instructor asks, usually regarding curriculum content, to elicit a student response. The use of questioning in EMS programs is a very effective method to increase student participation by soliciting responses from individual students. Questioning is useful in promoting interaction between instructors and students and in providing students with an evaluation method for testing knowledge levels, thought processes, retention of material, and problem solving abilities.

Purpose of Questioning

Questioning is used for multiple purposes in the classroom. Following are a few examples of its uses.

To initiate discussion

Group discussions often focus around answering a question. For example, "What are the logistics of dealing with a multi-vehicle accident?" or "What is the difference between angina pectoris and a myocardial infarction?" When using questions to initiate a discussion, make certain the topic is focused. Questions should not be too general, or so specific that a yes/no answer would suffice.

> When using questions to initiate a discussion, make certain the topic is focused.

To tie in a previous lesson

When a topic relates directly to a previous topic, it is helpful to ask students questions in order to make the new topic more relative and provide a smoother transition. Questions also indicate to the instructor that prerequisite information has been learned so that instruction can be presented in a manner which is more relevant and meaningful. For example, when covering the cardiac arrest portion of a CPR class, students should already be proficient at airway obstruction and respiratory distress. An opening question might be, "Today we are going to cover the C of the ABCs. What do A and B stand for?" If nobody can answer that question, remedial training is necessary before the planned session can continue.

To assess knowledge or past experiences

At the beginning of a class, it is useful to question students to ascertain whether they have read the required material. During a lecture, questions increase student participation and make certain that students are attentive. Inquiring about past experiences relevant to current subject matter increases retention of information by making it more meaningful for students.

To evaluate instructional effectiveness

When providing a summary of a lesson, questions can determine whether any learning has taken place. Questions can be asked in the form of a review, quiz, or drill. Questions often work well as a summary or wrap-up of a session to reinforce key material. In some situations, providing a quiz at the beginning of class and again at the end of class will demonstrate how effective the training session was.

To involve nonparticipants

Student learning increases with participation. If students are not participating actively, recruit them by asking questions.

Student learning increases with participation.

To deter the problem student

If a student is disruptive in class, asking him a question will let both the class and the student know that you have identified a problem. Chances are the student has not been paying attention and will not know the answer. Either way, asking a question will probably deter the student from future disruptions, at least for a while.

To assist the instructor in lecture presentation

During a lecture, all of the material does not need to come from the instructor. In adult education, the onus of learning is on the student. They should be prepared for class by reading required material. Therefore, instead of stating "There are seven cervical vertebrae," ask the class "How many cervical vertebrae are there in the body?" This type of questioning involves the students, and will increase their retention of that material and keep them awake for the session. It will also increase the likelihood of students being prepared for class.

Students often remember items emphasized by instructors through recitation.

To stress key points

Students often remember items emphasized by instructors through recitation. As a class summary, ask questions regarding the most important aspects of a lesson.

To motivate the group and maintain attention
Questioning students will keep them attentive during a lesson and motivate them by interaction.

Types of Questions

Questions generally fall into two categories: factual and cognitive. Factual questions require students to regurgitate information previously presented. Cognitive questions, on the other hand, require students to engage in a higher thought process in order to develop a response. Questions are asked to elicit three response categories:

Recall

These questions require memorization of content material. An example of a recall type question would be "What is 2×2" or "What is the medical term for thigh bone?" The answers are simply facts.

Application

These questions require the use of content without analysis: if this, then that. An example of an application question is "What do you do if you encounter a person who is conscious but choking?" There is only one answer to this question.

Problem-solving

These questions require the use of content material in new situations. This type of question is very useful to elicit discussions. An example question is "You arrive first at an automobile accident. The car is unstable and there are six victims. What would you do?" There could be multiple responses to this question since the responder has many tasks to complete.

Questions that require students to think through the answer, as well as those that require regurgitation of information are both useful in their own context. The challenge is to use each type of question to its best advantage.

The challenge is to use each type of question to its best advantage.

Keys to Effective Questioning

When asking a question, remember a few key points.

- **Ask specific questions that have a specific answer.** Students cannot read your mind; they need to understand what it is you are asking.
- **Use the APC technique for asking questions**. The instructor **A**sks the question, **P**auses to allow for consideration of the question, and then **C**alls on a student for an answer.
- **Wait approximately 8 seconds for a response**. It takes approximately 8 seconds for a student to formulate a response. If there is no answer, ask the rest of the class if anyone knows the answer.
- **Do not let one student dominate when answering questions**. There are a variety of ways of choosing students to answer questions. You could proceed in order of the class, asking each student one question. Or you could pick students randomly. One strategy for asking questions is deciding when to pick a student. If you call on a student prior to the question, the rest of the class "turns off" because they know they are "safe" for the moment. The alternative is to ask the question and then pick a student. The second method ensures that the entire class is pay-

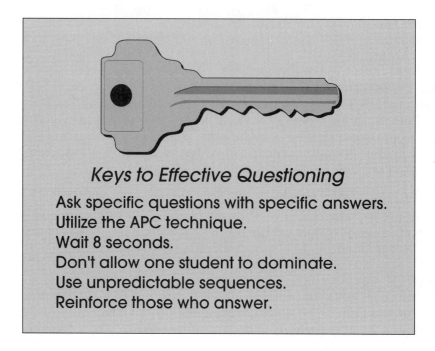

Keys to Effective Questioning

Ask specific questions with specific answers.
Utilize the APC technique.
Wait 8 seconds.
Don't allow one student to dominate.
Use unpredictable sequences.
Reinforce those who answer.

ing attention. If there is a disruptive student or one who is not paying attention, use the second method and call on that student.

- **Use an unpredictable sequence when asking questions**. Asking students in any pattern that may be obvious to the class will result in students spending more time figuring out the pattern in order to determine "their" question than listening to responses. The benefit of recitation is then lost for most of the class.
- **Reinforce those who answer**. Those students who make the initiative to offer a response should be rewarded. Make certain to acknowledge their responses.

Constructing Effective Questions

- **Avoid yes/no questions**. The goal of questioning is to get the student to think. A yes/no question provides little information and requires little thought. In order to make the discussion more meaningful if yes/no questions must be used, ask the student why he chose that answer.
- **Make certain the question is understandable**. Students need to know exactly what you are asking. It is best to ask questions with openings of why, what, or how. Students are able to understand exactly what response you are seeking when asking these types of questions. If the class cannot respond to your question, restate it; more than likely it is a poor question.
- **Limit each question to one main thought.** Do not confuse the students by asking multiple questions in one. Separate each idea into a new question.
- **Make certain the question is related directly to the subject matter.** Students get confused with questions that are so minute in detail that unless they were a genius they cannot answer. Do not ask questions in order to boast your knowledge. If students do not need to know something, do not ask the question. Likewise, if the question is not relevant to the subject matter at

hand, do not confuse the class. Wait until the question does relate before asking it.

The Process of Answering Questions

Answering a question requires the student to engage in the following five steps[1].

1) **Listening to the question as asked.** Students who are not attentive when a question is asked will not be able to answer the question, nor will they benefit from the answer.
2) **Deciphering the meaning of the question**. The student must determine what is being asked. It is sometimes difficult for students to understand what the instructor is asking because of the way a question is phrased.
3) **Thinking of a response.** Students need to think of an answer before they can put it into words. In order to think of a response, students must have the information available for recall, and must possess the cognitive abilities required to process such information.
4) **Generating a response to the instructor.** Just because a student develops an answer to a question does not ensure his delivery of the response. Students often compete for "air time" with other students.
5) **Revising the response, if necessary**. If the student's response is incorrect, he may need to rethink the answer.

Handling Student Responses

When students give correct answers, acknowledge their responses and reinforce the key points. Praise students for correct responses. If the student gives an incorrect answer, however, do not simply say he has the "wrong answer," especially if it is a shy student. Your objective as an instructor is to promote learning, not hurt students' feelings or degrade them.

Praise students for correct responses.

If the student gives a partially correct answer, give him credit for the answer, acknowledge the incorrect part as needing clarification, and provide the opportunity for the student to alter his response. For example, you ask "What is the correct ratio for compressions and ventilations for one-rescue CPR on an adult victim?" The student replies "15:1." You should reply, "You're right, you give 15 compressions, but how may ventilations?" This reinforces the correct statement while providing the opportunity for the student to "save face" and correct his answer.

If the student gives a totally incorrect answer, tact must be taken in preparing a reply. Again, if you can salvage the response and offer the chance for the student to correct the answer, try. For example, if the above student said "5:1," an incorrect answer, you could reply: "It's 5:1 for an infant, but what about for an adult?" thereby offering a second chance. There are two additional strategies for handling a student whose response is completely incorrect. One strategy is termed probing and the other prompting. *Probing* involves using every possible means for getting the student to the correct answer, without answering it yourself. You could also simply restate the question. *Prompting* involves giving the student hints to try to extract the correct response.

Prompting involves giving the student hints to try to extract the correct response.

Instructors can facilitate the learning process by providing explanations that clarify and correct student responses to questions. Learning is further enhanced by acknowledging correct responses and building new information on them.

Why is Recitation Effective?

Questions asked throughout a training session serve multiple purposes. Following are possible effects which cause questions to increase learning[1].

Practice and feedback effects

Students usually participate in questioning sessions following a lecture or reading of required materials. Recitation provides students the opportunity to practice recalling information previously presented. Through this process they receive feedback from the instructor regarding the accuracy and quality of their responses.

Cueing effect

> *Through recitation, key information can be brought out in a new context and with new meaning.*

Recitation may provide cues to focus students' attention on particular information contained in the textbook or from a lecture. Students sometimes pass over important content material, which they view as irrelevant or meaningless. Through recitation, key information can be brought out in a new context and with new meaning. Furthermore, students often perform better on exams that test items that have been previously discussed through recitation. This suggests that when students hear a question, they are more likely to rehearse the answer. Conversely, they are likely to discard information that has not been covered during recitations as being unnecessary to study.

Instruction and test similarity

> *The practice provided by recitation increases the student's ability to perform well on exams.*

The question-and-answer format of recitation parallels widely used testing formats. The practice provided by recitation increases the student's ability to perform well on exams. Constantly drilling students on key information leads to increased retention of information. In addition, asking the types of questions that will be seen on interim and final examinations will result in higher test scores.

Pitfalls of Questions

There are a few actions to refrain from in order to increase the effectiveness of questioning.

- **Allowing insufficient time to think.** Always allow at least 8 seconds for the student to answer a question. It will take this long to process the question and formulate a response.
- **Asking questions that are too simple.** Give students credit for knowing something. Asking questions that are too simple will alienate students and provide little information or motivation.
- **Answering your own questions.** Again, allow the student ample opportunity to answer the question. If he cannot produce an answer in 8 seconds, rephrase the question and try again. If the student still cannot answer the question, ask the rest of the class. As a last resort, provide the answer. Keep rhetorical questions to a minimum.
- **Calling on the same student.** Avoid calling on the same student repeatedly. Instructors tend to call on the person who knows the most because chances are he will provide the correct response. The person who knows the information does not need the benefit from questioning.

Questioning is an acquired art requiring practice and experimentation. When planning your lesson, remember this saying: "The novice concentrates on what to say. . . the pro on what to ask."

Handling Student Questions

The most important factors when answering student questions are honesty and sincerity. Remember, there is no such thing as a stupid question. If you degrade students who ask questions, you are robbing them of a very important part of the learning process. In addition, the rest of the class will be turned off by your attitude and will not ask questions. Be sure to answer the questions as honestly as possible. If you do not know the answer to a question, acknowledge that fact and promise to find the answer and report it at the next class. Then be sure to follow through with that promise. Otherwise, you have once again lost credibility with the class.

One method for handling student questions is to redirect the question to the rest of the class. For example, if a student asks, "What would you do if a patient is impaled on a fence post?" Your response could be, "What does the rest of the class think? How could we handle that situation?" This allows the opportunity for discussion and increased student participation.

> The most important factors when answering student questions are honesty and sincerity.

KEY POINTS

1. The selection and use of instructional strategies is the backbone of effective instruction.
2. The *law of primacy* states that what students learn in initial instruction, and the way they learn it is what they will remember. If initial information is incorrect, it will be more difficult for the instructor to teach new information because the initial information is still in the student's mind.
3. The *law of recency* states that what the student learns last is what he is most likely to remember. Consequently, instructors should reinforce key points at the end of a training session so that these items are discussed last.
4. The *law of vivacy* refers to the way in which information is presented. Making information more vivid in a student's mind increases the likelihood the student will remember it. The use of audiovisual materials help information appear more vivid.
5. *Instructional strategies* are various methods for organizing and presenting material during a course. It is important when choosing a method to keep the following in mind: instructor self-confidence, time and materials needed for preparation, availability of materials, classroom environment, size and makeup of the group, and the type of information being presented.
6. Instructional strategies commonly used in EMS training programs, alone or in combination, include ice breakers, lecture, group discussion, demonstration and practice, programmed learning, small group interaction, role play, simulation, brainstorming, consultation triads, case studies, and team teaching.
7. *Ice breakers* are short exercises designed to get students "warmed-up" on the first day of class, and serve as an introduction to class members. Specific ice breakers include the Name Game, Paired Introductions, Written Exercises, and the Scavenger Name Hunt.
8. When using group discussion exercises, it is essential for the instructor to keep the group focused on the task. Various strategies can help minimize problem groups and keep the discussion on track.
9. Questioning in EMS training programs is very effective in increasing student participation. It is useful in promoting interaction between instructors and students, and in providing students an evaluation method for testing knowledge levels, thought processes, retention of material, and problem-solving abilities.
10. The process of answering a question requires the student to engage in a five-step process, including listening to the question being asked, deciphering the meaning of the question, thinking of a response, generating a response to the instructor, and revising the response as necessary. This process usually takes 8 seconds.

REFERENCES

1. Gall M. Synthesis of research on teacher's questioning. *Educational Leadership.* 1984; November:40–46.
2. Courseware GP. *Designing and Maintaining Instructional Programs.* Columbia, MD; General Physics Corporation: 1983.

4 Components of EMS Instruction

Upon completion of this chapter, the reader will have sufficient information to:

1. Identify five basic characteristics of students who participate in EMS training programs.
2. Describe five guidelines for maintaining a positive attitude in the classroom.
3. List six factors to consider to increase instructor effectiveness through behavior.
4. Describe advantages and disadvantages to six variations of classroom seating arrangements.
5. Identify two environmental factors that should be considered when selecting a classroom facility.
6. Define communication.
7. Identify five differences between a facilitating instructor and a controlling one.
8. Describe nonverbal behavior that may affect learning.
9. List five types of noise that may interfere with the accurate transmission of a message.
10. Describe five possible outcomes of communication.
11. Describe nine principles to help increase effectiveness of communication.
12. Identify five possible roles of an EMS instructor.
13. Identify 10 expectations students have of instructors.
14. Identify 10 expectations instructors have of students.
15. Describe six strategies instructors should use to encourage student participation in the learning process.

KEY TERMS

Chunking Organizing information into small sections of material in order to make the delivery more easily understood and remembered

Communication The process by that information is exchanged between two or more students

Decoding The translation of a message into information the brain can process

Encoding The organization of thoughts and ideas into appropriate words and expressions as the first stage of communication

Excess baggage Outside problems that when brought into the classroom may distract the student from effective reception and processing of information, thereby minimizing learning

Noise Anything that interferes with the accurate transmission of a message

Paradigm A pattern, example, or model that describes the boundaries by which one lives; it is within such boundaries that a student looks at situations or ideas that are most comfortable; can be similar to "tunnel vision"

WHAT STUDENTS EXPECT FROM INSTRUCTORS

- **Instruction that is organized and easy to follow**
- **Recognition and praise for a job well done**
- **An interesting, informative, and worthwhile class**
- **Empathy**
- **Clear objectives, directions, and instructions so they know what is expected of them**
- **Evaluations that are fair and pertain to class objectives and information presented**
- **The opportunity to learn, develop, and apply knowledge and skills taught in class**
- **Continual feedback of how they are progressing in class**
- **Equal and fair treatment for all students**
- **Freedom of expression and the opportunity to participate actively in learning**
- **Protection from humiliation**
- **Pleasant and safe classroom conditions**
- **Consistency**
- **Honesty**
- **Conscientious grading of all work performed**
- **The enthusiastic presentation of all necessary content and the elimination of nonessential information**
- **Punctuality of class start and end times, including returning from breaks**
- **Breaks as necessary (15 minutes every 1½ hours is recommended)**
- **Protection against harassment**

INTRODUCTION

The instructional process consists of three basic components: the instructor, the student, and the content. In order for the student to understand the content, the instructor must communicate the material effectively and accurately.

It is important for instructors to understand students and what variables they bring to the classroom. It is equally important that instructors understand themselves and the characteristics they possess. By looking inward to what makes a good instructor or a bad one, the instructor can emphasize the positive and minimize the negative to increase the effectiveness of their training programs.

This chapter will provide information regarding characteristics of students in EMS training programs, what makes an instructor effective, and how to communicate information accurately and effectively.

CHARACTERISTICS OF STUDENTS

Participants of EMS training vary greatly in age, educational background, physical characteristics, and other features. Instructors must understand the diversity of students and take steps to use this diversity to develop a successful course structure.

Age

Students in EMT-Basic and first responder programs are usually the most diverse in terms of age, ranging from 16 to 70 years of age. Although actual statistics are not available, the majority of students seem to be between 18 and 40 years of age. Paramedic students, on the other hand, are often a relatively younger population, most likely due to the need to dedicate a large number of hours to training. Many take such training for career advancement.

Personality

Most students attending EMS training programs are dedicated to serving the community and helping others. They often use such training as a qualification to volunteer with an ambulance service. Others, however, attend these classes as a social event or under pressure from employers; they are often the students who present a challenge for instructors in the classroom.

It is the instructor's role to identify student characteristics that promote and inhibit learning, and to try to modify such traits in order to achieve maximum learning potential. Some students are inherently leaders, while others are followers. In an emergency situation, however, the follower may be required to take control of a scene. In order to boost his confidence in the ability to do so, it is often advantageous to pair an academically strong individual with a slower learner. Such pairs often work because the stronger student can assist with tutoring the slower learner and help instill self-confidence.

Physical Characteristics

With the implementation of the Americans with Disabilities Act (ADA) of 1990, new challenges have been placed on instructors and administrators. The ADA requires equal access for all students, regardless of any physical limitations they might have. While job requirements for EMS personnel may be physically demanding, the way in which specific tasks are accomplished may need to be modified to allow for physically challenged students.

The ADA prevents students from being excluded from participation in a training program or from becoming eligible for certification on the basis of a disability. While students with certain disabilities may be unable to perform all required skills, they should still be provided the opportunity to audit training programs and to receive certificates of attendance.

The ADA does allow students with disabilities to use performance aids readily available and easily accessible to them in the prehospital environment. It is the responsibility of the student to provide such aids, which may include an amplified stethoscope, glasses, or hearing aids.

In addition to instructional modifications that may be necessary because of the ADA, alternative access to training facilities may also be required. Wheelchair accessibility is required for most facilities. Such modifications may include ramps and/or elevators as well as bathroom facilities and doors that allow enough room to maneuver a wheelchair.

Regardless of any modifications provided during EMS training programs, at the completion of a course, the student must be able to perform the duties of the level of certification he will obtain (*eg*, First Responder, EMT-Basic, EMT-Paramedic), as identified in specific job descriptions. For example, the functional position description for an EMT-Basic requires the following qualifications for certification; the ability to:

- Hear, read, write, communicate and interpret instructions in the English language

- Demonstrate competency in handling emergencies using basic life support equipment in accordance with the objectives of the Department of Transportation National Standard Curriculum for the EMT-Basic

- Verbally communicate the status of a patient, in person and via telephone and telecommunications, to other EMS providers and hospital staff, and answer questions regarding such status

- Lift to a height of 33 inches and carry and balance a minimum of 125 pounds

- Use good judgement and remain calm in high-stress situations

- Read training manuals, books, and road maps

- Accurately discern street signs and address numbers

- Verbally interview patients, family members, and bystanders and hear their responses

- Document, in writing, all relevant information in a prescribed format

- Demonstrate manual dexterity, with the ability to perform all tasks related to quality patient care

- Bend, stoop, crawl, and walk on uneven surfaces

- Function in various environmental conditions such as lighted or darkened work areas, extreme heat, extreme cold, and moisture

Intellectual Development

As previously discussed, students attending EMS training programs vary significantly in age, background and other factors. Intellectual development for students also varies greatly. Educational background for

---

WHAT INSTRUCTORS EXPECT FROM STUDENTS

- **Attention during classroom presentations**

- **Active participation of all classroom activities**

- **Preparation for class by reading all homework assignments prior to each class session**

- **Attendance at all class sessions**

- **Honesty**

- **Consistency**

- **Preparation for examinations by studying, taking notes, and practicing**

- **Respect**

- **The enthusiastic reception of knowledge and information**

- **Protection from humiliation**

- **Punctual attendance (at the beginning of class and end of breaks)**

- **Desire to learn**

participants ranges from secondary school students to postgraduate degree recipients with a variety of academic backgrounds.

Some students are very affluent and well educated, while others have been raised in a culturally challenged environment and may require alternative teaching strategies. Identifying such differences and modifying instruction to accommodate them is the role of the instructor. As with personality characteristics, matching a more intellectual student with a slower learner may be beneficial.

Maturity

As with age and often intellectual development, the maturity levels of participants of EMS training programs vary greatly. While maturity is more closely related to age, some older students have been known to act immaturely in training sessions. Such immaturity may express itself in a variety of actions. Some students will disrupt the class, trying to impress classmates; others are simply shy and tend not to participate in activities.

More often than not, the immature student is the one who sits in back of the room, takes no notes, and disturbs class members as well as the instructor. It is essential that instructors let students know who is in charge from the onset in order to keep disruptive students in line and minimize any negative influence.

STUDENT SELECTION

The selection of students will vary from program to program and from state to state. Often, members of ambulance services are given priority over nonmembers. In some states, potential students are screened prior to acceptance into a training program. Such students can be rejected for various reasons.

Entrance evaluations provide valuable information to instructors and administrators.

Screening Examinations

Entrance evaluations provide valuable information to instructors and administrators. Whether they are used to eliminate potential students or not, they will provide a baseline by which to judge learning. An instructor can identify those students who may prove to be slow learners. This will provide a proactive approach to helping these students succeed in class, rather than waiting until they begin failing exams.

At a more advanced level of training, such as paramedic and nursing programs, screening examinations are often required for admission. Such evaluations may include English and math tests, psychological testing, and written and skills testing at the EMT level.

Interviews provide information such as reasons why students are interested in enrolling in a training program.

Interview Process

Interviews may also be used as an entrance requirement for certain training programs. Interviews provide information such as reasons why students are interested in enrolling in a training program. These reasons can help identify motivation factors and help instructors estimate success in such training. In addition, potentially difficult students can be identified, and attempts to minimize problems can be made.

CHARACTERISTICS OF AN EFFECTIVE INSTRUCTOR

While effective learning involves a multitude of factors, one of the most important is the ability of the instructor. An effective instructor prepares thoroughly for each lesson, uses a variety of materials and teach-

Characteristics of an Effective Instructor

Everyone can identify certain characteristics they remember about their favorite instructors, or those who have had the most profound effect on learning. The key is to combine all positive characteristics while minimizing negative ones. An effective instructor can be defined as one who:

Enjoys teaching
Is genuinely interested in student achievement
Is enthusiastic
Is polite and pleasant
Exhibits self-control
Is open to student suggestions and values
Is patient
Is concerned for students and calls them by their names
Is fair, impartial, and objective to students
Involves all students in instruction and decision-making
Does not put down students
Offers praise to students appropriately
Is encouraging
Is demanding but not overbearing
Is pleasant but business-like
Is knowledgeable of the subject matter
Is well organized and structures information appropriately for each
    specific audience
Individualizes instruction as necessary
Is flexible and adjusts to the unexpected
Identifies and provides remedial training for slower learners
Asks open-ended questions
Is interesting
Links accurate examples to information
Provides structure during class sessions, including closure at the
    conclusion of each class
Understands instructional design principles
Is skilled in content and instructional abilities
Is motivated to teach and motivates students to learn
Believes session content is important
Exhibits a professional attitude and appearance

ing methods, and has a sense of mastery over lesson content. The effectiveness of an instructor is also contingent on certain characteristics such as attitude, language, and behavior.

Attitude

An instructor's attitude has a definite effect on the learning process. Students attend and participate in training sessions for a variety of reasons, but primarily to learn. Instructors should promote such learning, not stifle it by a negative or overbearing attitude.

Instructors should remain open to student ideas. Because of the life experiences students bring to class, alternative methods for performing skills or meeting objectives may be identified by class members. The beliefs that all participants learn the same material, in the same sequence and at the same speed, or that the instructor always knows best, are hazardous to the learning process. The classroom should pro-

An effective instructor prepares thoroughly for each lesson, uses a variety of materials and teaching methods, and has a sense of mastery over lesson content.

The classroom should promote a cooperative environment where students feel free to express their own perceptions and beliefs.

mote a cooperative environment where students feel free to express their own perceptions and beliefs and add creativity to determine how objectives can be met effectively.

In order to maintain a positive learning environment, instructors should exhibit a positive attitude by adhering to the following guidelines[1].

- **View students as people** with certain needs. Care about them as students as well as human beings. They are not simply empty vessels in which to pour knowledge, but intricate learners with ideas, problems, beliefs, and needs that make them unique.

- **View students as a group of individuals**. A class is a group of individuals seeking to increase knowledge and skills through instructors. All students are not all alike.

- **Identify the positive as well as negative**. When an individual provides an incorrect answer to a question, identify some positive aspect in order to minimize the negative motivational effect.

- **View the learning process as a means to help learners** obtain knowledge and skill proficiency. To that end it is important to instill confidence within students. An attitude on the part of an instructor that portrays superiority or self-righteousness can halt the learning process because students may lose respect for the instructor.

- **View the classroom as an environment in which learning takes place**. It is the instructor's role to facilitate learning, not to control students. Box 4.1 identifies instructor actions and attitudes that promote both a facilitating environment and a controlling one.

Language

As with attitude, the language an instructor chooses can either facilitate or prohibit learning. In an attempt to improve learning, instructors should do the following:

- **Refrain from laying blame**. Statements such as "You should have known better" are counter-productive in a learning environment.

BOX 4.1 Characteristics of Instructors in Facilitating and Controlling Environments

FACILITATING INSTRUCTOR	CONTROLLING INSTRUCTOR
Encouraging	Impatient
Identifies indivual problems	Identifies group problems
Concerned	Annoyed
Responds to individual concerns and needs	Responds to group requests and needs
Seeks to correct reasons for inaccuracies	Corrects inaccuracies

Characteristics of instructors in facilitating and controlling environments (adapted from Margolis and Bell, 1986[1]).

- **Do not embarrass students or co-instructors** by your tone of voice, by body language or gestures, by ignoring an individual, or by confronting someone with a mistake. Praise in public; discipline in private. This is true with fellow instructors as well; if an instructor is teaching something wrong, take him aside. Do not confront the instructor in front of class members.

- **Use facilitating terms rather than controlling ones**. For example, "I want you to take notes," is a controlling statement that may turn off some students. "Taking notes will help identify important points that may help you study for exams," is a facilitating statement.

- **Never use language that will offend any individual within a class**. This includes humor, foul language, or slang terms. Humor should be used cautiously as to not offend anyone. Many individuals find jokes, especially those targeted toward a group of people such as women, members of ethnic groups, or handicapped individuals offensive, even if listeners are not members of these groups.

Behavior

In order to improve individual effectiveness, it is essential that instructors recognize the following:

- **It is alright to be nervous** before a session; everyone is. In fact, when an instructor is no longer nervous, it may be time to stop teaching. Such anxiety is essential for helping instructors do well in the preparation and presentation of information.

- **Most students attend training sessions because they want to learn**. As a result, they will most often respond, participate, and cooperate with instructors and the learning process.

- **Some students are simply not going to participate in class**, no matter what. An instructor cannot change people who do not want to be changed, nor can they teach an individual who does not want to learn. As long as instructors do their best and put every effort into the planning and delivery of each class presentation, they cannot blame themselves for those who do not learn.

- **Everyone has their own style and approach to teaching**. What works well for one instructor may be different from what works for another. It is important that instructors develop their own personal style, based on approaches that they like and work well for them.

  There are no rules on how to teach a session, what to do, or what to say, only guidelines for what usually works best. Instructors should experiment with recommended instructional and classroom management techniques until they find a style they like that has a positive effect on the class.

- **Control of the classroom is the responsibility of the instructor**. An instructor who exhibits greater control over the class generally elicits greater learning, to a point. An overbearing, over-controlling instructor, however, may cause dissension within the class, causing diminished learning.

- **Student involvement tends to result in higher achievement**. Interactivity between students and instructors is a key factor of academic excellence. Questioning students to

Encouraging Student Participation

Encouraging student participation is one of the more difficult but important challenges affecting instructors. Some individuals are inherently more comfortable sitting in the back of a room absorbing information while saying or interacting little. Others actively participate in learning and enjoy it. Still others are actively involved in being disruptive in the classroom. It takes skill and practice for an instructor to manage the classroom situation effectively to increase learning for all individuals.

ESTABLISH EXPECTATIONS

There are certain individuals who will only take notes, study, and remember the information they are required to learn. Consider the student who asks "Is that on the test?" or "Do we have to remember that?" These are the students who need structured guidance, direction, goals, and objectives.

Let students know what is expected of them. They will be more likely to take notes if they know which information is important. When possible, make class participation part of the course grade, such as extra credit points. This may cause more active participation on the part of those not doing well in class.

SELECT APPROPRIATE TEACHING STRATEGIES

By limiting class sessions that are straight lecture and including practice, games, or demonstrations, students are forced to participate in the learning process. If a class looks bored, tired, or uninterested, change the focus of a session to a guided discussion to gain participation, or ask the group questions such as in a quiz game like Jeopardy.

If the group looks bored, there must be a reason: either the instructor is indeed boring, in which case a new presentation method is necessary because information is not being received appropriately, or students already know the information. If the students know the information, throw control of the class back to them by determining exactly what they know and rearrange the class session accordingly.

CREATE A POSITIVE LEARNING ENVIRONMENT

If a learner does not feel comfortable participating, he will not participate. As was previously discussed, the learning climate must be comfortable in order to promote interaction. Select a seating arrangement that meets the learning objectives for a specific class session and remove any physical barriers that may exist.

The attitude of the instructor is very important for creating a positive learning environment. Instructors can quickly offend a group of students by portraying a superior image. Be enthusiastic but not overbearing. A loud, demanding, and aggressive instructor will not be well received and may only cause tension within the group. It is the instructor's responsibility to facilitate the learning process, not to cram information down students' throats.

USE PARTICIPANT FEEDBACK

When students offer information through a question, response, or suggestion, the instructor should let them know he was listening. When possible, use the suggestions that are offered, thereby reinforcing to students that you value their input. When an individual asks a question, answer it truthfully; never make up a response or students will lose respect and trust in your ability.

If a student offers an incorrect response to an answer, *never* say, "Eeh, wrong answer." Such a response will alienate the individual and prevent the other participants from ever answering questions for fear of similar humiliation. Instead, point out some portion of the response that was correct, or rephrase the question to give the student a chance to offer a different response.

CONTROL PARTICIPATION

In every class, there are individuals who over-participate in learning. Likewise, there are those who under-participate. Obviously, the goal of an instructor is to elicit more participation from those who quietly sit in the back of the room, and less participation from those who always answer or ask questions.

Students often like an over-participator because it takes pressure off themselves. They believe, "Well if he's going to answer the question, I won't have to study." If an over-participator offers the answer to a question, tactfully ask someone else for an answer. A statement such as, "Well I know John studied, but what about the rest of the class?" passes over the over-participator without putting him down.

Likewise, if an over-participator asks a legitimate question, redirect the response to the rest of the class to elicit more involvement. If the question is not legitimate, ask the student what he thinks the answer is. Chances are the student knows the answer but was either testing the instructor or trying to show the class how smart he is. Either way, throwing the question back to the student will let him know that the instructor is not "playing" the game.

CONTROL CONTENT

Students can be annoyed easily if an appropriate pace is not maintained throughout a course. Adult learners are easily disgusted with instructors who "waste" their time. Be careful not to add irrelevant information or allow too much time for activities. Maintain a tempo that promotes learning and elicits class participation.

When an individual asks a question that does not pertain to the topic at hand, offer to discuss it at a break. This will provide the opportunity for the student to get additional information without wasting the rest of the class' time. Try to refrain from going off on tangents.

promote a discussion is an excellent method to elicit such inter-activity.

THE LEARNING CLIMATE

One of the most important factors influencing the effectiveness of a training session is the environment surrounding a class. The *learning climate* is the atmosphere in which people are motivated to learn and are open and cooperative to the learning process.

This climate is set and maintained by the instructor. Factors influencing the learning climate include seating arrangements, room layout, and other environmental conditions.

Environment

Seating Arrangement

There are numerous arrangements for chairs and tables in a classroom. Much research has been conducted to determine which arrangements are more effective in which types of training situations.

Instructors should know how they want a classroom arranged, and be prepared to move furniture as necessary. Room arrangement has a significant effect on the climate, and, therefore, on the learning process.

Theater/Auditorium Style — As identified in Figure 4.1, this type of arrangement provides rows of chairs, and occasionally tables, that are arranged similar to a movie theater.

> The *learning climate* is the atmosphere in which people are motivated to learn and are open and co-operative to the learning process.

> Room arrangement has a significant effect on the climate, and, therefore, on the learning process.

ADVANTAGES:

☑ This type arrangement can fit the largest number of people in one room.

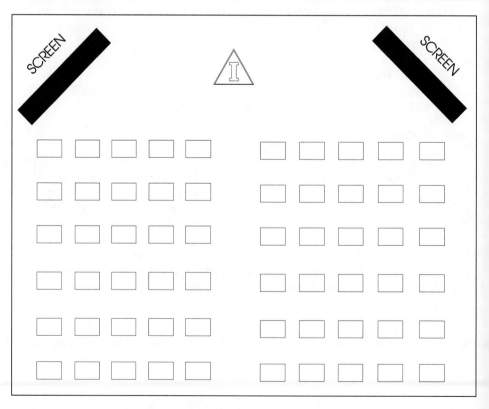

FIGURE 4.1 Theater Style Seating Arrangement

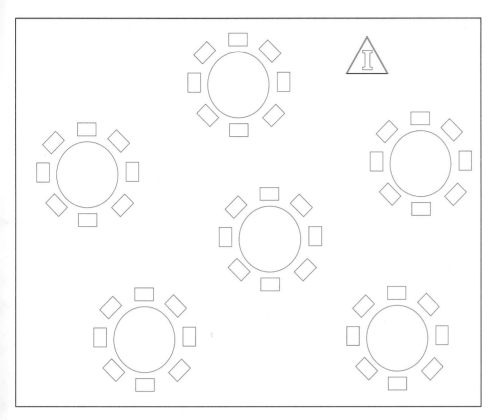

FIGURE 4.2 Round Table Style Seating Arrangement

DISADVANTAGES:

✖ Everyone is focused on the instructor and not on other students. The front of the classroom tends to be blocked by the heads of persons in front of each row of students. Tables and chairs often block the ability of instructors to move around, go up and down isles, and interact with students.

WHEN TO USE:

🍎 During large group sessions. When little student interaction is necessary.

Round Table Style — As identified in Figure 4.2, this arrangement provides round or rectangular tables for eight to 10 seats each.

ADVANTAGES:

☑ This type of arrangement provides ready-made small work groups, thereby saving set-up time.

DISADVANTAGES:

✖ People tend to get locked into one group and may miss interaction with other students.

WHEN TO USE:

🍎 When small work sessions are useful, *eg*, in certain games, such as Beat the Reaper, and in review or study sessions.

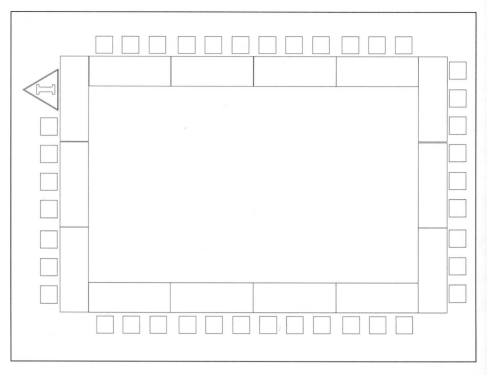

FIGURE 4.3 Open Square Style Seating Arrangement

Open Square-Conference Style — As shown in Figure 4.3, this arrangement places chairs around a square of adjoining rectangular tables. This seating style allows for approximately 20 to 60 chairs, depending on the size of the room. This arrangement is effective for meetings or active discussion since everyone is facing someone, and the focus of the room is the center of the square, not at an instructor in front of the room. In order to remove attention from himself, the instructor should sit off center at a side table when using this arrangement.

ADVANTAGES:

☑ This arrangement forces students to look at, and hopefully talk with, each other, thereby providing interaction.

DISADVANTAGES:

✖ The focus of attention is an empty square in the center, and some students may find it uncomfortable. Using audiovisual aids with this set-up is quite difficult since someone's back will always be toward a screen, board, flipchart, or other aid.

WHEN TO USE:

🍎 Use this type arrangement when student-to-student interaction is important. A square-shaped arrangement is more effective during meetings, where compromise and discussion are necessary and facing opposition is useful.

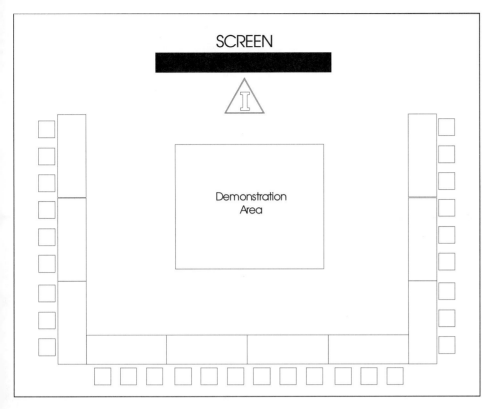

FIGURE 4.4 U-Shaped Style Seating Arrangement

U-Shaped Table Style — This type of arrangement provides chairs and tables in the shape of a "U," with the open end in the front of the room, as identified in Figure 4.4. With this arrangement, the instructor is usually in front of the room or in the center of the "U" providing information, performing a demonstration, or eliciting discussion.

ADVANTAGES:

☑ This type of arrangement focuses attention toward the center of the room, allowing for effective demonstration of equipment and treatment techniques. Ample room is available for demonstration purposes.

DISADVANTAGES:

✖ This set-up limits the number of seats available. It is not conducive to discussion or cohesion since one side is left unmatched.

WHEN TO USE:

🍎 This arrangement is most useful for demonstration sessions.

Circle Style — Like the square conference style arrangement, chairs are placed in one large circle. This arrangement is effective in promoting discussion, as pictured in Figure 4.5.

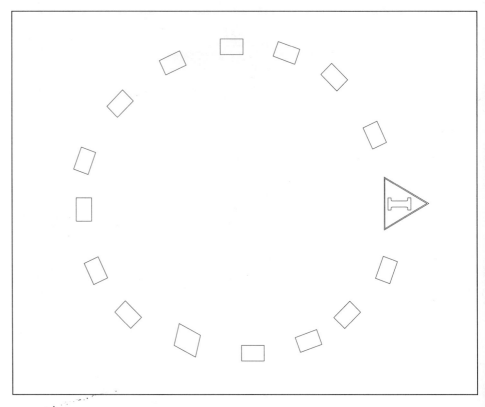

FIGURE 4.5 Circle Style Seating Arrangement

ADVANTAGES:

☑ This arrangement provides student-to-student interaction and promotes an informal environment.

DISADVANTAGES:

☒ Students who take copious notes may feel uncomfortable since they do not have a writing surface area. Some students feel uncomfortable without the "barrier" of a table and feel somewhat exposed, physically and mentally.

WHEN TO USE:

🍎 This arrangement should be used for demonstration sessions when the floor is needed, such as for practice scenarios, since the view of the floor may be obstructed when using other arrangements.

🍎 A circle of chairs is also beneficial for ice-breaking sessions and certain games such as the Introduction Name Game.

Classroom Style — One of the most productive arrangements of tables and chairs for learning is the classroom arrangement, as identified in Figure 4.6.

ADVANTAGES:

☑ This type of arrangement allows the instructor to walk up and down the isles to interact with all students and allows students an unobstructed view of the front of the room. It allows

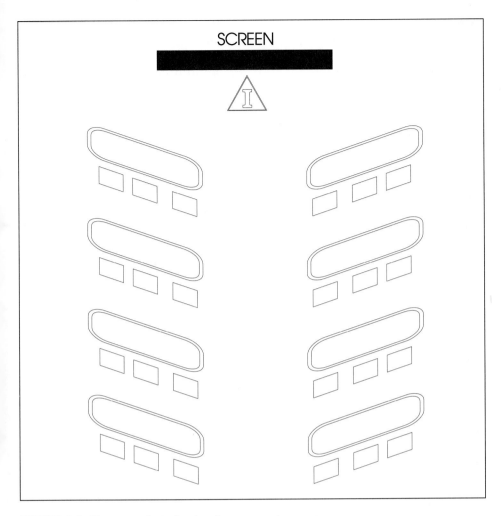

SCREEN

FIGURE 4.6 Classroom Style Seating Arrangement

for a fairly large number of students in a room while still allowing them a writing table on which to take notes.

DISADVANTAGES:

- This arrangement places students on only one side of the tables, that which faces the front of the room. Consequently, the room layout can only accommodate a small number of students.
- Learner attention is focused on the instructor in front of the room; therefore, interaction among students is virtually nonexistent.

WHEN TO USE:

- This room arrangement is best for lecture presentations.

Room Arrangement

How a room is arranged with regard to equipment, audiovisual aids, and other materials is also important when trying to improve the learning climate, and ultimately the effectiveness of instruction.

> It is important that students be able to see all aspects of instruction clearly at all times.

> An unobstructed view of the instructor, equipment, and audiovisual materials is essential for effective learning to take place.

Room Layout

It is important that students be able to see all aspects of instruction clearly at all times. This means tables and chairs should be moved during demonstrations, or demonstrations should be done on a platform. Regardless of the seating arrangement selected, audiovisual materials should be free from obstruction for all students.

In addition, tables and chairs should be placed far enough apart to allow students room to maneuver, place personal belongings, and take notes without feeling confined.

Many instructors use multiple forms of audiovisual aids at the same time. A common combination is the use of a board and a screen (for either slides or transparencies). Most often, however, the screen is placed in front of the board, making it difficult to use both forms without retracting the screen to see the blackboard.

The most beneficial room layout allows all students to see all aspects of instruction. An unobstructed view of the instructor, equipment, and audiovisual materials is essential for effective learning to take place. As identified in Figure 4.7, the screen should be placed diagonally in the corner of the room, with the board in the center. This layout allows instructors to use both the board and the screen simultaneously, allowing for better instruction. In addition, a screen in the

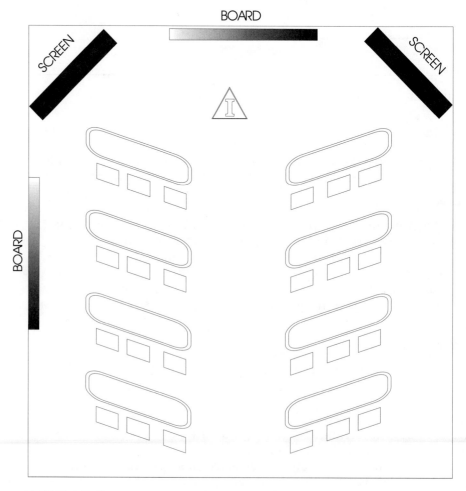

FIGURE 4.7 Classroom Layout

corner is more visible to all students. When multiple slide projection or overhead units are used simultaneously, one should be placed in each corner of the front of the room.

Equipment

Equipment should be placed so that its view is not obstructed for any student and is within the line of focus. For example, if the layout focuses students' attention toward the front of the room, demonstrating the use of a hare traction splint from the back of the room would not make sense, nor would using a blackboard located where students would need to reposition themselves to view its contents.

When demonstrating the use of equipment or other emergency techniques, instructors should do so in the center of the room whenever possible, allowing every student to see. Doing this on a table may be necessary so that students can stay in their seats and take notes.

Environmental Factors

Other factors that affect the learning climate include the setting, room temperature, lighting, outside noise, instructional techniques, and language used. Instructor treatment of students should also be taken into account when determining an effective room arrangement.

ROOM SETTING

The room itself, including the colors of the room, the walls, and the carpet can have an effect on learning. For example, dark walls may promote drowsiness, while lighter walls help brighten the room and promote increased attention.

The room itself can have an effect on learning.

Items on the walls can also cause a distraction if they are not relevant to a class session. Students may become bored with a topic and begin scanning the room to look at wall hangings, thereby disrupting the learning process.

TEMPERATURE

The room temperature should be comfortable in order to maintain student concentration. Rooms that are too warm tend to cause drowsiness, and those that are too cold cause students to become more concerned with keeping warm than with learning.

Maintaining a comfortable climate may be difficult during classes held outdoors. It is important, however, to take measures to ensure the safety of students. Providing cold liquids (*eg*, ice water or juice) during hot days and warm liquids (*eg*, coffee or tea) during cold days will provide some relief.

Having a room or van nearby that can offer relief during inclement weather is also useful. When students are not participating actively in hands-on training, they can rehabilitate in the room.

LIGHTING

Good lighting is important. Lights should be dimmed when appropriate for audiovisual materials, and should be well lit so all students can see demonstrations and take notes.

COMMUNICATION PRINCIPLES

There are three primary reasons for communicating: to express oneself, to learn and grow, and to enlist the cooperation of others[2]. Communication is a two-way process, resulting in the building of interpersonal relationships. In education, communication is the basis for learning; it is through communication that information is exchanged.

The ability to communicate is one of the most important characteristics of an effective instructor. Quite simply, communication is the process by which information is exchanged and understood by two or more individuals. Communication requires active participation for a mutual exchange of facts, thoughts and opinions by both the presenter and the receiver of information. Without participation, communication cannot occur.

Communication occurs when two or more individuals interact through the exchange of a message and requires at least two people. These messages can be verbal or nonverbal in nature.

The communication process in EMS training depends heavily on verbal behavior. In most such training sessions, messages are exchanged primarily through the spoken word, although demonstration is certainly important.

Types of Communication

Verbal

There are several variables that influence verbal communication, including the choice of vocabulary, instructor's intention and tone when speaking, context of what is being said, experiences of learners, and feelings and attitudes of instructors and students when a message is sent.

In addition, clarity of speech is important when presenting information. An instructor with a speech impediment may be distracting to students, causing a learning barrier. While an instructor may be extremely knowledgeable, if students cannot understand him, it can be very detrimental to learning.

Each instructor has a unique method of verbal communication. In order to ensure effective processing of information, it is essential that instructors use effective verbal communication, characterized by:

- Effective quality and dynamics of voice
  - Appropriate syntax and sentence patterns
  - Appropriate emphasis on certain words
  - Positive tone or emotional level
  - Appropriate volume and inflection of voice
  - Minimal outside noise or interference
  - Appropriate speed of information delivery
- Distinct pronunciation
- Appropriate vocabulary
- Enthusiasm
- A flowing style

Nonverbal

What is heard by learners is also influenced by nonverbal behaviors. *Nonverbal behaviors* are thoughts and feelings that are transferred from one individual to another through gestures, facial expressions, and physical contact. Such nonverbal communication often informs learners of the instructor's attitude about what he is teaching, and may influence students attitudes of what they are learning.

BOX 4.2 Nonverbal Communication Features and Indications

BEHAVIOR	INDICATION
Eye contact and movement	
Wandering eyes	Boredom
Raised eyebrows	Skepticism or disbelief
Looking at individuals	Understanding and attentive Listening
Looking at clock	Boredom
Vacant stare	Confusion
Gestures and body language	
Head resting on hand	Boredom or disinterest
Leaning on desk or lectern	Inattentive
Hand and foot movement	
Scuffing feet	Impatience and boredom
Fiddling with hands	Anxious
Tapping or toying with objects	Anxious or nervous
Scratching head	Confused
Silence	Lack of understanding or tired
Pace	
Fast	In a hurry
Slow	Tired or disinterest
Attire	
Neat and clean	Professional
Wearing a uniform	Egocentric
Dirty or unkept	Disinterest
Facial expressions	
Smiling	Enthusiastic or understanding
Frown	Disagreement or lack of understanding
Yawn	Boredom
Posture	
Leaning	Boredom or disinterest
Looking down at students	Egocentric
Arms folded	Cold, bored, or resistant

Nonverbal communication features and indications.

The most effective communication occurs when the instructor sends a consistent message with both verbal and nonverbal cues. If discrepancies exist, the effectiveness of communication is diminished.

Nonverbal communication is an integral part of the total communication process for both instructors and students. The instructor's unspoken attitudes will effect the students' own attitudes and perceptions. Nonverbal behaviors and what they indicate are identified in Box 4.2.

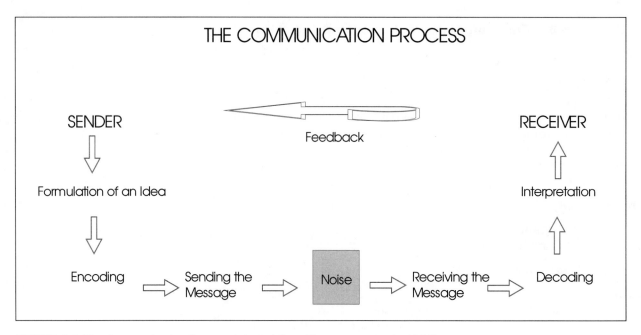

FIGURE 4.8 The Communication Process (adapted from Zimmerman et. al., 1980).

The Communication Process
For an instructor, communicating information is the basis for teaching. Some instructors lack the ability to "get the point across" to learners regardless of how intelligent the instructor may be. Unless the knowledgeable instructor can express ideas clearly, maintain student interest, and make himself understood, the instructor will not be effective.

As identified in Figure 4.8, communication follows a distinct process and encompasses many factors[2]. Problems at any phase of the process may result in communication not taking place, or incorrect information being processed.

Formulation
The sender of information must first clearly formulate the information to be communicated and determine the best channel for delivery. Factors such as audience characteristics, appropriate vocabulary, and available media for communication should be taken into account.

Encoding
Encoding is the organization of a message into a deliverable format and it includes choosing words or images used to present the message. When encoding the message, it is important to take into account audience characteristics and background knowledge to determine the appropriate language and channel for communication.

Sending the Message
Once encoded, an idea becomes a message in the form of a memo, letter, speech, presentation, or other medium. The message is then sent via one of the five senses that channel such information (*ie*, sight, sound, taste, smell, and touch). The primary channels for communication in education are seeing and hearing.

Once the information is delivered by the sender, its outcome is dependent on two factors: noise and the receiver. During this phase of communication, noise may interfere with the accurate transmission of a message. It is important for instructors to minimize noise in an attempt to ensure accurate communication.

Noise
Noise includes anything that interferes with the accurate transmission of a message. Such noise may be auditory, visual, or physical in nature[3]. Any noise interferes with communication, although the negative extent of such interference varies. Instructors should minimize noise to every extent possible.

Receiving the Message
After the transmission of a message, it is up to the receiver to actually receive and process a message. In order to receive information, the receiver must be able to hear a verbal message, read a written message, or make arrangements for alternatives (*eg*, sign language, audiotapes).

Once the information is delivered by the sender, its outcome is dependent on two factors: noise and the receiver.

Instructors should minimize noise to every extent possible.

AUDITORY NOISE
- Voices heard in the hallway
- Activation of scanners or pagers
- Talking within the room
- The humming of a fluorescent light
- Students tapping pencils or fingers on the table
- Extraneous words from the instructor ("uhh," "umm," or unfamiliar jargon)
- The fan from an overhead or slide projector
- Inaccurate or conflicting information presented by multiple instructors
- Accents or incorrect grammar ("ain't" or "y'all")

VISUAL NOISE
- People passing by in the hallway
- A flickering light
- Nonverbal communication (appearance, behavior, and gestures on the part of an instructor and/or participant)
- Ineffective audiovisual materials (too much information on one visual, text not large enough for students to read)

PHYSICAL NOISE
- A vibrating floor from music next door or a dance class downstairs
- An ineffective seating arrangement
- A negative tone of the classroom environment
- Hunger or the need to use restroom facilities
- "Excess baggage" of outside problems learners bring into the classroom
- Individual characteristics including, paradigms, past experiences, intellectual development levels, cultural background, and personalities
- Coughing, sneezing, or clearing throat
- Verbalizing emotions such as "I do not want to be here"

Decoding is the transla-tion of a message, by the receiver, into a form the brain can process.

Decoding

The message must then be decoded by the receiver. *Decoding* is the translation of a message, by the receiver, into a form the brain can process. The receiver processes information through the senses and must be able to listen to or read information. The same factors that effect encoding by the sender are also influential in the decoding of a message (*ie*, communication skills, attitudes, knowledge, and cultural beliefs).

The personality and perception of the receiver play an important role in communication. If an instructor is sending a message with a certain set of beliefs and perceptions, and the learner has a separate set of beliefs and perceptions, miscommunication is likely.

Interpretation

The decoded message must then be interpreted by the receiver. Such interpretation involves assigning meaning to a message that has been decoded. It is at this step that the receiver applies past experiences, knowledge, attitudes, expectations, and feeling in order to interpret the message.

Feedback

The sender of the original message then asks for feedback to ensure the correct message was received. If the correct message was not received, then the process must begin again.

Possible Outcomes of Communication

There are various possible outcomes of communication, depending on factors occurring within the process. Here are some possible outcomes:

1) The intended message is received.
2) The actual message sent was received; this message may be different from the intended message due to an error in encoding.
3) The message received is distorted due to noise.
4) The message received differs from the intended message due to an error in decoding.
5) The actual response to the message differs from the anticipated response due to an error in interpretation.

Instructors have little control over how a message is received, decoded, or interpreted. What they can control, however, is how a message is formulated and sent. During the formulation of a message, it is important that information be presented in a manner that is clear, concise, and accurate.

Instructors have little con-trol over how a message is received, decoded, or inter-preted. What they can control, however, is how a message is formulated and sent.

The instructor must then receive feedback from the student to determine whether the information received is correct. If not, regardless of the cause of inaccurate communication, it is essential the instructor re-send the message in a different form.

HOW TO COMMUNICATE EFFECTIVELY

Everything an instructor does affects communication. If an instructor fails to communicate effectively, he will fail to teach effectively. Therefore, it is important to adhere to certain guidelines in order to make a training session informative and allow learners to meet their objectives. These guidelines are as follows[4]:

🍎 **Formulate a clear message using simple language**. A message is clear when it is free of jargon and is unambiguous in meaning. It must include enough information to result in the receiver accurately interpreting the message; critical aspects of a message should not be left to assumption. There should be only one way to interpret a clear message.

- **Use short sentences to formulate a concise message**. A concise message is one that uses the minimum number of words necessary to communicate effectively. If the message can be stated in five words, the instructor should not use 10. Shorter sentences are easier to follow since longer ones may be too wordy or difficult to understand.

- **Present information in a clear, organized flow**. The message should follow a logical path, building on past messages. Information can be "chunked" as a method of organizing ideas for learners. Group and communicate information on a specific topic or idea in its entirety before moving to the next section rather than providing segments of one topic through a training session and leaving the organization to the learner.

  In addition, make certain all prerequisite information has been provided. For example, it is important to cover patient assessment techniques prior to a lesson on shock (hypoperfusion syndrome) in order to provide a basis for which students will understand the signs and symptoms of shock.

  Likewise, prior to teaching AED, students should be knowledgeable in CPR. Otherwise, the AED session may be quite confusing to the student. When prerequisite skills are needed, it may be useful to offer a quiz to assess the knowledge levels of students and provide the instructor with a baseline on which to judge learning.

- **Avoid speaking in jargon**. Teach important "EMS jargonese" and forget the rest. At the conclusion of an EMT class, students will understand the meaning of terms such as ACLS, AED, FEMA, BTLS, PALS, KED, CID, and others. Do not overwhelm them at the beginning of a program by using jargon. When such jargon is important for the learner to understand, fully explain the meaning of each.

- **Do not bury important information** by providing lengthy discussions on trivial information or telling too many war stories. Use only examples and exercises that directly relate to course objectives. If a case history provides a clear explanation of a certain principle, use it; if not, do not. Students are often turned off by too many war stories.

- **Identify key points within a lesson** to focus learner attention toward important information and away from trivial knowledge. At the conclusion of a session, summarize important information students should remember and understand.

- **Make certain information is accurate, complete, and free of errors in spelling, meaning, or information**. It is much more difficult to retrain a student after providing inaccurate information, and misinformation instills doubt of instructor qualifications.

- **Provide information at an appropriate pace**. If learners quickly understand the information presented, move to the next section. If not, provide a means of review and remediation until the information is understood.

PHYSICAL RESPONSES TO "STAGE FRIGHT"

- Sweating
- Increased heart rate
- Increased respiratory rate
- Increased peristalsis
- Dry mouth
- Quivering voice
- Stomach cramps
- Shaking

PSYCHOLOGIC RESPONSES TO "STAGE FRIGHT"

- Flight of ideas
- Speeding up (talking fast)
- Mind racing
- Blanking out (choking)

WAYS TO MINIMIZE "STAGE FRIGHT"

- Relaxation exercises
  - Deep breaths
  - Squeeze and relax muscles
  - Let mind go numb
- Rational emotive therapy (self-talk: "It will be OK" or "I'll be fine")
- Directed focus (focus on anything except instructing)
- Mental gymnastics (visualize the audience in their underwear to make them less intimidating)

🍎 **Channel nervousness**. It is alright to be nervous, as long as it is not noticeable. All responsible instructors have some level of anxiety when facing an audience. This anxiety generally subsides after the initial 30 seconds of instruction. Through preparation and practice anxiety becomes stimulation to do well.

LISTENING PRINCIPLES

Exhibiting good listening skills is very important to the learning process. Letting students know the instructor is listening assures them that the instructor is interested in what they have to say.

Listening to students allows the instructor the opportunity to determine if they understand the information being presented. Feedback is only useful if instructors take time to listen to it and take it into account in order to modify the remainder of a program as well as future training programs.

While individuals may try to listen attentively, it is sometimes difficult. The average speaker delivers approximately 140 words per minute, yet the average listener can comfortably comprehend messages delivered at up to 300 words per minute[5]. When information is comprehended at a speed of less than that at which it is delivered, learners tend to fill "dead space" (ie, time) by doodling, staring around the room, or thinking of other things. It is then necessary to get the individual back on track.

CROSS-CULTURAL COMMUNICATION

As previously mentioned, EMS training programs consist of individuals from a variety of backgrounds. Such backgrounds can cause obstacles in learning and include the following:

- Race
- Religious customs

> Listening to students allows the instructor the opportunity to determine if they understand the information being presented.

- Language barriers
- Social customs
- Ethnic backgrounds
- Previous associations

These backgrounds can instill biases that interfere with the learning process. For example, religious customs may prohibit a student from attending training on Saturdays, Sundays, or certain religious holidays. In addition, race still plays a factor in society and although instructors may try to minimize this fact, racial bias and stereotyping may occur.

Social customs may also surface in training programs. Some cultures direct individuals not to speak unless spoken to, thereby preventing the ability to ask questions openly. Other cultures require that a certain type of clothing be worn which may impede the effective performance of certain skills. In some cultures burping is a positive reaction, in others it is viewed as rude. In some cultures, "personal space" must be respected, while in others it is acceptable to stand very close to another individual.

Obviously, language barriers can prevent learning. A student who speaks little English will have a difficult time understanding lectures. Likewise, certain jargon may be common to one type of background and cause a disadvantage for learners from another.

All these factors should be taken into account when orchestrating a training program. Developing alternative teaching methods to handle diverse cultural backgrounds is necessary to allow all students an equal opportunity to succeed in a training program. Alternatives may include a more advanced learner or instructor tutoring a disadvantaged student, or, when possible, pairing individuals with someone of the same cultural background.

RESPONSIBILITIES OF THE INSTRUCTOR

An instructor is much more than simply the presenter of information. While students enter the training environment to learn, they also look to the instructor for guidance, reassurance, knowledge, and direction.

Regardless of the role an instructor is filling, it is essential to maintain focus of the student, not the instructor, as the center of a learning experience. The students are the customers and it is the instructor's responsibility to analyze and fulfill their needs.

Responsibilities of the instructor are many, depending on a particular training institute's organizational makeup. Some instructors hold more of an administrative role, while others serve as instructional designers or consultants. All instructors, however, have a greater responsibility than simply presenting information.

Students look to the instructor for guidance, reassurance, knowledge, and direction.

Role as an Instructor

The main responsibility of the instructor is to deliver accurate information in a form that can be understood by the student. It is essential that instructors continually evaluate whether students understand the information being presented and clarify confusing information as necessary.

The instructor must be thoroughly prepared to teach. Preparation may include researching information in order to understand the content, developing lesson plans and audiovisual materials, and practicing presentation techniques. For every hour of actual instruction, an estimated 3 hours of preparation is required. Once a lesson is fully de-

The instructor must be thoroughly prepared to teach.

ROLES AND RESPONSIBILITIES OF INSTRUCTORS

Instruction-Related Roles

- Presenter
- Motivator
- Coach
- Trainer
- Evaluator
- Facilitator
- Leader
- Tutor
- Academic adviser
- Warden
- Referee
- Audiovisual repair specialist

Instructional Design-Related Roles

- Curriculum designer
- Innovator
- Planner

Administration-Related Roles

- Counselor
- Organizer
- Examiner
- Record keeper
- Manager
- Budget specialist
- Coordinator
- Scheduler

Consultation-Related Roles

- Support person
- Resource specialist

Role Model-Related Roles

- Subject matter expert
- Mentor

veloped, however, required preparation time is drastically reduced for delivery of the same topic in subsequent courses.

Preparation also includes arranging materials for a class session. This includes arrangement of furniture, placement of audiovisual equipment, and ensuring that equipment is in working condition. Figure 4.9 provides a sample checklist for ensuring that instructors are properly prepared for a training session.

To be effective, the instructor must accurately know his audience,

INSTRUCTOR PREPARATION CHECKLIST

ITEM		YES	NO
FACILITY			
Keys	Do you have keys to the facility? (If appropriate)		
Equipment Overhead Projector Slide Projector TV/VCR Remote Controls Film Projector Screens Remote Projection Stand Video Projection Unit Training Equipment (manikins, oxygen) Extension Cord Laser Pointer Accessible Spare Equipment, (*ie,* bulbs, parts)	Is necessary equipment available and in working condition?		
Logistics	Do you know the location for: Restrooms Snack Area Smoking Area Fire Escape Route Fire Extinguishers		
Room Arrangement Lighting and Switches Ventilation Accessibility Space Seating Arrangement AV Location Electrical Outlets	Is the room set up adequate?		

FIGURE 4.9 Instructor Preparation Checklist

ITEM		YES	NO
MATERIALS			
Curriculum			
Lesson Plan			
Slides			
Transparencies			
Videos			
Films			
Handouts			
Easel and Pads			
Markers			
Chalk and Eraser			
Extra Supplies	Do you have these "nice to have" items, just in case?		
Markers			
Pens and Pencils			
Paper			
Tape			
Glue			
Staples			
Pencil Sharpener			
Scissors			
Index Cards			
3 Hole Punch			
Screwdriver			
Thumbtacks			
Blank Transparency Film			

FIGURE 4.9 continued. Instructor Preparation Checklist

what information they have already learned, and what is next in the curriculum. Only then can he effectively insert specific information for that session in a meaningful fashion. If the group is confused about a topic discussed at the previous session, the instructor must clarify and ensure that students understand the information prior to beginning a new presentation. Otherwise, learners may not fully understand subsequent information.

During a class session, it is also the instructor's responsibility to regulate the class tempo. If the group does not seem to understand a particular concept, provide remedial training. Likewise, if they quickly grasp information, move on to the next session or spend time reviewing and practicing. The difficult task, however, is handling a group comprised of both fast and slow learners. In this situation, it may be beneficial to split the group and provide a "quiz" or game for those who understand the information and remedial training to those who do not.

One of the more creative responsibilities of an instructor is motivating students to learn, participate, and practice. If a student is not motivated, little learning will take place. While some learners are motivated internally, with little need for instructor intervention, others need constant external motivation.

To be effective, the instructor must accurately know his audience, what information they have already learned, and what is next in the curriculum.

One of the more creative responsibilities of an instructor is motivating students to learn, participate, and practice.

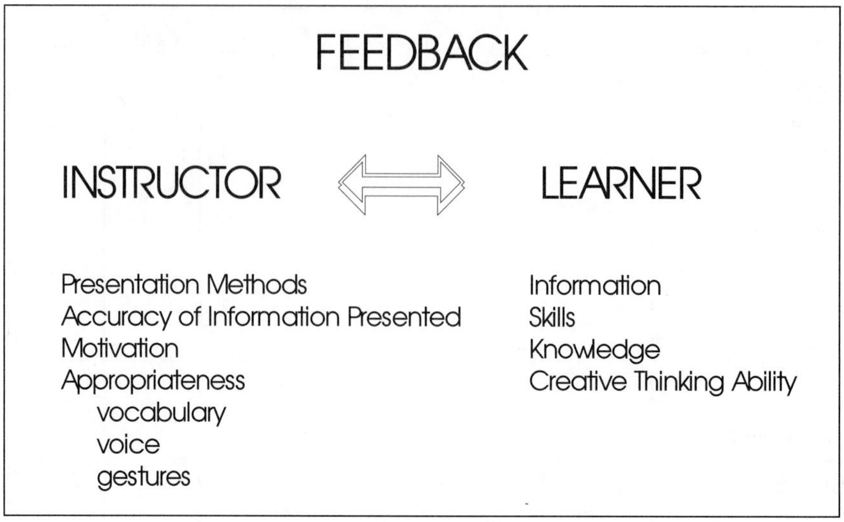

FIGURE 4.10 Two-Way Communication Feedback Process

At the conclusion of a classroom presentation, instructors should summarize information and identify key points. It is important that students feel closure at the end of each class session and understand what is next. Identifying what the learner should now understand and discussing how to prepare for the next class session provides a sense of continuity within a long training program and ensures students they are moving along at the correct pace.

In addition to presenting information, the instructor must evaluate the effectiveness of instruction and provide feedback to the students. Feedback should occur throughout a training session. By asking the group whether a particular presentation method is effective, the instructor can modify what he is doing to meet the needs of the class. At the end of a session, the instructor must evaluate the effectiveness of the program by determining if educational objectives were mastered.

Continual feedback is essential for both learners and instructors. As identified in Figure 4.10, feedback is twofold: instructors must evaluate students to determine whether learning took place, and students should evaluate the instructor to identify the effectiveness of a training session and instructor presentation skills. There is no such thing as a perfect instructor; there is always room for improvement. Attempting to identify and modify flaws within a presentation will only improve the program for the next time.

Role as a Designer
Some instructors choose to be involved with instructional design and curriculum development. As a designer, the instructor is usually concerned with identifying training needs and developing training programs to meet those needs.

The challenge in instructional design is to find new or innovative approaches to learning techniques. If a particular training module does not work following currently designed lesson plans, modifications to the approach can result in increased learning. For example, if students consistently find anatomy and physiology a difficult subject to grasp, modifying the program to require students to participate in an autopsy or view a video of an autopsy may provide the necessary pre-lesson information to assist them in meeting lesson objectives.

> There is no such thing as a perfect instructor; there is always room for improvement.

> The challenge in instructional design is to find new or innovative approaches to learning techniques.

Role as an Administrator

One of the least favorite tasks of instructors is paperwork. While most instructors understand the importance of paperwork, it is often time-consuming. This can result in a relaxed attitude for completing paperwork and cause instructors to put it off until the end of a program.

Administrators are very concerned with record keeping. Records are the basis for which lawsuits can be won or lost. Records such as criminal history forms, exam results, attendance rosters, student skills sign-off forms, incident reports, student counseling reports, instructor schedules, and payment rosters should remain with each class file for future reference.

Records prove invaluable when evaluating the effectiveness of a training program. If the majority of a class fails a particular subject, instructor records can identify who taught that particular lesson. If a student blames the instructor because he was not taught certain information, the instructor can look at attendance rosters to show that the student did not attend class on the day the material was presented.

Incident reports and counseling forms are important should legal action be sought against an instructor or training facility. It is essential that instructors document counseling sessions accurately to include what was discussed, student reaction, plans for future work, and a time line for improvement or remediation. Incident reports should include an exact summary of what happened. For example, was anyone injured, was the incident reported to anyone, and what was the end result?

Another administrative role in a training program is ensuring that regulatory requirements have been met. This responsibility is often shared with a Course Coordinator. Requirements such as instructor to student ratios, instructor qualifications, and the amount of equipment available must be considered. In addition, certain paperwork (*eg*, course applications, rosters, examinations) may need to be filed with state or regional regulatory agencies.

Financial concerns are also included in the administrative role of instructors. While the manager of a training program is more likely to develop an actual budget, staying within that budget or requesting additional materials may be the responsibility of instructors and coordinators.

Instructors should understand that although something may be beneficial to a training project, it may not be possible due to budget constraints. For example, a one-to-one student instructor ratio may be optimal, but in reality the cost for administering such a program would be astronomical. Likewise, giving students duplicate materials such as books or pocket masks because they lost theirs would prove costly and could make a training project go over budget.

The downside to budgetary constraints is a negative effect on learning. Obviously if a student loses his books, he will not be able to study and may fail the program. In this situation, a library loan program may be beneficial.

Another financial consideration is instructor pay scales. While paying instructors additional money may result in a higher-quality or a more professional instructor, this increase may also result in an increase in tuition, which may prevent students from attending the training program.

One of the most difficult and time-consuming roles for the administration of a training program involves the scheduling and general logistics of training. It is important for instructors to understand that much time, effort and thought goes into a training program. Schedul-

> Records prove invaluable when evaluating the effectiveness of a training program.

ing classroom facilities, ensuring the appropriate number of instructors, maintaining equipment in working condition, and ensuring that materials are available when needed (*eg*, books, pocket masks, skills sheets, handouts) is very time-consuming and often quite exhausting.

Role as a Consultant

Consultants are often concerned with performance problems after training. They provide ongoing support and encouragement to students and serve as a resource to students as well as to other instructors. Consultants are concerned with finding creative solutions to training and performance problems.

The Instructor as a Role Model

The student enters a training environment open to learning new information. Just as a child mimics his parents, students often mimic their instructors. If the instructor has an "I don't care" attitude, vulnerable students may reflect that same attitude.

A professional image on the part of an instructor is essential,.

The manner in which an instructor presents himself is very important for the integrity of EMS training. A professional image on the part of an instructor is essential, not only to instill a higher level of training and increased respect from students, but also to improve the level of professionalism in EMS in general.

KEY POINTS

1. Students entering EMS training programs are from a variety of ages, personalities, physical characteristics, intellectual development, and maturity levels. These student characteristics must be taken into account when planning and presenting a lesson.
2. Screening exams and interviews help identify potential problems and motivation factors of individuals enrolling in training programs. Exams can also provide a baseline from that to evaluate learning.
3. The attitude, language, and behavior an instructor exhibits can promote or prevent learning. An instructor should maintain a professional image using appropriate language that students do not find offensive or embarrassing. They should exhibit a positive attitude by viewing individuals as learners and as people. Students attend training to grow and learn. For an instructor to gain respect from the student, he must first respect the student.
4. There are multiple seating arrangement variations for the classroom, each with its own positive and negative features. Instructors should take the time to select the most appropriate arrangement for each training session and feel free to rearrange furniture as necessary.
5. The formality of the educational setting affects learning. In an informal setting, students are more open to actively participate in learning. In a formal setting, on the other hand, students are less willing to experiment or try new ideas. Instructor and learner attitudes, behaviors, language, and appearance help to determine whether the setting is formal or informal.
6. The environment of the classroom itself greatly affects learning. If a student is too cold or too hot, he is less likely to pay attention to the instructor. Likewise, if breaks are not provided at regular intervals, the student may lose interest in the class.
7. If there is excessive noise in the room, the student will tune out the information being provided. Such noise includes distractions from other students talking, pagers or scanners, useless jargon, and poor instructor habits (ie, playing with change in pockets, saying "uh,"), and anything else that interferes with learning.
8. Communication is a two-way street, resulting in the building of interpersonal relationships.
9. Communication involves a sender, message, channel, and receiver. The method by which the message is transmitted is through one of the five senses (sight, smell, hearing, touch, or taste). The primary channels for communication are seeing and hearing the message.
10. The sender and receiver of a message each have factors that can promote or impede the effectiveness of communication. Such factors include communication skills, attitudes, knowledge, and cultural beliefs. If there is a significant conflict between these factors in the sender and the receiver, effective communication may be halted.
11. During communication, each person takes a turn serving as both the sender and receiver of information.

KEY POINTS continued

12. The process of communication involves a clear formulation of the idea to be communicated, encoding the message, sending the message via a channel, receiving the message, and decoding and interpreting the message.

13. Nonverbal communication includes gestures, eye contact, body language, pacing of a presentation, attire, posture, and facial expressions. It is essential that the instructor send messages that match both verbally and nonverbally. If an instructor sends the message that he is not interested in the class or in what he is teaching, learning will be diminished.

14. Instructors have more responsibility than simply the presentation of information. Students look to instructors for guidance, support, assurance, information, feedback, assistance, motivation, and a variety of other needs. In addition, many instructors have at least a small amount of responsibility for the administrative end of training such as coordinating, scheduling, adhering to budgetary constraints, submitting paperwork, and counseling students.

REFERENCES

1. Margolis F, Bell C. *Instructing for Results.* San Diego: University Associates, Inc. Pfeiffer & Co., and Minneapolis: Lakewood Publications; 1986.
2. Zimmerman G, Owen J, Seibert D. *Speech Communication,* 2nd ed. St. Paul, MN: West Publishing Company; 1980.
3. International Association of Fire Fighters (IAFF). *Hazardous Materials Instructor Training.* Washington, DC: IAFF; 1993.
4. Carliner S. The six deadly sins of educational communication. *Performance & Instruction.* 1991, November/December:29-32.
5. Zemke R. Learning to listen to trainees. *Training.* 1977, July:76-83.

5 PLANNING FOR INSTRUCTION

OBJECTIVES

Upon completion of this chapter, the reader will have sufficient information to:
1. Develop instructional goals for training programs.
2. Describe the difference between instructional goals and objectives.
3. List the benefits of instructional objectives to both instructors and students.
4. Develop accurate instructional objectives consisting of performance, condition, and criteria.
5. Provide an instructional objective for each level of each of the three domains of learning.
6. Develop a lesson plan.
7. Describe the stages involved in the learning process.
8. Describe the four levels at which most information is learned, and the instructional processes needed for students to learn such.
9. List behavioral terms for objectives based on each of the domains of learning.

KEY TERMS

Criteria The element against which a student is judged to determine whether he or she has successfully met the terms of an instructional objective

Condition Part of an instructional objective that describes any materials, restrictions, or requirements placed on a student when attempting to meet such objectives

Instructional goals Statements describing the major purpose of a training program

Lesson plan A detailed outline of the objectives, content, procedures, and evaluation methods of a single instructional session

Metacognition Knowledge of one's own cognitive processes and the ability to regulate such processes

Objective A statement regarding the specific changes educators intend to produce in student behavior as a result of instruction

Performance The behavior a student should be able to accomplish as a result of training, relative to instructional objectives

INSTRUCTIONAL GOALS

Instructional goals are statements that describe the major purpose of a training program or class session; they provide direction for the selection of course objectives, content, and materials. While goals provide direction for the overall course, they do not provide information regarding specific skills or tasks students should be able to perform as a result of training, nor do they provide information regarding the process for achieving or assessing competency.

Instructional goals provide direction for the development of instructional objectives. Objectives, on the other hand, specify the steps necessary to meet these goals. According to the 1994 EMT-Basic National Standard Curriculum[1], the course goal is "to instruct a student to the level of Emergency Medical Technician-Basic, formerly the EMT-Ambulance, who serves as a vital link in the chain of the health care team. . . This includes all of the skills necessary for the student to provide emergency medical care at a basic life support level with an ambulance service or other specialized service. Specifically, after successful completion of the program, the student will be capable of performing the following functions at the minimum entry level:

- Recognize the nature and seriousness of the patient's condition or extent of injuries to assess requirements for emergency medical care
- Administer appropriate emergency medical care based on assessment findings of the patient's condition
- Lift, move, position, and otherwise handle the patient to minimize discomfort and prevent further injury
- Perform, safely and effectively, the expectations of the job description[1]"

These goals provide the overall basis of the EMT-Basic curriculum. And, while they provide direction, it is difficult to establish specific lesson plans from these goals. Likewise, it is difficult to judge when a learner has successfully completed the training program, since specific, measurable tasks that the individual should be able to perform are not part of these goals. Therefore, while a goal provides the overall objective of a training program, instructional objectives provide a list of specific behaviors that students should be able to perform at the conclusion of instruction. It is from these objectives that instructors can develop lesson plans and materials to effectively present information.

DEVELOPING INSTRUCTIONAL OBJECTIVES

Objectives are descriptions of behaviors a student should be able to exhibit at the end of instruction; they are the anticipated result of a training program. It is essential that a training program consist of instructional objectives to assist both instructors and students.

For Instructors (Instructional Objectives)
- Provide the basis for the selection of instructional materials, content, and methods
- Provide direction for training and a goal to know when the student has completed the learning process
- Provide a method of communicating expectations to students
- Provide a basis for creating test questions and monitoring learner progress and achievement of training goals
- Provide a contract between instructors and students

For Students (Instructional Objectives)
- Provide an understanding of what is expected of them within a training program
- Provide a logical framework to organize their efforts toward accomplishment of training goals

🍎 Provide the opportunity for self-assessment throughout a training program

ELEMENTS OF AN OBJECTIVE

An effective objective is comprised of four key elements that answer the following questions:

1) Who must complete the task? (audience)
2) What task must the individual accomplish? (performance)
3) Under what conditions must the task be accomplished? (condition)
4) How well must the task be performed in order to be successful (criteria)?

The Audience

The "who" element indicates that the audience should be able to accomplish the objective. In most training programs, the "who" is usually the student, as shown below:

- With the use of a rigid board splint, *the student* will be able to adequately stabilize a deformed femur.
- Given a chart of human anatomy, *the student* will be able to identify the major bones of the body.
- When provided with necessary examination tools and a victim, *the student* will be able to perform a patient assessment.
- Given a list of signs and symptoms, *the student* will be able to accurately identify the illness or injury of a patient.
- Given an illness or injury, *the student* will be able to list all steps of treatment.
- Given a stethoscope and blood pressure cuff, *the student* will be able to auscultate a blood pressure within +/− 10 mm Hg of the actual measurement.

> The "who" element indicates that the audience should be able to accomplish the objective.

The Performance

The "what" element is the behavior that the student should be able to perform at the end of a training session. The behavior must contain an action- or behavior- oriented verb that explains exactly what it is the individual must be able to perform. Such behavioral terms should be observable, although objectives written for the affective domain may be difficult to judge. Observable behavioral terms include the following:

- Identify
- Describe
- Define
- List
- Compare
- Correctly answer
- Write
- Solve

Less observable terms, which should be avoided, include the following:

- To know
- To appreciate
- To believe
- To understand
- To enjoy
- To have faith in

> The "what" element is the behavior that the student should be able to perform at the end of a training session.

The Condition

The "how" element of instructional objectives is often referred to as the condition. Such conditions include any restrictions or requirements placed on learners as they attempt to meet the objective. This might include time constraints placed on an individual or tools, equipment, or supplies that can or cannot be used. Examples of such conditions might include the following:

- *With the use of a rigid board splint*, the student will be able to adequately stabilize a deformed femur.
- *Given a chart of human anatomy*, the student will be able to identify the major bones of the body.
- *When provided with necessary examination tools and a victim*, the student will be able to perform a patient assessment.
- *Given a list of signs and symptoms*, the student will be able to identify the illness or injury of a patient accurately.
- *Given an illness or injury*, the student will be able to list all steps of treatment for each.
- *Given a stethoscope and blood pressure cuff*, the student will be able to auscultate a blood pressure within +/− 10 mm Hg of the actual measurement.

The Criteria

The "how well" element of instructional objectives identifies the criteria against which the individual will be judged in order to determine if he has successfully met the terms of the objective. Examples of such criteria include the following:

- With the use of a rigid board splint, the student will be able to stabilize a deformed femur adequately, *as outlined in the National Standard Curriculum.*
- Given a chart of human anatomy, the student will be able to identify *at least eight* major bones of the body.
- When provided with necessary examination tools and a victim, the student will be able to perform a patient assessment *within 2 minutes.*
- Given a list of signs and symptoms, the student will be able to identify the illness or injury of a patient *accurately.*
- Given an illness or injury, the student will be able to list *all steps of treatment for each.*
- Given a stethoscope and blood pressure cuff, the student will be able to auscultate a blood pressure *within +/− 10 mm Hg of the actual measurement.*

If the degree to which a behavior is to be accomplished is not stated, it is expected that the student accomplish the objective 100%.

There are times when several objectives are written for the same audience. In these cases, it may be easier to write the objective using one statement at the beginning of a list of behaviors, as identified below:

Upon the completion of this presentation, the student will be able to do the following:

- With the use of a rigid board splint, adequately stabilize a deformed femur, as outlined in the National Standard Curriculum.
- Given a chart of human anatomy, identify at least eight major bones of the body.
- When provided with necessary examination tools and a victim, perform a patient assessment, within two minutes.
- Given a list of signs and symptoms, identify the illness or injury of a patient accurately.
- Given an illness or injury, list all steps of treatment.
- Given a stethoscope and blood pressure cuff, auscultate a blood pressure within +/− 10 mm Hg of the actual measurement.

> The "how well" element of instructional objectives identifies the criteria against which the individual will be judged.

OBJECTIVES WRITTEN TO THE DOMAINS OF LEARNING

As described in Chapter 1, there are three domains of learning: the cognitive, psychomotor, and affective domains. Just as teaching is designed to incorporate the three domains, instructional objectives should also be written for all areas of instruction. The 1994 EMT-Basic National Standard Curriculum provides objectives at three levels for each domain of learning: the knowledge, application, and problem-solving levels. Tables 5.1 and 5.2 provide a listing and description of each level based on the domains of learning.

- The *knowledge level* is targeted toward helping students comprehend facts, procedures, and feelings.
- The *application level* is targeted toward the integration and execution of principles, procedures, and values within specific situations.
- The *problem-solving level* is the highest level and involves the analysis of information, procedures, and feelings in order to modify and adapt specific tasks depending on specific situations. In the affective domain, this level also involves making judgements about the value of these procedures and information.

TABLE 5.1 Domains of Learning

LEVELS OF OBJECTIVES	DOMAINS		
	COGNITIVE	PSYCHOMOTOR	AFFECTIVE
Knowledge	Recalling Comprehending	Imitating Manipulating	Receiving Responding
Application	Applying	Precision	Valuing
Problem-solving	Analyzing Synthesizing Evaluating	Articulating Naturalizing	Organizing Characterizing

Levels of objectives based on the three domains of learning (adapted from TIPS[2]).

TABLE 5.2 Domains of Learning

LEVELS OF OBJECTIVES	DOMAINS		
	COGNITIVE	PSYCHOMOTOR	AFFECTIVE
Knowledge	Involves the student memorizing and recalling facts, ideas, and principles	Involves the student observing a more experienced individual perform an activity	Involves a student's willingness to receive and respond to stimuli
Application	Involves the student applying previously learned information into new situations	Involves the student practicing skills under supervision until reaching proficiency	Involves the student exhibiting a consistent feeling, value, or belief
Problem-solving	Involves the student dissecting a problem to identify its parts, resynthesize the parts into a new form, and make judgements about the problem	Involves the student observing and imitating a skill performed by someone else, until perfection is attained	Involves the student bringing complex values into a harmonious relationship

Description of levels of objectives based on the three domains of learning (adapted from TIPS[2]).

Table 5.3 provides a list of behavioral terms for objectives based on each level of the domains of learning. An example of behavior terms used in instructional objectives for each level and domain of learning, based on the 1994 EMT-Basic National Standard Curriculum, are provided in Boxes 5.1- 5.3.

USING LESSON PLANS

A written plan provides organization and structure to a presentation.

A lesson plan is an outline of information that the instructor intends to present in order to ensure the completeness and accuracy of a training session. A written plan provides organization and structure to a presentation and will ultimately add to the continuity and professionalism of a program.

TABLE 5.3 Behavioral Terms for Objectives

LEVELS OF OBJECTIVES	DOMAINS		
	COGNITIVE	PSYCHOMOTOR	AFFECTIVE
Knowledge	Define	Demonstrate	Assist
	Describe	Imitate	Attend to
	Discuss	Observe	Be interested in
	Explain	View	Comply with
	Identify		Differentiate
	Indicate		Listen
	Label		Practice
	List		Volunteer
	Name		
	Recall		
	Recite		
	Recognize		
	Record		
	Repeat		
	Report		
	Restate		
	Review		
	State		
	Show		
	Summarize		
Application	Apply	Demonstrate	Advocate
	Classify	Draw	Approve
	Compute	Employ	Be convinced of
	Demonstrate	Illustrate	Believe
	Determine	Locate	Challenge
	Employ	Measure	Criticize
	Find	Operate	Persuade
	Operate	Perform	Value
	Perform	Practice	
	Predict	Record	
	Schedule	Use	
	Solve	Set Up	
	Use		
	Write		

TABLE 5.3 continued			
Problem-solving	Analyze	Adjust	Advocate
	Assess	Design	Approve
	Compare	Experiment	Assess
	Compose	Master	Challenge
	Construct	Modify	Change
	Create	Perfect	Characterize
	Design		Defend
	Differentiate		Formulate
	Distinguish		Judge
	Establish		Manage
	Evaluate		Resist
	Examine		Resolve
	Invent		Revise
	Judge		
	Organize		
	Plan		
	Prepare		
	Rate		
	Select		
	Synthesize		

Behavioral terms for instructional objectives based on the three domains of learning (adapted from TIPS[2]).

The Learning Process
As discussed in Chapter 1, information is processed through various stages before it is learned, as identified in Figure 5.1.

The Lesson Design Process
Most information is learned on one of four different levels[3]:

- **Memorizing information** is the most superficial level, requiring rote learning and memorization.
- **Understanding relationships** requires the integration of new information with existing knowledge.

BOX 5.1 Cognitive Domain	
Knowledge Level	At the completion of this lesson, the EMT-Basic student will be able to describe the anatomy and function of the following major body systems: respiratory, circulatory, musculoskeletal, nervous, and endocrine
Application Level	At the completion of this lesson, the EMT-Basic student will be able to determine whether a scene is safe to enter
Problem-solving Level	At the completion of this lesson, the EMT-Basic student will be able to differentiate between a strong, weak, regular, and irregular pulse

Instructional objectives for the cognitive domain (adapted from 1994 EMT-Basic NSC).

BOX 5.2 **Psychomotor Domain**

Knowledge Level	At the completion of this lesson, the EMT-Basic student will be able to observe various scenarios and identify potential hazards
Application Level	At the completion of this lesson, the EMT-Basic student will be able to demonstrate general steps for assisting patients with the self-administration of medications
Problem-solving Level	(Note: The 1994 EMT-Basic National Standard Curriculum does not identify any objectives at this level. The following is an example of a psychomotor problem- solving objective). At the completion of this lesson, the EMT-Basic student will be able to, given a variety of typical situations and patient conditions, demonstrate the ability to make necessary changes in CPR procedures

Instructional objectives for the psychomotor domain (adapted from 1994 EMT-Basic NSC).

- **Applying skills** requires the transfer of a skill to various situations (mental and physical).
- **Higher-level thinking** is the most complex form of learning and involves thinking skills and metacognition.

Instructional strategies for each level can vary due to the way in which each type of information is encoded. It is important that instructors understand the different levels in which information is processed and develop lesson plans that assist the student in obtaining proficiency at the level necessary to meet course goals and objectives. Each level of learning skills will be discussed on the pages that follow.

Memorized Information

The memorization of information is often termed rote (non-meaningful) because the information has no relation to prior knowledge.

The memorization of information is often termed rote (non-meaningful) because the information has no relation to prior knowledge. An ex-

BOX 5.3 **Affective Domain**

Knowledge Level	At the completion of this lesson, the EMT-Basic student will be able to recognize and respond to the feelings patients experience during assessment
Application Level	At the completion of this lesson, the EMT-Basic student will be able to explain the value of performing the baseline vital signs
Problem-solving Level	At the completion of this lesson, the EMT-Basic student will be able to defend the need for obtaining and recording an accurate set of vital signs

Instructional objectives for the affective domain (adapted from 1994 EMT-Basic NSC).

Information Stimulus

- Information is received by one of the five senses.
- Input is either ignored or processed.

⇩

Short-Term Memory

- Only a few items (plus or minus seven) can be stored in short-term memory at one time.
- Information is lost quickly unless it is rehearsed.

⇩

Long-Term Memory

- Information is encoded and can usually be retrieved and used at a later time.
- Information not encoded is lost.
- When information is "encoded" it is said to be learned.

FIGURE 5.1 The Communications/Learning Process

ample of this level of learning includes the knowledge of different types of shock.

- Information is obtained through the senses (the student reads the information or hears the instructor list the various types).
- The information is transferred to short-term memory.
- Unless the student rehearses the information, it will be lost. If rehearsed, the information will be encoded in long-term memory.

For difficult information, memorization can be enriched by the following tactics:

- Chunking information
- Using mnemonics, rhymes, or acronyms
- Repetition
- Using flash cards

Understanding Relationships

Understanding is a gradual process that requires the student to view information as meaningful and be able to relate new information to prior knowledge in order to explain how something works. Strategies to enhance understanding include:

Understanding is a gradual process that requires the student to view information as meaningful.

- Paraphrasing information
- Elaborating on information provided

Paraphrasing information is simply the rewording of the meaning of a concept. This strategy provides for the superficial level of understanding known as comprehension. Elaborations provide detailed information linking a new concept or idea with relevant prior knowledge. Elaborations can take various forms including analysis, case studies, drawing analogies, and comparing, or contrasting information.

The application of skills occurs in three ways: applying concepts, procedures, and principles.

Applying Skills

The application of skills occurs in three ways: applying concepts, procedures, and principles.

Applying concepts requires the grouping of objects, events, or ideas. It is generally a two-part process:

- The memorization of a label and characteristics
- The application of information to generalize skills to various examples or situations

The application process requires the use of various examples and nonexamples so the student becomes familiar with the wide range of instances of the concept. An example of this process is the recognition of an unconscious patient. Learning this information requires the following:

- Memorization of
  The label (unconscious)
  The characteristics (the patient is unarousable with the use of verbal or painful stimuli).
- The use of examples and nonexamples to effectively learn the application of concepts for identifying an unresponsive patient:
- Examples:
  A patient who is lying on the ground and is unarousable
  A patient who cannot be awakened
  A patient who does not respond to painful stimuli
  A patient who does not respond to verbal stimuli
- Nonexamples:
  A patient who moves his arm upon painful stimuli
  A patient who staggers when walking

Applying procedures involves following steps in order to perform a task (physical or mental). To learn this process requires:

- A memorization aspect such as the student remembering specific steps and the order in which the steps are to be performed so that a goal can be achieved
- An application phase, whereby students use skills in various situations
- The presentation of goals, the steps to attain such goals, and the order in which steps must be performed
- The presentation of a variety of demonstration scenarios to help students apply skill in new situations.

Applying principles requires the use of knowledge to solve problems, make predictions, and provide explanations. It requires an understanding of changes that occur, and why. To learn and apply principles requires:

- Memorization of processes or cause-and-effect relationships.
- Application of generalizations of a skill to various conditions or situations. To do this, students should be taught the phases, order of phases, and cause-and-effect relationships.
- Practice of skills in a variety of situations.

Higher-Level Skills

Higher-level thinking involves the use of skills that can be applied across multiple subjects and domains. It tends to take longer to acquire these skills. This level may require the following:

- Memorization of several sequences of skills
- An understanding aspect, which is necessary to transfer skills across various domains
- An application aspect in which learned skills are applied to previously unencountered situations.

To assist learners with the acquisition of higher-level thinking skills, it is necessary to identify more simple procedures and understandings that comprise such, and build upon them. Specific strategies for teaching higher-level skills include:

- Providing a simple-to-complex sequence for the higher-level skill
- Analyzing each skill to be taught based on the level of complexity, breaking it into simple components, and then teaching each component individually and then integrally

DEVELOPING LESSON PLANS

A lesson plan identifies how information will be presented in order to gain maximum benefit from the learning experience. The plan is generally divided into three sections; the introduction, body, and closing.

Introduction

The first few minutes of instruction are extremely important. The instructor should use this time to prepare students for the class session and to introduce them to the lesson. Specifically, the introduction should provide an overview of the content to be covered, establish a positive climate for learning, motivate the students to the topic, state the instructional objectives for the lesson, describe how the topic relates to other course content, and state why it is important.

When developing the introduction, it is useful to begin with something to gain the learner's attention. It is then important to relate the lesson to the content area learner's have previously learned or will study in the future. By the end of the introduction, students should know exactly what is expected of them and what they can expect from the lesson.

Body of the Lesson

This part of the lesson plan should reflect the main part of the session topic. It indicates how the instructor plans to present key information to ensure maximum learner interest and comprehension. When determining how to present information in the most effective manner, it is important to maintain interest and motivation and challenge learners through various instructional strategies.

When developing the body of a lesson plan, maintain organization and clarity of information and provide variations in instructional strategies. Outline key points, list any questions that should be asked during the class session, note supplementary materials necessary to provide, and indicate instructional media to be used.

Closing

At the conclusion of a class session, it is necessary for the instructor to deliberately plan time for closure. This time should provide a sense

Higher-level thinking involves the use of skills that can be applied across multiple subjects and domains.

By the end of the introduction, students should know exactly what is expected of them and what they can expect from the lesson.

of finality and cohesiveness that instructional objectives have been met. The lesson plan should identify a review or summary of key points covered within the lesson.

New content should not be introduced during the closing, but the instructor should build interest for the next class session by providing reading assignments or explaining how the current topic relates to subsequent training sessions.

New content should not be introduced during the closing.

LESSON PLAN FORMATS

The general design of a lesson plan can take one of three main formats: a sentence outline form, a two-column format, or a three-column

SOFT TISSUE INJURIES

LESSON OUTLINE

Introduction
1. Introduce topic - Soft Tissue Injuries
2. Peak interest
3. Establish knowledge base - ask questions about the last session and survey knowledge of the current topic.
4. Inform students of lesson objectives.

Body of Lesson

1. Types of injuries

    a) Closed

        1) Contusion
        2) Hematoma
        3) Crushing injuries
        4) Rupture or hernia

    b) Open

        1) Abrasion
        2) Incision
        3) Laceration
        4) Puncture wound
        5) Avulsion
        6) Amputation

2. Treatment of Soft Tissue Injuries

    a) Closed wounds

        1) Monitor airway - watch for vomiting
        2) Position patient appropriately
        3) Treat for shock
        4) Administer high flow oxygen

FIGURE 5.2 Sample One Column Lesson Plan

format. The sentence outline format provides single-line statements of what information is to be provided. The two-column format provides one column for the lesson outline and the other for notes or instructional media to be used. The three-column format provides one column for the lesson outline, a column for notes or questions, and a column for instructional materials or activities to be used.

Figures 5.2–5.4 provide sample lesson plans based on each of the three formats.

SOFT TISSUE INJURIES

LESSON OUTLINE	NOTES/MEDIA
Introduction 1. Introduce topic - Soft Tissue Injuries 2. Peak interest 3. Establish knowledge base - ask questions about the last session and survey knowledge of the current topic. 4. Inform students of lesson objectives.	Coroners' Slides 1–4
Body of Lesson 1. Types of injuries	Overhead #1
a) Closed	
1) Contusion 2) Hematoma 3) Crushing injuries 4) Rupture or hernia	Slide #5 Slide #6 Slide #7 Slide #8
b) Open	
1) Abrasion 2) Incision 3) Laceration 4) Puncture wound 5) Avulsion 6) Amputation	Slide #9 Slide #10 Slide #11 Slide #12 Slide #13 Slide #14
2. Treatment of Soft Tissue Injuries a) Closed wounds	What is the most common form of a closed wound?
1) Monitor airway - watch for vomiting 2) Position patient appropriately 3) Treat for shock 4) Administer high flow oxygen	What is the least serious form of an open wound?

FIGURE 5.3 Sample Two Column Lesson Plan

SOFT TISSUE INJURIES

QUESTIONS & NOTES	LESSON OUTLINE	MATERIALS & ACTIVITIES
	Introduction	
	1. Introduce topic - Soft Tissue Injuries	
	2. Peak interest	Coroners' Slides 1–4
	3. Establish knowledge base - ask questions about the last session and survey knowledge of the current topic.	
NSC objectives	4. Inform students of lesson objectives.	
	Body of Lesson	
	1. Types of injuries	
What is the most common form of a closed wound?	a) Closed	Overhead #1
	1) Contusion	Slide #5
	2) Hematoma	Slide #6
	3) Crushing injuries	Slide #7
	4) Rupture or hernia	Slide #8
What is the least serious form of an open wound?	b) Open	
	1) Abrasion	Slide #9
	2) Incision	Slide #10
	3) Laceration	Slide #11
	4) Puncture wound	Slide #12
	5) Avulsion	Slide #13
	6) Amputation	Slide #14
What type of wound carries the greatest chance of infection?	2. Treatment of Soft Tissue Injuries	
	a) Closed wounds	
	1) Monitor airway - watch for vomiting	
	2) Position patient appropriately	

FIGURE 5.4 Sample Three Column Lesson Plan

KEY POINTS

1. Instructional goals are statements that describe the major purpose of a training program or class session. They provide overall direction for learning, but do not provide information regarding specific skills or tasks the student will learn.

2. An instructional objective is a description of specific behaviors an individual should be able to exhibit as a result of instruction. These objectives provide the basis for selecting instructional materials, content, and methods of teaching; communicating expectations to students; and providing a basis for creating test questions and monitoring student progress.

3. An effective objective is comprised of four key elements: the audience, performance, condition, and criteria. The audience indicates who should be able to perform the objective; the performance indicates what behavior the individual should be able to exhibit; the condition indicates under what circumstances the task should be performed; and the criteria identifies against what the individual will be judged.

4. Objectives in the 1994 EMT-Basic National Standard Curriculum are provided at three levels for each domain of learning. The knowledge level is targeted toward helping learners comprehend facts, procedures, and feelings; the application level is targeted toward the integration and execution of principles, procedures and values within specific situations; and the problem-solving level involves learner analysis of information, procedures, and feelings in order to adapt specific tasks to alternative situations.

5. A lesson plan is an outline of information that the instructor intends to present during a training session. It provides organization and structure to a presentation and ultimately adds to the continuity and professionalism of a program.

6. When designing a lesson, it is important to determine at what level the information is being presented. Memorizing information is the most superficial level, requiring rote learning of facts. Understanding relationships requires the integration of new information with existing knowledge. Applying skills requires the student to transfer the use of skills to various situations. Higher-level thinking is the most complex level of learning and requires the use of skills across multiple domains.

7. A lesson plan consists of three sections: the introduction, body, and closing. The introduction is designed to prepare and motivate students for the class session, establish a positive climate for learning, and present instructional objectives for the lesson.

8. The body of a lesson plan should reflect the key points to be presented during a lesson. It indicates how the instructor plans to present key information to ensure maximum student interest and comprehension.

9. It is important to include a closing within the lesson plan to allow time to provide a sense of closure and cohesiveness that instructional objectives have been met and to review key points presented during the lesson.

10. There are three primary formats for lesson plans. The sentence outline format provides single-line statements for what information is to be provided. The two-column format provides one column for lesson information and the other for notes and comments. The three-column format provides one column for lesson information, one for notes and questions, and the third for instructional materials or activities to be used.

FOLLOW-UP ACTIVITIES

1. Develop three complete instructional objectives for each level of each of the three domains of learning.
2. Develop an instructional goal for the First Responder and EMT-Paramedic training programs.
3. Develop a complete lesson plan for one of the lessons included in the 1994 EMT-Basic National Standard Curriculum utilizing the one-, two-, or three- column formats.

REFERENCES

1. *1994 EMT-Basic National Standard Curriculum;* Lexington, KY: Department of Transportation; 1994.
2. *Teaching Improvement Project Systems For Health Care Educators (TIPS).* Center for Learning Resources, College of Allied Health Professions, University of Kentucky, Lexington, KY.
3. Leshin C, Ploock J, Reigeluth C. *Instructional Design Strategies and Tactics.* Englewood Cliffs, NJ: Educational Technology Publications; 1992.

6 Instructional Media

Upon completion of this chapter, the reader will have sufficient information to:

1. State the importance of audiovisual aids in education.
2. Define media.
3. Explain seven benefits of media in the learning process.
4. Describe the two main channels for communication.
5. List at least eight criteria for selecting the most appropriate form of media.
6. Describe the advantages and limitations of eight types of media as well as tips for their use.
7. Describe techniques for producing slides and overhead transparencies.
8. List four sources of media or materials to produce media.
9. Describe design considerations for producing effective and efficient visuals.
10. Define multimedia.
11. Define interactivity.
12. Describe three uses for computers in education.
13. List equipment requirements for linking technology with education.
14. List the most effective type of media to meet objectives in the psychomotor, cognitive, and affective domains.
15. Identify the three primary causes for audiovisual equipment failure.

KEY TERMS

Beta A 1/2-inch videocassette format not compatible with the VHS format

Bullet In text, a circle, star, or other symbol used to emphasize a line or word

CD-I (compact disc-interactive) An interactive product that delivers still images, audio, graphics, and data; a closed-system box designed to connect to a home television or some other monitor, similar to that of a VCR

CD-ROM (compact disc-read only memory) A format of standard laser disc that stores a large amount of information and requires a CD drive in a computer system; each 4.72-inch disc stores approximately 650 megabytes of digital data. Information cannot be written to or stored on the disc

Computer-aided instruction Instruction that uses the computer as its medium

Computer based instruction A stand-alone training program using the computer as the medium

Interface A card that, when installed into a computer, allows for information contained on a videodisc or videotape to be viewed on a computer screen

Interactivity A balance of control of learning between instructors and students, resulting in some type of interaction from both

Interactive video The use of a videotape player and a computer interface to function in coordination in order to provide interactive training

KEY TERMS continued

LCD panel A device that allows text and graphic information to be displayed from a personal computer onto a large screen or wall, using a standard overhead projector as the light source; it allows large groups of people to view the computer display and images at one time

Megabyte One million bytes of information

Megahertz (MHz) Millions of cycles per second; referring to the speed of a microprocessor unit of a computer

Multimedia The integration of more than one form of medium, often referring to the use of multiple forms of media centrally controlled and coordinated, usually by a computer

Multi-screen The projection of images onto several image areas

Resolution The clarity or graininess of a video or computer image as measured by lines or pixels; the smallest resolvable detail in the image

Slides A piece of film usually containing an image, which, when projected through a light source, is enlarged and viewed from the screen; refers to the traditional 2 × 2 inch 35-mm or overhead transparency film

Slide-show presentation A feature offered by some presentation software packages that allows for slides to be shown automatically on the computer screen, in either a predetermined sequence or at random

Storyboard A visual outline of media design

S-VHS (super-VHS) A videotape format that provides for better resolution and less noise than standard VHS tapes

VHS (video home system) The most popular 1/2-inch consumer videotape format

Videoconferencing The use of a specialized audiovisual system along with satellite telecommunications, which allows for groups at remote locations to participate in the same meeting or seminar at the same time

Virtual reality An extensive gamut of technologies used in an attempt to merge physical senses and actions with computer-generated images in order to create a perception of realism

INTRODUCTION

Education has advanced in leaps and bounds since the days when chalk and a chalkboard were the key ingredients for teaching. The modern world stresses that the medium is as important as the message, and presentation is everything.

With the great proliferation of media in recent years, instructors may feel overwhelmed and intimidated when faced with the smorgasbord of instructional materials available. It is important to understand, however, that media does not necessary equate with high technology or expensive equipment. The basic chalkboard, in fact, is a valuable form of media.

There is nothing magical about media, and unless it is properly used, media will not enhance the learning process. Media does not relieve the instructor of the burden of teaching nor does it replace the instructor-student relationship in the classroom setting. It is, however, a very useful tool to assist instructors and the learning process.

Media is a vehicle for education. When appropriately selected and properly used its use can greatly enhance the learning process, resulting in greater student achievement. Such media should reinforce an instructor's presentation and further the instructional objectives of a training program.

The terms instructional media and audiovisual aids are often used interchangeably. In general, media refers to anything that illustrates an idea, process, or theory, or demonstrates the mechanics of how something works or a procedure for performing a task.

Instructional media enhances learning by targeting multiple senses. Research has shown that the more senses used in the learning process, the greater chances for the retention of information. This chapter will describe various types of audiovisual aids and provide tips for designing appropriate materials and effectively using them.

Media does not relieve the instructor of the burden of teaching nor does it replace the instructor-student relationship in the classroom setting.

WHAT IS MEDIA?

Instructional media is the means of transmitting instruction. It is a way to convey information. Examples of media include overhead projectors, slide projectors, chalkboards, VCRs, and tape players.

Instructional material is what carries the message. In simple terms, instructional material contains the information that is transmitted by media. Examples of instructional material include overhead transparencies, handouts, slides, and worksheets. Together, material and media can dramatically improve the presentation of information, thereby facilitating the learning process. For our purposes, media and materials are used interchangeably.

If used correctly, media can play an important role in education, since the use of media augments a presentation. It is imperative, however, that instructors be knowledgeable about the media they will use, and do not use it as a "crutch." Using any type of media as a replacement for preparation can be fatal. An instructor who reads verbatim from a slide will not only put students to sleep, but may cause them to become hostile and feel that attending class is a waste of time.

In addition, if the media does not relate to the topic at hand, it should be omitted. Although students may enjoy watching a video of the latest "Rescue 911" series, if it does not reinforce the information presented during class, it is a waste of time. Our job is to educate students, not to entertain them.

Using any type of media as a replacement for preparation can be fatal.

MEDIA AND THE LEARNING PROCESS

The use of media has recently become more widespread by presenters and educators. Instructional media is useful for reinforcing and illustrating the spoken word by appealing to more than one sense. There are many benefits from the use of media in the classroom setting.

Motivation
Media makes instruction more interesting. By augmenting a lesson with instructional media, students take on a more active role in the learning process. Students prefer classes that provide information that cannot be obtained by reading a textbook. Students are often "turned off" by the instructor who stands in front of the class and lectures directly from a book. Instructional media provides a change of pace, thereby maintaining student interest, attention, and motivation.

Standardization
Media can provide a means for standardization of lessons. The American Red Cross uses videos as a means of presenting their standard first aid courses. By doing this, instructors simply open the class, review objectives, and play the video. While this method of instruction is not recommended, videos can be used to enhance a lesson or provide standardization for lessons that should be taught the same way, regardless of who the instructor is. Such lessons might include CPR and patient assessment, which are two of the most important skills an EMT must learn.

Videos can be used to enhance a lesson or provide standardization for lessons that should be taught the same way, regardless of who the instructor is.

Review
Media is also beneficial as a form of review. Quizzes, tests, or games can be used to provide feedback to both students and instructors.

For example, after the lesson on medical emergencies, a short video of a simulated ambulance run (start to finish) for a patient suffering from chest pain will help the student "put it all together."

Remediation

Media is useful for helping students who are slow learners. Providing extra videos, films, tapes, or worksheets to students who need academic tutoring lets them review, study, and learn at their own pace. It also provides a mechanism for students who were absent from a class to make up a lesson without causing an inconvenience to the instructor.

Time Saver

Media can reduce the length of a lecture. Through the use of media, instructors can present essential material concisely. During a lecture, instructors have a tendency to go off on tangents. The use of media helps keep instructors on track, leading to a more efficient use of class time for both instructors and students.

Quality Improvement

Instructional media can improve the quality of instruction. When lessons are carefully planned, integrating pictures and words, instruction becomes more clearly defined and organized. This way, instructors present specific information while emphasizing key points.

Instructional media can improve the quality of instruction.

Provide Vivacy

Consider the saying "A picture is worth a thousand words." This is especially true in education. A visual aid can often present information more clearly, thoroughly, quickly, and effectively than simply using words. The student will remember the information given in a vivid presentation.

In order to receive these benefits, careful planning and development of instructional media must take place. Certain educational principles are incorporated into the design of instructional materials as well as to the selection of media. They must be of high quality, meet specific program objectives, and become an integral part of the instructional process. Finally, instructional media must be relevant to the material being presented. No matter how good the medium, if it is irrelevant to course content, it will divert student attention.

Instructional media must be relevant to the material being presented.

CHANNELS OF COMMUNICATION

Communication takes place when a message is transmitted from a sender to a receiver. In education, the sender is the instructor and the student the receiver. The message can be transmitted by various means including written texts, lectures, and videos. How the message is transmitted directly correlates with the amount of information students retain.

Communication occurs through various channels. Students use their senses to receive information. Auditory and visual channels are the most common and most effective means of communication. Students may also use the senses of smell and touch in the learning process, primarily during casualty simulations to identify injuries.

Using a medium that deals with one sense is referred to as *single-channel communication*. Examples of single-channel media using audio

14 Tips for Improving Instruction through Media

1. Make a conscientious effort to incorporate media into each lesson.
2. Identify objectives of instruction.
3. Based on those objectives, identify what form of media will have the most positive impact on the audience.
4. Look for available materials that can be used or modified; if specific material is not readily available, consider designing new materials.
5. Modify existing materials to meet the specific needs of your audience.
6. Identify local sources of materials such as national, state, or local government organizations, EMS organizations, libraries, colleges and universities, or other organizations.
7. Review audiovisual materials and equipment prior to using them; avoid unexpected problems.
8. Use storyboard cards to assist with media planning, design, and development.
9. Identify what equipment is available at the training facility in order to determine what materials can be used.
10. Practice setting up and operating various audiovisual equipment in order to become comfortable with it.
11. Expand the media horizons; experiment with materials that are not often used.
12. Evaluate materials after every use. Include a self-evaluation as well as an analysis of their effectiveness relative to the student's attitudes, motivation, and/or academic achievement. Modify any errors or problems identified. Store materials in a dry, cool room.
13. Develop and maintain files of materials including evaluation sheets. Keep a master copy of original materials in the event that those in use become worn, damaged, or lost.
14. Constantly search for additional forms of media, materials, or techniques for improving instruction.

include cassette tapes, reel-to-reel tapes, and phonograph records. Single-channel visual media include overhead transparencies, slides, photographs, posters, and the chalkboard.

The use of two or more senses is *multichannel communication*. Multichannel media includes videos, slide or tape presentations, or films that use both audio and video channels for communication. Audiovisual presentations greatly enhance the quality of information being provided in the classroom setting.

Impressions that are created by combining pictures, words, and sounds are retained by students significantly longer than those made by just listening or reading alone. Therefore, the more channels of communication an instructor uses, the greater the impressions that will be made on students and the more information students will be able to remember and recall when needed.

Many people rely on visual input as their primary source of information. Research has indicated a significant impact of visual aids on the comprehension and retention of information in adult learning[7]. In

Impressions that are created by combining pictures, words, and sounds are retained by students significantly longer than those made by just listening or reading alone.

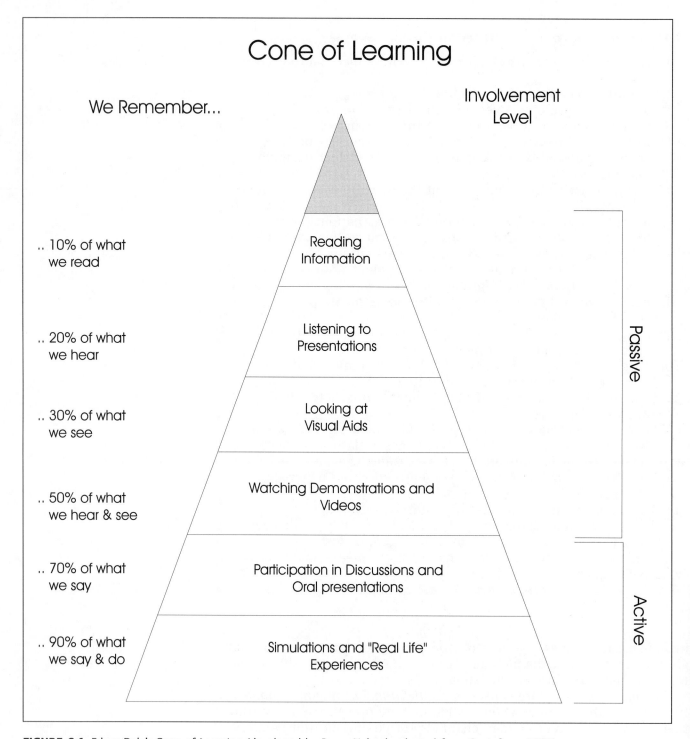

FIGURE 6.1 Edgar Dale's Cone of Learning (developed by Bruce Nyland, adapted from Gustafson, 1985).

fact, a notable study conducted by Dr. Edgar Dale measured the retention of skills and knowledge 3 days after training. As shown in Figure 6.1, the study found that students remember:

- 10% of what they read
- 20% of what they hear
- 50% of what they hear and see
- 70% of what they say
- 90% of what they say as they do

Although these percentages vary according to sources, the general concept remains that students comprehend and retain information at a significantly higher rate when instructional adjuncts are used in classroom training.

I see, I forget
I hear, I remember
I do, I understand
I practice, I master
I master, I enjoy

CRITERIA FOR SELECTION

Prior to the selection of any form of instructional media, it is essential that the lesson plan developed includes course objectives. The course objectives should dictate appropriate media, not vice versa. While some lessons may require minimal media in the form of handouts or a chalkboard, others may demand more advanced forms such as video or simulations.

What form of media an instructor uses depends on various factors, including cost, availability, and relevance to course content[6]. It is important when evaluating various media that instructors look past the "bells and whistles" and concentrate on meeting educational objectives. When selecting media, consider the following factors:

What form of media an instructor uses depends on various factors, including cost, availability, and relevance to course content[6].

Availability
The primary determining factor of what form of media to use is what types are available for the training program. This may require a phone call to the facility hosting a program to determine if the room is normally equipped with a chalkboard, screen, video monitor, or other equipment.

In addition to equipment, availability includes access to materials to produce instructional media as well as availability of already produced material. Local hospitals, universities, and training centers may have the ability to produce instructional materials and be willing to lend these resources to instructors.

Relevance to Learning Objectives
It is essential when selecting instructional media to make certain the material is directly relevant to course content. Using material that is not relevant may have negative effects on learning.

Likewise, the nature of objectives may require alternative forms of media. While cognitive objectives may only require a written form of media such as handouts, charts, or overhead transparencies, psychomotor and affective objectives may require a more visual form of media such as slides, video, or simulations.

For purposes of media selection, learning objectives are divided into five groups: psychomotor skills, knowledge of facts, knowledge of procedures, use of concepts and principles, and attitudes. As identified in Figure 6.2, the type of objective suggests which type of media should be used.

Psychomotor Learning
Psychomotor skills are those involving the use of physical manipulation based on a mental decision. Such skills include the application of a traction splint or the set-up and administration of oxygen. In fact, the majority of training programs for emergency response personnel involve primarily psychomotor skills.

Psychomotor skills are best learned by doing. Hands-on experience, when efficiently and safely available, is optimal. When such real experiences are prohibited, by expense or hazardous condition, simulations are a valuable training alternative.

Psychomotor skills are best learned by doing.

MEDIA BASED ON OBJECTIVES

MEDIA   **OBJECTIVE**

	Psychomotor	**Cognitive**			**Affective**
		Facts	**Processes**	**Concepts**	
Audiotapes	-	* +	-	-	*
Boards, Charts, etc.	-	**	*	*	-
Computers	*	**	**	**	**
Equipment (Demonstrations)	**	-	**	*	*
Handouts	*	**	*	**	*
Simulations	**	*	**	**	**
Transparencies	-	**	**	*	*
Video & Film	**	*	**	**	**

+ Through repetition.

-	Not very effective
*	Effective
**	Very effective

FIGURE 6.2 Selection of Instructional Media Based on Learning Objectives (adapted from GP Courseware, 1983).

Cognitive learning involves mental processes for the acquisition of knowledge.

Cognitive Learning

Cognitive learning involves mental processes for the acquisition of knowledge. Such cognitive learning can be classified as facts, procedures, and concepts and principles.

Facts involve a rote memorization process that can be accomplished through a single-channel medium. Learning the names of certain bones in the body or parts of a blood pressure cuff can be accomplished through the use of diagrams and flash cards.

Procedures normally involve motion, and often require memorizing facts in a specific order and repeating them appropriately. Such procedural activities include CPR, patient assessment, and AED use. Media that uses motion such as video, film, or demonstration are best for meeting this type objective.

Concepts and principles involve abstract ideas regarding relationships between facts. One example of such concepts involves hazardous materials. Without using knowledge of principles regarding hazardous materials, an emergency responder may enter a contaminated area without proper protection and succumb to vapors within that environment. When presenting concepts, it is useful to display cause-and-effect relationships. This type of objective is best presented through the use of multichannel media such as video, film, or role play.

Affective Learning

Affective learning involves the alteration of an individual's attitude, and often includes motivation of learners. The use of instructional media is extremely effective for meeting the objectives of affective learning; video and multiscreen slide or tape presentations can be very motivational.

Affective learning involves the alteration of an individual's attitude.

Student motivation and attitudes greatly affect the learning environment. Instructional materials that are boring, ineffective, or confusing may decrease motivation and interest in a training program. Instructors must develop and use media that is appealing, accurate, and relevant.

Time Constraints

Time constraints occur in two forms, the first of which is the time necessary to develop materials. Some forms of media are much more time consuming to create than others. This may result in instructors using a "canned presentation," which may not be designed for a specific audience but generally meets objectives, or using a different form of media.

The second time constraint involves the time needed to play back or use instructional materials. Often the instructor finds a suitable video but runs out of time for the session, cuts short the lecture, fails to properly introduce the video, or has no time to provide closure after viewing the video. This scenario is an injustice to students since they are unsure of what they are watching and why it is important.

Cost

The fourth factor for consideration is cost relative to media selection, development, and use. Various factors play a role when determining cost, including start-up equipment, supplies, and production costs. These costs should be considered based on a cost-benefit model, *ie*, does the benefit of such materials outweigh the cost?

Various factors play a role when determining cost, including start-up equipment, supplies, and production costs.

Equipment generally refers to playback devices including the chalkboard, overhead projector, screen, slide projector, VCR, television monitor, and computer. Some equipment is quite costly and may limit the availability of that form of media, while other equipment is relatively inexpensive.

Supplies and production costs refer to the cost to develop instructional materials. Production costs may include those for additional equipment, such as a laser printer, color printer, copier, computer and software, slide generator, camera, video camera and recorder, or poster maker. Supplies refer to those disposable materials needed to produce media such as transparency film, markers, easel paper, slide film, or videotape.

Most forms of media require a one time cost for the purchase of the equipment as well as the ongoing purchase of supplies. Some additional costs may be the purchase of already produced material such as videos, slides, transparencies, and charts. These materials are frequently costly and may not meet specific needs. However, they are a good alternative if producing specific materials is cost-prohibitive.

Experience

When selecting a form of instructional media, it is important to take into account the learner's experience and knowledge level. Instructional videos, slides, or scenarios that present advanced concepts may be difficult for students to understand and may cause confusion. Likewise, playing games that test information to which students have not yet been introduced may cause aggravation and decrease motivation and confidence.

Instructor Characteristics

How an instructor views his role as an educator may influence the selection of instructional materials. Some instructors are comfortable with a certain form of medium; others prefer not to use any form of media.

Learner Characteristics

As indicated in Chapter 1, students learn in different ways and usually have some preferred method for learning information that is either visual, auditory, or kinesthetic. Specific learning styles of an audience should be taken into account when selecting instructional materials.

In addition to learning styles, other characteristics of the audience should be taken into account such as their ages and performance levels. It is important that instructional media fit the characteristics of the individuals in order to be effective. Showing adult learners cartoons may prove an insult and inhibit learning.

> It is important that instructional media fit the characteristics of the individuals in order to be effective.

Control of Delivery

Another consideration when selecting media is the need to control the delivery rate of instruction through the media. Some content can be presented at a fixed rate and sequence such as a videotape or film. However, it may be necessary to select a format that permits more control such as slides or overhead transparencies.

Quality

Obviously, quality should be considered when selecting instructional media. Important factors to consider include readability, reliability, and repetition of key points.

Readability refers to whether materials can be easily read by the audience. For example, are words printed in a size large enough and presented in a font that is easy to read? Reliability is also an essential aspect of quality. If the media does not provide accurate or consistent information it is not only useless but may be harmful to the learning environment.

Repetition of key points is also an important factor when considering the quality of materials. Students learn best when they know what material is important for them to remember. Therefore, instructional media that highlights key points and repeats them in summary form is more beneficial than those that do not.

Additional factors that should be taken into account when evaluating the quality of instructional materials are the design features used during their production. Such design features will be discussed later in this chapter.

> Instructional media that highlights key points and repeats them in summary form is more beneficial than those that do not.

Room Layout

Finally, the size of the audience may influence the appropriate form of media. If the group is large (*ie*, more than 20 students), it is necessary to select a medium that can be seen or heard clearly by all par-

MEDIA	GROUP SIZE	LIGHTS	FLEXIBILITY
Flipcharts	1 - 20	On	Bulky Non-electric Portable
Overhead Transparencies	10 - 100	On	Portable
Slides	1 - 100 *	Off	Portable Universal Equipment
Video	1 - 20 with 19" Screen	On	Tapes Portable Format Specific Equipment
Video with Projection	10 - 100	Dim	Portable or Fixed

* For larger audiences, use multiple screens.

FIGURE 6.3 Audiovisual Selection Tips

ticipants. The use of one 20-inch television monitor, a small model, mannequin, or flipchart may not meet the needs of a large group. The use of slides, overhead transparencies, and/or a video projection unit may be necessary to meet the needs of this group.

Figure 6.3 provides a summary for different types of audiovisual materials based on audience size and room format.

TYPES OF AUDIOVISUAL AIDS

Audiovisual aids vary from extremely simplistic to highly technical. Different types of materials are used for various reasons and include handouts, charts, equipment, video, computers, and mannequins. How one chooses and uses various media will determine its effectiveness.

Chalkboard

Chalkboards, as well as the more common version whiteboards, have been an integral part of training for many years. Since elementary school, students have been accustomed to writing down whatever appears on the board.

The chalkboard can be used to list key points, compare and contrast information, or highlight important material. In addition to written words, the chalkboard is also a good medium for identifying key elements of diagrams.

The chalkboard can be used to list key points, compare and contrast information, or highlight important material.

Advantages

- ☑ It is simple, inexpensive, versatile, and reusable.
- ☑ It seems to be drilled into everyone's head that if it appears on the board, it must be important; thus students are more likely to take notes.
- ☑ A chalkboard or whiteboard is usually readily available in any classroom environment.
- ☑ The use of a board does not require lights to be dimmed.
- ☑ It allows spontaneity in presentation, and changes can be made very easily.
- ☑ The whiteboard can be used as a screen, allowing the instructor to highlight information on slide photographs, charts, or graphs, by writing on the board.

Limitations

- ☒ Instructors often talk to the board, making it difficult for students to hear important information.
- ☒ Writing on the board is often time consuming.
- ☒ It may be difficult for students in the back of the room to see the board.
- ☒ Diagrams can be difficult to draw effectively.
- ☒ Boards become dirty easily from excess residual chalk or markers.
- ☒ Colored chalk does not easily erase without washing the board.

Chalk/Whiteboard Tips

- 🍎 Do not talk to the board, talk to the audience. After stating key information, write it on the board. Complete writing as quickly as possible, then return full attention to the audience.
- 🍎 When it is necessary to write a large amount of information on the board, do so prior to the class session.
- 🍎 Be sure to write using big letters (at least 3 inches in height).
- 🍎 While colors add a certain effect, be careful not to use too many colors or dark colors that may decrease visibility for students in the back of the room.
- 🍎 Limit writing to key words; it is not necessary to write complete sentences.
- 🍎 Neatness and clarity are important. Be sure writing is legible and dark enough for everyone to see.
- 🍎 Try not to block anyone's view while writing. Stand to the side of the board at a 45° angle for best visibility while writing.
- 🍎 When finished writing on the board, place chalk in the tray. It may be distracting to students if the instructor keeps the chalk in his hands and plays with it.
- 🍎 Use a pointer, rather than a finger, when referring to what is on the board.
- 🍎 After the material written on the board has served its purpose, erase it. When no longer useful it can be distracting. Before erasing it, however, be sure to allow enough time for students to copy the information.
- 🍎 Take time to thoroughly clean the board after each class session.

Flipcharts

The flipchart usually consists of an easel to which a large pad of paper (usually 34 × 28 inches) is attached. Felt-tipped markers are then used for writing on the paper. Uses for the flipchart are similar to those of the board, but erasing is not necessary because pages are not reused.

In general, flipcharts are a useful alternative to the chalkboard as a means of listing key points or collecting the thoughts of a group.

Additional charts such as anatomic charts and other medical charts are available. These charts provide detailed diagrams of various organs, the skeleton, and parts of various body systems such as the reproductive and respiratory systems. While these diagrams may be difficult for students to see during a lesson, hanging them around the room for use during breaks may be quite effective.

Flipcharts are a useful alternative to the chalkboard as a means of listing key points or collecting the thoughts of a group.

Advantages

- ☑ Flipcharts are relatively inexpensive, light-weight, portable, and readily available. Some units fold into a small size for increased portability.
- ☑ Use of flipcharts does not require lights to be dimmed.
- ☑ Pages can be prepared in advance and reused.
- ☑ Pages can be posted around the room for reference and review during breaks.

Limitations

- ☒ Easels are relatively bulky, although smaller portable units are available.
- ☒ Each page accommodates only a limited amount of information.
- ☒ It is time-consuming to write information on pages.
- ☒ The instructor's back is usually toward the audience while writing on pages.
- ☒ Students may find notes illegible.
- ☒ Viewing distance is limited relative to the size of print used.
- ☒ Complex illustrations or diagrams may be difficult to reproduce effectively.
- ☒ Mistakes cannot be erased.

Flipchart Tips

- Have a participant write on the pages so the instructor can face and interact with the audience.
- Use two flipcharts to contrast points or develop several ideas simultaneously.
- Use symbols and abbreviations to conserve space and time.
- Use wide-tip, dark colored markers to increase visibility of writing.
- To keep information understandable, use only four to five words per line and no more than three columns per page.
- Make certain writing is large enough for students to read. Generally, text should be at least 3 inches high.
- Stand to the side of the flipchart and use a pointer to emphasize key words.
- Use a variety of colors to highlight or contrast text as necessary.

Handouts

Handouts cover a wide range of materials. They can range from very simplistic handouts such as a lesson outline with space to take notes, to exercises, problems, and case summaries or supplemental reading material such as journal articles or sample quizzes.

Handouts cover a wide range of materials.

Advantages

- ☑ Handouts provide structure for the student.
- ☑ They allow for emphasis of key points.

☑ Use of handouts can decrease the amount of time students spend writing, thereby increasing the time they are attentive to the instructor.

☑ They can serve as instant review material for students.

Limitations

☒ It may be time-consuming to prepare, duplicate, and distribute material.

☒ Items may be bulky to carry around.

☒ Students may lose handout material.

☒ It can be costly to reproduce materials for entire class.

☒ Some instructors find it difficult to know when to distribute materials.

- If given out at early in the program participants may lose the material or read ahead and risk becoming confused or miss vital information the instructor is providing while they are reading.
- If given out only as needed, there may be a alteration in momentum during the delay in presentation for distributing the material.
- If given out at the end of a session, the benefit of decreased note-taking is minimized. Even if instructors advise them that handouts will be provided, the highly motivated or anxious student will most likely take notes "just in case" material is insufficient.

Handout Tips

🍎 The preferred distribution method is to divide handout material into chunks that will be used during a specific time frame and give out the material immediately prior to each section. This will allow minimal time to review the information and still provide participants with the other benefits of handouts.

🍎 Make certain there are enough copies for each student. Shared handouts are not nearly as beneficial. If only some students are required to share because there were not enough, those students may feel slighted, resulting in decreased motivation.

🍎 Make certain the information is relevant to course content. Providing handouts solely to say it was done is a waste. Content should relate directly to specific subject matter or a relationship should be provided to tie in some benefit for reading the material.

🍎 Handouts should be accurate, neat, and attractive. Make certain they are accurate for information, sequence, content, grammar, and spelling. Otherwise, learners may question the validity of course content in general as well as the instructor's capabilities and qualifications.

🍎 Prepare material according to the lesson plan. Handouts should follow the same sequence as the lesson.

🍎 Handouts should be easy to read, with lines double-spaced and an extra line between paragraphs. Margins of 1 to 1.5 inches on either side as well as the top and bottom of a page should be used to allow for students to write notes. Keep them clean and professional. Do not overuse fonts and icons; these can distract from the information you are attempting to present.

🍎 Distribute all handouts on 3-hole punched paper to allow students to immediately insert papers in a notebook, which minimizes the chance of material getting lost.

Audiotape Recordings

Audiotapes are a valuable tool when used appropriately. In order to assess lung sounds and blood pressure effectively, it is essential that students understand what it is they are looking for. What better way to learn then by listening to actual sounds in order to differentiate normal from abnormal?

Audio recordings are also useful for slow readers. Some students have difficulty reading various textbooks, yet when they listen to an audiocassette version of the text they are able to take notes and learn information. Exams on audiotapes can also be a useful tool for the student who has difficulty with tests or a reading disability. Be sure to check your state policy on reading certification exams to students. It is unfair to read course tests if this option is not available for the final exam.

Advantages
- ☑ Actual sounds can be heard to help students with assessment skills.
- ☑ Audiotapes are reusable.
- ☑ Important sections of a tape can be replayed to highlight key sounds.
- ☑ Audiotapes of lessons can be a useful tool to review and study important information.
- ☑ Audiotapes can be played back on any tape player.
- ☑ Students can listen to audiotapes of class notes or other information in the car, thereby enhancing the learning process.

Limitations
- ☒ Audiotapes use only one sense—hearing. Visual students may find it difficult to focus hard enough to find this tool useful and may "tune out" early in the session.
- ☒ The volume must be loud enough for all students to hear the tape. Unfortunately, when a tape is played back on an inexpensive player with the volume turned up, sounds may be distorted by extra "noise."
- ☒ The quality of an audiotape may decrease after significant use.

Audiotape Tips

- 🍎 Attention spans are relatively short, usually 7 to 8 minutes, for this type of medium. Therefore, use audiotapes in moderation, primarily when learning audiobased skills such as those identified above, and only when it is certain they will be effective. Otherwise, a video that incorporates audio with visual media is more effective since multiple senses are used and motivation is increased.
- 🍎 Only use professionally produced audiotapes.

Equipment

By far, the most effective way to learn a skill is by doing. Therefore, hands-on demonstration of actual equipment is a vital audiovisual aid in educating emergency responders. It is far less productive to teach students how to apply a traction splint without actually using a splint, or how to take a blood pressure measurement without using a blood pressure cuff.

Additional essential equipment includes teaching tools such as intubation and CPR mannequins, skeletons, or intravenous arms. These adjuncts are vital for allowing students to practice essential skills without harming potential victims.

Audiotapes are a valuable tool when used appropriately.

Hands-on demonstration of actual equipment is a vital audiovisual aid in educating emergency responders.

Advantages

☑ Use of equipment allows hands-on experience with actual instruments students will use in the field.
☑ They provide the visual key to allow students to incorporate knowledge with skills.

Limitations

✖ Equipment can break and students get frustrated when trying to use equipment that is not functional.
✖ Various types and models of equipment are available. The model used in a training session may be different from what participants use at their station, thereby causing some confusion.
✖ Small pieces of equipment may be difficult for students to see during a demonstration.

Equipment Tips

● Check equipment prior to the start of class to make certain it is in working condition.
● Be sure there is enough equipment to accommodate small groups.
● Obtain various types and models of equipment so students can practice with they same devices they will use at their stations.
● Have spare equipment on hand in case of any unforseen problems.
● When using small equipment such as an oral airway or anatomic organs, pass pieces around the room so students can see them first hand.

Overhead Transparencies

Overhead transparencies use a clear film on which, when light is projected through them via an overhead projector, the image on the film is enlarged and sent out to a screen. Transparencies have become one of the more common forms of medium for training due to their relative ease of preparation and use.

Transparencies have become one of the more common forms of medium for training.

Advantages

☑ Transparencies can be viewed with the lights on, so students can take notes.
☑ Overheads can be used with small groups as well as larger ones.
☑ The production of transparencies is easy and relatively inexpensive.
☑ Transparencies can be copied and used as handouts.
☑ Transparencies can set a pace for instruction through revealing key points in an appropriate sequence.
☑ Instructors can alter transparencies, highlight an item, underline text, and make comments by writing directly on the film. Such writing can be permanent or easily removed depending on the type of pen used.
☑ Transparency film can become a "portable chalkboard" by using a clear piece of film and markers.
☑ Because of the way the projection unit works, instructors can face the audience and make eye contact with students, thereby maintaining momentum and focus with the group while reading the transparency.

Preparing Transparencies

There are three methods for producing transparencies. One requires the use of a thermal machine and another uses a copier, while the third method is accomplished by drawing directly on the transparency film.

A thermal machine is a dry copy machine that creates transparencies through a heating process. A special type of thermal-sensitized sheet of acetate film and a high-carbon photocopy of the artwork are placed through the machine to create an overhead. The sheets are exposed to infrared light that heats the carbon and bonds to the acetate.

When finished, most of the carbon is transferred from the photocopy to the transparency. Colored acetate film is available for thermal copies that can be placed through the machine in stages to add color to a transparency.

With the copier, the ability to prepare overhead transparencies is greatly enhanced. In fact, the copier has almost replaced the thermal machine for the production of transparencies. With this method anything on a sheet of paper can be copied onto a piece of transparency film. Acetate especially made for copiers is available in various colors or clear film.

To create a transparency from a copier, create a visual using a computer graphic package or word processor, or cut and paste to produce a final "master" copy, and print it onto plain white paper. Then place the master onto the copier and place the transparency film into the paper tray or sheet feeder. The machine will make a copy of the visual onto the film and leave the master sheet intact. The master should then be placed in a file for future use.

The direct method for creating transparencies can be accomplished in two ways. The first requires the use of permanent or erasable transparency markers that are available in multiple colors. With such markers, drawings, charts, diagrams, and letters can be drawn directly onto transparency film.

The second direct method can be accomplished through the use of a computer and laser printer. Transparency film specifically for laser printers or copiers can be used. By placing the film in the paper tray, the printer prints the visual, text, or graphics directly onto the film. Color printers can also be used by this process provided the correct type of transparency film is used to produce color transparencies.

Regardless of the manner in which transparencies are developed, once prepared they should be protected with a frame. Two common types of frames include a rigid frame usually made from cardboard and a plastic looseleaf frame.

With the cardboard frame, the transparency film is attached directly to the frame with tape. The looseleaf frame is a plastic cover, the side of which is three hole punched; the film is inserted between the plastic cover for protection. Both types allow for instructor notes on the outside area and are available at most office supply stores.

☑ Equipment necessary to create and use transparencies is generally readily available.

☑ Instructors can use overhead transparencies as note cards of key information to present.

Limitations

☒ Equipment may fail. The primary problem with equipment is a burned out light bulb or lack of an available power source (outlet or extension cord).

☒ Equipment may be bulky. A classroom with a screen installed in or on the wall is preferable. Portable screens are available but are usually smaller, have a more noticeable glare, and are bulky to carry. Projection units were originally big and bulky, however, lighter, portable units are now available.

☒ Glare from light focusing on the screen may be tiring.

☒ The transparency may become a distraction if projected too long while the instructor is discussing a topic.

☒ If not properly designed, a transparency can hinder, rather than help, the learning process.

☒ The projected image may be distorted if the screen is not properly tilted.

Overhead Tips

🍎 Place the overhead projector on a low table near where you will be standing. Use the remaining table to spread out and organize notes and transparencies.

🍎 Stand away from the screen as to not obstruct the students' view. If students still cannot see the screen, ask them to move.

🍎 Be sure the transparency is focused.

🍎 Watch out for the hazards of Murphy's Law:

- Always carry a spare bulb.
- Always have a backup form of medium.
- Number the transparencies in case they fall or otherwise get mixed up.
- Check the order of transparencies before beginning a lesson.

🍎 Tilt the top of the screen forward in order to prevent image distortion.

🍎 For a clearer image, dim the lights nearest to the screen.

🍎 Do not project a blank screen any longer than necessary. Turn the projector off when changing transparencies.

🍎 Use colorful markers or print for emphasis of key points.

🍎 Use some type of mounting technique to protect transparencies and ensure proper placement on the projector unit.

🍎 Place a piece of tape on the glass of the projector to serve as a guide for where to place the film.

🍎 Make notes on the transparency frame to serve as a guide for key information.

🍎 Use some type of pointing device (pointer, pen, or pencil) to identify information on the transparency. Point directly on the film rather than on the screen.

🍎 Turn off the projector when control of audience attention is necessary.

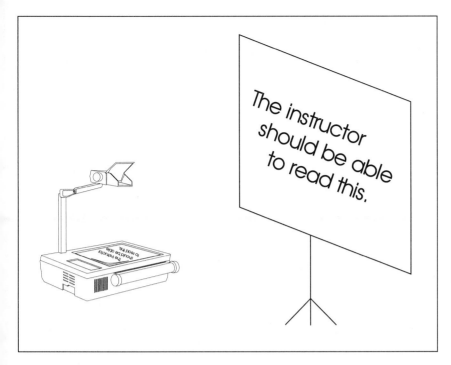

FIGURE 6.4 Placing the Transparency onto an Overhead Projector

- Make certain the transparency is carefully designed for optimal impact.
- Place the transparency on the overhead projector unit so information can be read while facing the audience. As shown in Figure 6.4, the instructor should be able to read the transparency from the projector while facing the audience.

Slides

Slides are usually 35-mm film mounted on 2-inch square cardboard. Since they can be projected, slides are useful for large audiences provided they are of good quality and relevant to the session content. Slides can create a formal, polished, and well-prepared image to a presentation.

Slides can create a formal, polished, and well-prepared image to a presentation.

   In order to be effective, a slide presentation requires a great deal of preparation and practice. In addition, it is important that slides be selected carefully so they meet specific course objectives adequately; slides must be relevant to course content.

Advantages

- ☑ Slides are compact and relatively easy to use.
- ☑ Playback equipment (*ie*, slide projector and screen) is generally readily available.
- ☑ Slides have a high visual impact.
- ☑ Production, reproduction, and editing for a specific audience is generally easy and inexpensive, provided equipment is available.
- ☑ Slides of incidents create interest and gain attention.
- ☑ Slides are useful for illustrating or identifying objects.

Limitations

- ☒ Student passiveness is greatest with the use of slides.
- ☒ Lights must be dimmed, making it difficult for students to take notes.

Preparing Slides

There are multiple ways in which to prepare 35-mm slides for educational purposes. The first method requires the use of a 35-mm camera and standard slide film. If slides are of items such as equipment, people, or outdoor scenery (*eg*, animals, trees or accident scenes) simply take pictures as usual. When the film is developed, it will be prepared into slides.

The second option, still using the 35-mm camera and slide film, is the use of a photocopy stand such as that identified in Figure 6.5. This method is useful for making slides of small models or equipment, text, artwork, or photographs from books or magazines. To make these slides, attach the camera to the holder in the center of the stand and place the item (model, photograph, *etc*) onto the base of the stand, facing up.

Next, make certain the lights are shining at 45° angles and do not reflect a shadow on the item. When the item is properly aligned and centered in the eye of the camera, snap the picture. Again, when the film is developed it will be processed as slides.

The third method for creating slides is through the use of a computer and slide generator. Visuals are created on a graphics program such as Harvard Graphics, Corel Draw, Aldus Persuasion, or Power Point, and then saved to a file in slide format. With the use of a slide generator, the file is transferred to slide film. Some universities or EMS training centers have this type of equipment. There are also organizations that offer the conversion of slides from a computer disk, or via modem, to slides as a professional service.

Most film processing centers develop slide film, and many offer 2–5 hour service for slide film developing. This is quite useful for last-minute presentation preparation.

☒ Dim lights may cause students to lose interest or fall asleep.
☒ Eye contact between the instructor and audience is difficult.

- If the instructor faces the group, he must turn to see the screen to identify which slide is showing.
- If the instructor is in the back of the room, next to the projector, he is facing the screen as well as the backs of the audience.

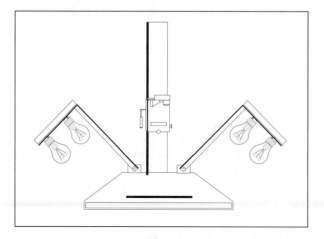

FIGURE 6.5 Photocopy Stand

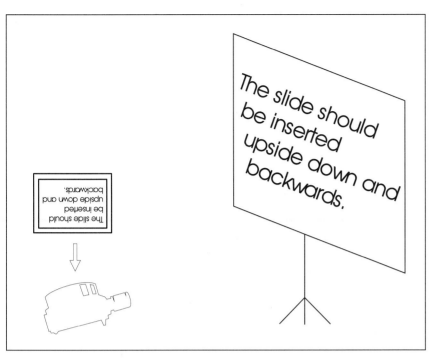

FIGURE 6.6 Placing Slides into a Carousel

The following technical problems are common with equipment:

- Light bulbs burn out.
- Slides get stuck in the projector.
- An outlet or extension cord is not readily available.
- The carousel does not fit the projector.
- The screen is obstructed for some students.

Slide Tips

- Make certain slides are in the correct order and position. As shown in Figure 6.6, slides should be placed in the carousel upside down and backwards.
- Set up the projector and screen in advance to make certain equipment is in working order. If the carousel does not fit, find an alternative. Generally, carrousels can hold either 80 or 140 slides.
- Plan and rehearse what should be said for each slide. Slides should only be used if they are **directly** relevant to lesson content. They should not be used just because they are funny or gross. If it is not readily apparent what the purpose of a slide is, it should not be used.
- Dim only those lights directly in front of the screen in order to brighten the image without darkening the entire room. If necessary to view notes, obtain a light for the lectern.
- Position the screen in an area easily visible to the entire class. The best place for a screen is usually in the front left corner of the room at least 4 feet above the floor.
- Allow enough time for students to study the information on the slides. In general, allow 10 to 20 seconds per slide.
- Place slides in a logical sequence according to lesson objectives and course content.

- Use some type of pointing device (laser pointers are ideal) to focus student attention on specific items on the screen. The finger should not be used as a pointer because the body may cast a distracting shadow.
- Provide a review slide to summarize key points at the conclusion of a slide presentation.
- Avoid using too many slides since a rapid succession of slides can be ineffective.

Video

Videotapes are commonly used to augment training. Videotapes come in two formats: beta and VHS. VHS is the most popular form of videotape and is available in two sizes: 3/4 inch and 1/2 inch. Professional production of videos is usually accomplished on 3/4-inch tapes and then reproduced on 1/2-inch tapes, which is the more common size of playback equipment.

Video has various uses including training, simulation, broadcasting conferences, evaluating student performance, critiquing drills and exercises, and advertising training programs or equipment.

Videotapes are commonly used to augment training.

Advantages

- ☑ Video can introduce students to environments that would ordinarily be too difficult or expensive to explore.
- ☑ Video can bring motion and real life situations into the classroom setting.
- ☑ Video has a high interest factor and is ideal for motivating students.
- ☑ Commentary is usually incorporated into the video, leaving the instructor free to complete other functions, such as retrieving equipment while the video is playing.
- ☑ Scenes can be replayed and shown in slow motion to drive home key information such as scene safety, assessment techniques, and placement of vehicles.
- ☑ Videotaping student performances during exercises provides excellent, immediate feedback.
- ☑ Students relate well to video since television is a common visual medium in most lifestyles.
- ☑ VHS playback equipment is common, relatively inexpensive, and usually available in training environments.
- ☑ Video provides one-on-one detailed instruction for remedial training.
- ☑ Videotapes are reusable and easy to use.

Limitations

- ☒ Producing a video program can be very expensive.
- ☒ Watching videotapes can be time-consuming.
- ☒ If not readily available, playback equipment can be bulky and difficult to transport.
- ☒ The quality of videotapes can be poor unless they have been professionally produced, and professionally produced videotapes can be expensive to purchase.
- ☒ Poor-quality videotapes can be detrimental during a training session.

- Videotapes are difficult to update. When standards change, the decision has to be made whether to stop using a tape or highlight the errors from the beginning.
- Audience size is limited unless the classroom has multiple monitors or or a video projection unit available.
- Although visibility is improved when lights are dimmed, this can lead to that "dim light phenomenon"—drowsiness.
- Videotapes can decrease in quality with significant use.

Video Tips

- Set up video equipment in advance to check operation, visibility, and sound levels before class begins.
- When only using a portion of a tape, fast forward to the proper location before class so the students' time and motivation is not wasted.
- Make certain all students can see and hear the videotape. If not, suggest that they move.
- Only use videotapes that complement or support a training session. Be sure there is a purpose for showing the tape that helps meet an educational objective of the course.
- Preview videotapes to determine the usefulness and identify any discrepancies in accuracy or regional protocols.
- Prior to showing a videotape, instruct the audience on the purpose of the tape in order to guide their learning. List questions they should be able to answer at the conclusion of the tape.
- At the conclusion of a video, provide a follow-up by summarizing key points that students should remember.
- Wait until after class to rewind videotapes.
- Make a duplicate copy of the videotape for use and leave the original on the shelf as a "master" copy. When the tape becomes worn from significant use, make a new copy from the master (refer to copyright laws first).

Other Audiovisual Aids

A flannel board is a piece of flannel stretched over a board or frame to which words or pictures with a flannel backing can be hung. These boards can be portable or permanent and they permit a step-by-step reusable presentation. Since items are removable, they can be shifted or changed easily to show variations of ideas from different angles. Flannel boards are not commonly used in adult training programs.

A magnetic board is useful for demonstrating tactical information such as position and movement strategies during a rescue operation or staging during a disaster incident. Many whiteboards are magnetic, allowing magnetic backed shapes to stick to the board and be moved around as necessary to demonstrate various processes.

Many whiteboards are magnetic.

As described in Chapter 7, games are extremely effective as a form of instructional media. Games can increase motivation and greatly enhance the retention of information. Almost any topic can be developed into a game, and students benefit from the competitive nature of games.

Games can increase motivation and greatly enhance the retention of information.

A film is a moving picture, usually accompanied by a sound track, similar to a videotape, that is played back through a film projector. While film is generally of greater quality than video, it is much less common in current educational programs. Some of the more classic

GENERAL DESIGN HINTS

1. **Keep it simple. Each visual should stress only one idea. Use simple, direct words that are easy for viewers to read.**

2. **Use headlines to "chunk" information into meaningful segments and provide a method for orienting viewers to the screen.**

3. **Align elements at the left.**

4. **Leave a lot of white space between lines and around the borders of the screen.**

5. **Keep the information organized through appropriate layout, colors, grouping, and framing of key elements.**

6. **Create a pleasing path for the eye.**

7. **Divide space on the screen in an interesting way.**

8. **Use visuals to explain text, *not* to display it as you read.**

9. **Use a maximum of six words per line and six lines per visual.**

10. **Be consistent with page orientation whether portrait or landscape.**

11. **Select the best media for the presentation situation and the size of the group.**

Troubleshooting

Regardless of how well prepared an instructor is, there will always be instances when equipment fails. It is important, therefore, for instructors to always have a backup form of media.

When a projection system is not functioning properly, instructors can perform a few simple checks to try to rectify the problem. Give the students a short break while troubleshooting audiovisual equipment failures as follows:

- When the projection unit does not work, check to make certain:
  1. The projector is receiving electrical power (*ie*, it is plugged into an electrical outlet and the switch controlling the outlet is turned on).
  2. The light bulb is not defective; change the bulb as necessary.
  3. The power switch is turned on.

- When the projection unit is on, but materials are not projected effectively, check for:
  1. Proper placement of the transparency or slide try on the projection unit.
  2. Proper insertion of the remote control plug.
  3. A clean projection lens.
  4. Proper focus of the object through the lens.

films, however, may not be available on video, resulting in the need to use a 16-mm film projector.

A filmstrip is a series of still pictures in a roll of film, played back through a filmstrip projector. While heavily used for training in the 1970s and 1980s, with the common use of videotapes, filmstrip use has greatly declined for adult education programs.

DESIGN CONSIDERATIONS

The layout for a slide, overhead transparency, chart, computer screen or any other form of media has a tremendous impact on the effectiveness of training materials. When designing a screen layout, the following should be considered.

Visuals and Learning

The goal of learning is to retain and be able to retrieve information and apply it to new situations. Psychologists believe that students learn by the following process.

First, a stimulus is presented by the instructor and perceived by the student. A small portion of that perception is then transferred to short-

Presentation of Stimulus

▼

Perception of Stimulus by the Learner

▼

Entry into Short-Term Memory

▼

Coding of Stimulus

▼

Entry into Long-Term Memory

term memory, most likely that which was most vivid or meaningful, with everything else being lost.

Researchers believe short-term memory can only hold about seven units of information. Unless rehearsed or repeated, information in short-term memory is usually lost after approximately 10 seconds. In order to move information from short-term memory to long-term memory, it must first be "coded" and stored as words or images[1].

Eye Motion

Viewers scan a screen in a very definite pattern, usually starting at the upper left corner, scanning down vertically, and ending at the lower right corner as identified in Figure 6.7. Scanning is usually done so students become visually oriented before settling into reading text. After a general scan of a screen, readers of western languages view the text in a top-down, left-to-right reading pattern as identified in Figure 6.8.

Instructors can exploit this scanning pattern during the development of visuals in order to improve the effectiveness of materials. Since students view the upper left corner first, the most important orienting information, title, or instructions should be placed there.

Since it takes students a few seconds to perform an initial scan of a screen, it is best that sequential screens not be altered dramatically in style or screen layout.

Since students view the upper left corner first, the most important orienting information, title, or instructions should be placed there.

Page Orientation

Page orientation refers to whether a visual is developed vertically or horizontally. A visual *portrait* in orientation is created with the page vertically; a horizontal format is *landscape* in orientation. Page orientation has an impact on the overall design of a visual. Since visuals in the form of paintings, photographs, and video usually present objects in a frame that is wider than it is high, students are accustomed to a landscape orientation.

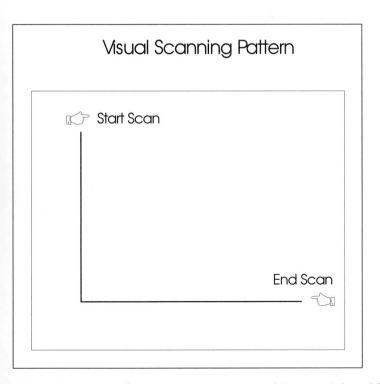

FIGURE 6.7 Pattern of Eye Movement During Visual Scanning (adapted from Strauss, 1992).

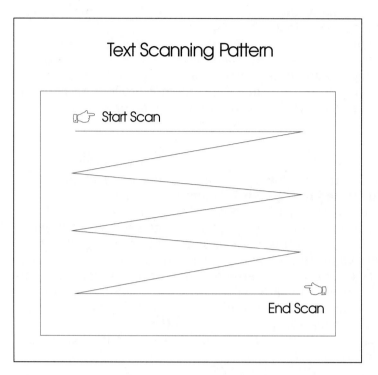

FIGURE 6.8 Pattern of Eye Movement for Reading Text

A visual that is portrait in orientation will appear long and narrow compared with a landscape visual. Consequently, a smaller amount of information can be presented on each line, and a smaller font size is usually necessary to fit all desired information on one screen. When using a portrait orientation, it is important for instructors to avoid the tendency to fill a page with more information simply because extra space exists.

Figure 6.9 demonstrates a common error with the design of visuals in a portrait orientation. Font size is smaller in order to fit words into the narrow space, and more lines are added to fill what would be open space at the bottom of the visual. The landscape orientation, however,

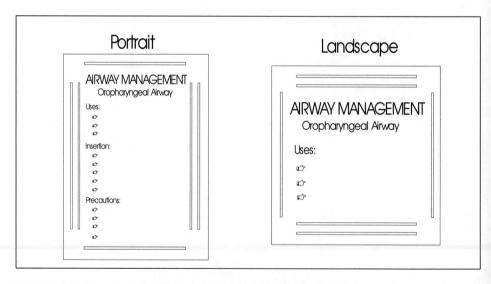

FIGURE 6.9 Portrait vs. Landscape Page Orientation

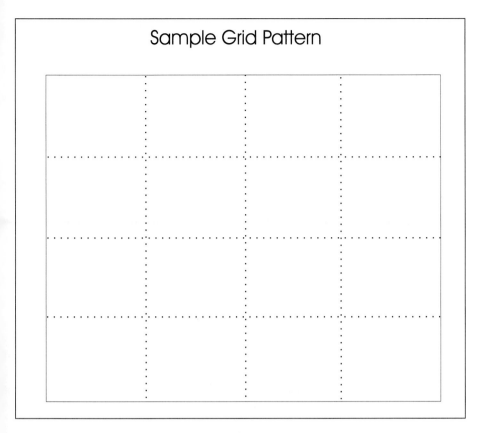

FIGURE 6.10 Sample Grid Pattern for Consistent Visual Design

allows for the presentation of one "chunk" of information per visual with the use of larger fonts.

Whether an instructor chooses to develop visuals in landscape or portrait orientation is generally a personal preference, but it is recommended that landscape presentation be used whenever possible. It is essential to remember, however, to maintain sound design principles and be consistent throughout an entire series of visuals.

It is recommended that landscape presentation be used whenever possible.

Use of a Grid

A grid, such as that illustrated in Figure 6.10, is the basic tool for graphic design and screen layout. It is beneficial for arranging and balancing graphic and textual components of a screen. Using a common grid for all screens allows an instructor to create a consistent style.

Use of Borders

Borders are important in visuals as a means for framing information. Borders help promote a sense of balance and consistency throughout a series of visuals. It is important that the border does not draw attention away from the content of the screen but rather enhances the overall look of the visual. Once a border has been chosen, it should be used for the entire series of screens to add consistency.

Borders help promote a sense of balance and consistency throughout a series of visuals.

Use of Colors

A viewer's eyes are attracted to various areas of a screen due to color. Hotter colors such as reds, yellows, and pinks attract the eye and tend to "pop-out," while cooler colors such as blues, greens, and browns do not attract the eye and tend to recede on a screen.

The following techniques will help instructors use color appropriately when developing visuals:

- Limit colors to two or three per visual. Too many colors may create a visual that looks like abstract art rather than a tool for learning.
- When more than three colors are necessary in one visual, use variations and shades of those colors rather than additional completely different colors.
- Use colors consistently from visual to visual. If a number of visual elements (graphics, titles, background, borders, symbols) are used, they should appear in the same color on all visuals.
- Use dark colors such as black or dark shades of purple, red, green, or blue, for key words, titles, and captions. Use bright colors to introduce a major change or to highlight key words.
- Men and women remember colors best as follows:

Men	Women
Dark blue	Dark blue
Olive green	Yellow
Yellow	Yellow
Violet	Red

- As identified above, dark blue, olive green, and yellow are viewed best by both males and females and should, therefore, be the colors of choice when designing visuals.
- Eighty percent of the adult male population is red/green color blind[2]. Therefore, avoid red/green combinations such as green text on a red background, or vice versa.
- Background colors should be cool colors that recede and do not vie for the viewer's attention. Use olive green, grays, blues, browns, or dark purples.
- Foreground colors such as those used for text should be hotter, lighter colors such as yellow, pink, orange, or red.
- The best combination for high color visibility occurs with the following color combinations of text on background colors. In order of effectiveness[4], they are:
  - Black on yellow
  - Green on white
  - Red on white
  - Blue on white
  - Black on white
  - White on blue

Use of Fonts

The ease of readability of text is essential for an effective visual. A visual that is hard to read not only annoys and frustrates students, it also lessens the overall impact of the instructional media.

A *font* is the style of letters of text. Desktop publishing and word processing programs offer a large selection of types, styles, and sizes of fonts. Letters can appear italicized, underlined, bold, outlined, or shadowed. The most easily read font type is sans serif or its equivalent. Courier text, the common font of most typewriters, is fairly unpleasing to the eye, and script text is difficult to read on a screen.

The ease of readability of text is essential for an effective visual.

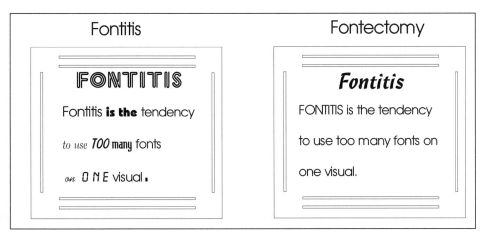

FIGURE 6.11 "Fontitis" and the Cure

When selecting a font, it is essential that instructors avoid "fontitis," the tendency to use too many fonts on one or sequential visuals[2]. It is best to use a maximum of three different fonts including various sizes or styles as shown in Figure 6.11.

As Figure 6.12 shows, it is easier to read words that appear in both upper and lower case letters than those that appear entirely in upper case letters[2]. Words written solely in capital letters should only be used occasionally in order to emphasize key words.

One of the most important factors when selecting a font is the size. On a computer, font size is generally expressed in point size. The minimum size for any visual being projected onto a screen is 1/4 inch, and for charts, chalkboards, and posters, a minimum text size of 3 inches is recommended. Font sizes are comparable as follows:

$$72 \text{ points} = 1 \text{ inch}$$
$$54 \text{ points} = 3/4 \text{ inch}$$
$$36 \text{ points} = 1/2 \text{ inch}$$
$$18 \text{ points} = 1/4 \text{ inch}$$

Use of Graphics

Graphics are used for illustrating points, providing for simulations, providing motivation, and organizing information. Instructional graphics need to be designed to attract and hold student attention. If a

Instructional graphics need to be designed to attract and hold student attention.

Upper Case

TEXT THAT APPEARS ENTIRELY IN UPPER CASE LETTERS IS DIFFICULT TO READ BECAUSE VIEWERS QUICKLY RECOGNIZE WORDS BASED ON SHAPE, NOT NECESSARILY BY READING EACH LETTER.

Lower Case

Lower case letters are easier to recognize because they offer more variation in shape.

FIGURE 6.12 Use of Upper Case vs. Lower Case Letters

graphic compels a student to concentrate on a screen, more information will most likely be extracted from the visual.

Use graphics appropriately. Effective graphics allow for the compression of information. The saying "A picture is worth a thousand words" is very true. A picture should present a visual description of words on a screen. Only graphics that offer a pictorial description of an item or idea should be used. Using pictures or graphics that are cute or funny are counterproductive if they do not directly relate to the idea of the visual.

Graphics should not distract from the overall meaning or purpose of a visual.

Graphics should not distract from the overall meaning or purpose of a visual. A colorful picture in the corner of a screen with small text in small black letters will distract the viewer's attention. While the viewer may be able to recall the picture, the information presented on that screen will be lost.

Finally, graphics are effective for providing an element of balance to a visual, providing it is relative.

Rule of Six

The "rule of six" is a general guideline to consider when designing visuals.

> Thou shalt not use more than:
> - six lines per page
> - six words per line

While this rule is a guideline, research has shown that students can retain only a small amount of information at one time. To present more information is counter-productive because students tend to "tune out" too much information.

Maintaining Consistency

Consistency refers to a common look and feel across multiple visuals.

Regardless of the font, colors, graphics, text, or borders used in a visual, it is essential that consistency be maintained throughout all screens of a lesson. *Consistency* refers to a common look and feel across multiple visuals. Screens with a consistent design are perceived to have a greater quality and a more professional appearance than those that have an unnecessary variety of backgrounds, colors, graphics, or layout across multiple screens.

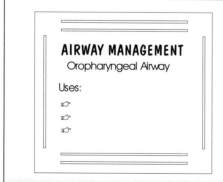 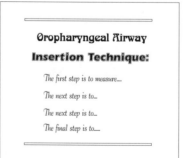 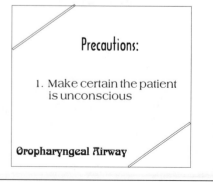

FIGURE 6.13 Inconsistent Sequential Screens

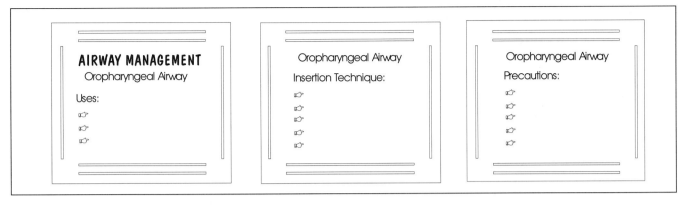

FIGURE 6.14 Consistent Sequential Screens

Consistency also decreases development time since common elements such as backgrounds, borders, and fonts do not need to be chosen for each sequential screen. An inconsistent format not only increases development time, but also forces viewers to re-orient themselves as each screen appears, distracting them from the actual subject matter of a screen. Figures 6.13 and 6.14 demonstrate the impact of consistency through a sequence of visuals.

Focusing Attention
Various principles can be used to focus student attention and perception toward a specific idea or concept within a visual[3].

Novelty
When an item needs attention, it can be highlighted in many ways. Use of colors, shading, or an alteration in appearance for a specific item will draw attention to it. It is important to choose only the most important features to highlight because if everything is highlighted nothing will stand out. Figure 6.15 illustrates the use of this principle.

Moderate Complexity
Providing extra detail to a specific element within a visual will draw attention to that element. Such complexity can occur by providing more detail through outlines, shades, or other visual enhancements. Figure 6.16 shows the use of this principle.

Visual Cues
Visual cues such as arrows, stars, and pointers can be used to direct learner attention when a visual follows a path that conflicts with logic. It is important to limit the need for visual cues except when it is necessary to highlight an idea or follow a logical sequence. Figure 6.17 identifies the use of this principle.

Relative Size and Accuracy
When an image is of an unfamiliar size to the audience, display an object of known size next to it to allow learners to provide a visual comparison. See Figure 6.18 for an example. Likewise, when highlighting key differences among multiple objects within a visual, keep all non-key items the same as to not confuse the learner.

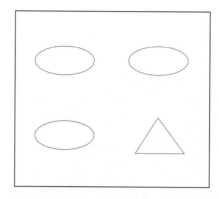

FIGURE 6.15 Novelty

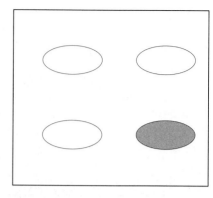

FIGURE 6.16 Complexity

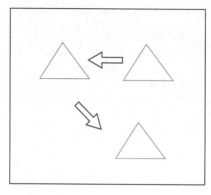

FIGURE 6.17 Visual Cues

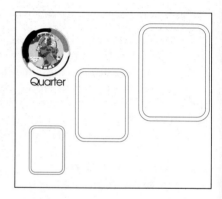

FIGURE 6.18 Relevance of Size

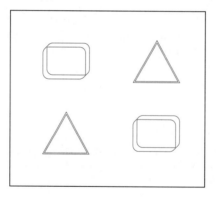

FIGURE 6.19 Visual Similarity

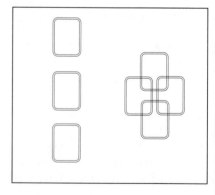

FIGURE 6.20 Spatial Proximity

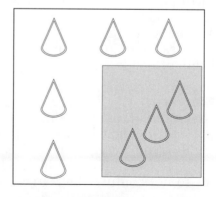

FIGURE 6.21 Framing

Visual Similarity

In order to "chunk" information, similar objects, concepts, or elements, should be identified within a single visual as well as subsequent visuals by using the same colors, shapes, and general design as identified in Figure 6.19. While this principle is true regarding total presentation organization, it is also important to group like elements by color, shape, or patterns within each visual.

Spatial Proximity

The page layout of a visual is very important for providing organization for the viewer. When elements of a visual are linked in some manner, it should be identified by grouping like objects together or overlapping like objects as shown in Figure 6.20. Labels or captions should be placed near the elements they describe.

Framing

Like similarity and spatial proximity, framing like objects by shading or geometrical frames promotes organization within a visual. By separating objects that go together from those that do not through the use of a border, learners are able to better grasp the organization of a visual and its meaning as seen in Figure 6.21.

How a visual is designed directly influences its effectiveness. Following these guidelines will allow instructors to develop the most effective instructional media possible in order to improve learning. When properly developed, such materials can greatly enhance the retention of information and help insure instructors meet specific course objectives.

How a visual is designed directly influences its effectiveness.

LINKING TECHNOLOGY AND EMS EDUCATION

Technology is emerging in education as a powerful tool. Learning systems combining computers, video, and satellite equipment provide an ultimate adjunct to the educational process.

Multimedia

What is multimedia? The answer to that question often varies. Literally the term multi-media is redundant since media is the plural of medium (an audiovisual adjunct), and multi also means more than one. In the eyes of most laymen, multimedia involves a means of combining two or more types of medium.

Multimedia in the future will most likely be referred to as:

- Still or motion video,
- Text,
- Graphics,
- Audio, and
- Animation all controlled by a computer

Multimedia implies some form of interactivity with the audience. Interactivity can vary from simple discussion sessions to more advanced forms of computer-based training programs that branch off, dependent on learner responses.

Interactivity

When reviewing instructional materials available for EMS instruction, it is helpful to understand certain factors that increase learner reten-

One of the best methods for increasing learning is by increasing interactivity.

tion of information. One of the best methods for increasing learning is by increasing interactivity within the classroom setting or within the instructional medium itself.

What constitutes interactivity? Interactivity allows an individual to move from being a passive to being an active participant in the learning process. Until recently, however, little interactive media was available for education. While some interactivity does occur through the active role of students through role playing, classroom discussions, and group dynamics and exercises, such interaction is very limited. Modern technology, through the use of computers and other systems, allows for a much greater opportunity for student interaction.

When reviewing instructional media for interactivity, it is important to look for the following elements[5]:

- **Immediacy of response** - If students need to know additional information about an item, they should be able to find the information immediately.
- **Nonsequential access of information** - Instructional media that allows students to access information as needed rather than when the designer decided it was relevant is much more effective.
- **Adaptability** - Students enter a learning environment with different experiences, knowledge, and skills. An effective interactive program should be adaptable to these individual differences, providing remedial training to those individuals who require it without boring those who do not.
- **Feedback** - As with all training, feedback within an interactive program is the information that lets learners know if they are successful in accomplishing lesson objectives. If feedback is not provided, learners do not know if modifications to their actions are necessary.
- **Learner control** - Interactivity implies that some degree of control over a learning experience is given to the student. By giving students greater control over various aspects of instruction, such as the pace at which they progress through the program or the sequence in which they proceed, training is tailored to the student's own style of learning. This leads to improved motivation and more effective and enhanced learning.

While some learner control increases motivation and learning, a total shift in control from one party to the other decreases interactivity. For example:

- In one class, an instructor presents a lecture and leaves the room.
- In another class, an instructor simply listens to students present information and then leaves.
- In the third class, the instructor and students discuss issues, react to, and learn from each other.

Students in the third class will have the greatest experience because of the balance of control, where interactivity is the greatest. When locus of control is entirely shifted from the instructor to the students, interactivity is lost and learning effectiveness compromised. There must be a balance of control for learning to be enhanced.

Types of Interactive Media

Basic forms of media including flipcharts, overhead transparencies, video, slide presentations, and others have already been discussed in this chapter. While very effective in augmenting a training session, these forms of media rely heavily on the instructor rather than on the student.

The trend in education now is to let students take control of their own education. Computers were introduced into the school system in the 1970s and have been become increasingly sophisticated in the tasks they can accomplish. While some adult learners may be afraid initially of such technology, many of those in EMS education today have used computers either in school or at the workplace.

Various forms of computer use in education include interactive videos, computer-based instruction, computer disc-interactive, simulations, and virtual reality. These types of media will be discussed from most simple to most complex.

Computers

The computer has become a very popular audiovisual device. Technology is an ever changing field with new advances and improvements. Today, the value of computers in medical education is enormous.

Computer-aided instruction uses computers as an adjunct to learning. The more common form of computer-aided instruction is in the form of both automatic and interactive "slide show" presentations. Numerous graphics packages are available to assist instructors in creating effective presentations. Such programs include Harvard Graphics, Power Point, Corel Draw, Draw Perfect, and Aldus Persuasion.

A slide show presentation can stand alone during an open house, by providing general information. Screens can be timed to change automatically by the computer. Audio, in the form of digitized text or music, can accompany these screens.

A slide show can also be useful as a replacement for overhead transparencies. With the use of an LCD panel, anything on the computer screen can be projected through on overhead projector onto a large screen, as identified in Figure 6.22.

Another use for computers in education are computer-based training (CBT) programs that provide stand-alone training as an interactive

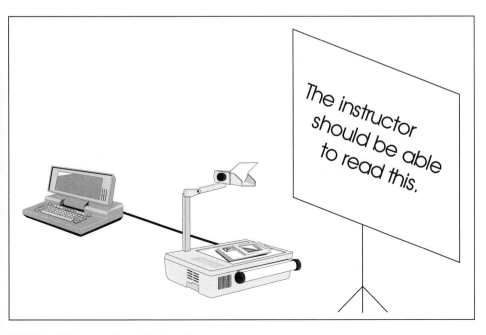

FIGURE 6.22 Use of an LCD Panel

Computer software is available for EMS training, including test bank programs, simulation programs, and database programs.

learning experience. Such programs are available in EMS training to provide a one-on-one learning experience in various topics such as CPR, AED, and Haz-Mat training. Additional programs can be developed easily using computer-based training authoring software such as Assymetrix' ToolBook or IBM's Linkway Live. Hypercard provides CBT authoring capabilities for Apple formatted computers.

Additional computer software is available for EMS training, including test bank programs, to generate examinations and quizzes; simulation programs, which place students in certain environments to test their ability to assess and treat various patients; and database programs, which allow for better coordination and management of training programs.

Advantages
☑ CBT provides highly motivatonal one-on-one training.
☑ CBT programs allow learners to progress at their own speed, depending on individual needs.

Limitations
✘ Initial costs for the purchase of equipment can be expensive.
✘ Some students may be anxious about using a computer.
✘ It may be difficult to know whether students are using a CBT program, except during evaluations.
✘ The availability of CBT programs specifically targeted to EMS are limited.

Equipment
The following equipment is necessary for optimal use of computers in education:

- IBM-compatible computer (processing speed greater than 386 MHz is recommended)
- VGA monitor (SVGA is recommended)
- 4 Mbyte RAM (8 Mbyte is recommended)
- A sound card and speakers
- Programs available on CD require a CD-ROM drive.

Interactive Video
Video is a useful medium for the delivery of subject content requiring motion or for content involving complex relationships. In order to increase the interactive aspects of learning, a videotape can be interfaced with a computer, thereby creating interactive video.

A videotape can be interfaced with a computer, thereby creating interactive video.

The purpose of the computer in interactive video is to manage the program, including directions, student control, textual information, and testing opportunities. The videotape player presents audiovisual material in segments as directed by the computer. The videodisc player provides random accessibility to information contained on the disc and is, therefore, preferred over the videotape player.

Advantages
☑ There is a greater retention of learning due to interactivity between the student and subject matter.
☑ Standard video equipment can be used.

Limitations
✘ Access time for the VCR to move to a specific portion of the videotape may be slow, and can potentially cause student attention to wander.
✘ With extensive play, the quality of a videotape may decrease.

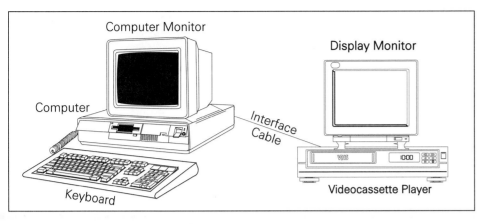

FIGURE 6.23 Interactive Video Equipment

Equipment

As shown in Figure 6.23 and Figure 6.24, in order to use an interactive video system, the following equipment is necessary:

- Computer system (complete with monitor and keyboard), which serves as the "brains" of the operation. This system receives signals from the learner, processes the information, directs playing of video segments, and outputs a display to the monitor.
- Computer interface card, that fits into the computer and allows the transmission of data between the computer and VCR in order to locate and play various segments of the videotape.
- Videocassette player, on which video segments are played at the command of the computer.
- Video monitor, which is the display unit for program information, video images, and sound.

There are some computer software programs that negate the need for a second video monitor by using a section of the computer monitor. With these programs, the computer sends a signal for the VCR to begin playing a section of tape and the tape is viewed through the computer monitor.

Compact Disc-Interactive

Compact Disc-Interactive (CD-I) is a closed-system unit that is connected to a home television or other type of monitor. It has the capacity to store large amounts of images, graphics, audio, text, and compressed full-motion video on a CD-ROM.

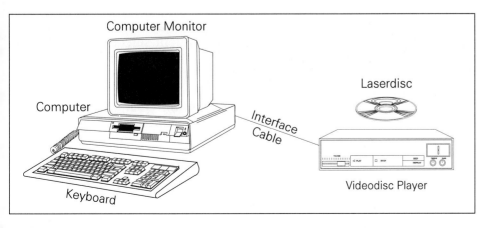

FIGURE 6.24 Interactive Laser Disc Equipment

A CD-I unit does not interface with a computer; it is a stand-alone unit that operates similar to a video game such as a Sega Genesis Unit. There are currently a few CD-I educational programs available for EMS education and certainly more are on the way.

Telecommunications

Two forms of telecommunications have been used widely in recent years. Teleconferencing links individuals from various regions to share information or ideas through the use of telephones. Videoconferencing provides interactivity through the use of video projection by satellite dishes, augmented by teleconferencing in which students can ask questions.

Various organizations offer emergency services training programs via satellite targeted toward fire, police, and EMS personnel. Such programs include classroom type lectures and demonstrations as well as panel discussions from various groups. The Federal Emergency Management Agency conducts panel discussions and offers regular training sessions via satellite as does the Volunteer Fire Insurance Service and other organizations.

Simulations

Simulations are primarily a re-creation of an environment or situation as a means of training. They provide the opportunity for students to apply knowledge and skills without potential risks.

Simulations can produce powerful experiences and provide insight and skills for learners, causing a change in future behaviors. If a student acts in a manner that causes a patient to die during a simulation experience, chances are he will not act the same way next time a similar situation is encountered.

Simulations are effective because of their motivational impact. When students are asked to take action and become totally involved in an exercise, rather than just talking about what they should do in a particular situation, they are more likely to learn.

Simulations have been around since World War II when "War Games" were commonly used for training. While they are currently used heavily for training emergency responders, the link with computers over the past few years has provided a new level of simulations for training purposes.

A computer-generated simulation generally reacts to student input. One such program available for advanced cardiac life support (ACLS) training allows learners to decide in what order to perform skills such as ABCs, endotrachial tube insertion, administration of medications (type and dosage), and cardioversion. Some programs allow students to finish the session and then review what they did right and wrong.

A more realistic simulation automatically changes a scenario based on student response. For example, if the student selects cardioversion prior to clearing the area the responder may die, thereby terminating the simulation. If the student administers the wrong dosage of medication, the patient may go into a different cardiac rhythm.

Such simulations are invaluable for training emergency providers. Obviously, students cannot perform certain skills on live patients until they are proficient at them and a patient requiring such skills is available. Simulations provide the next best training situation while limiting liability risks.

Virtual Reality

By far, the most realistic training environment, next to a real situation, is experienced through the use of virtual reality. Through the use of

---

Teleconferencing links individuals from various regions to share information or ideas through the use of telephones.

Simulations can produce powerful experiences and provide insight and skills for learners.

By far, the most realistic training environment, next to a real situation, is experienced through the use of virtual reality.

the computer and additional highly sophisticated technology, a student is able to become a participant in an abstract space. The hardware combination includes, at a minimum, a head-mounted display, data glove and tracking device.

The head-mounted display contains sensors to track the motion of the head as it moves, and the data-glove provides hands-on interaction with the virtual world. Sensors then report the position of the goggles and glove to the computer, which performs calculations and displays a three-dimensional image on the LCD screen located within the headset in front of the viewer's eyes.

The availability of the technology for virtual reality, although increasing in society, is far from the realm of EMS education although not that far away for medical education in general. Programs allowing medical students the experience of performing an autopsy, without encountering an actual body, are available. As this technology advances, prices will decrease to become somewhat affordable, leading to a greater availability for the use of virtual reality in the classroom.

SOURCES OF MATERIAL

Locating appropriate audiovisual materials may be difficult for some instructors, while others have a vast resource of available media at their disposal. Once a form of media is selected, it is necessary to locate and prepare the materials.

The first place to look for material is within the organization or institution for whom you are teaching. Many training centers and other educational institutions have a central resource center available to instructors. Other valuable resources are colleagues who have accumulated media such as slides, overhead transparencies, charts, and games that they have developed for a similar program. Regional and State EMS organizations can also serve as a resource for materials.

Should they not have such materials available, these organizations can often refer you to others that do. Some states have developed statewide resource manuals that include materials developed and submitted by other instructors.

Other government agencies such as the Environmental Protection Agency, Department of Energy, Nuclear Regulatory Commission as well as certain EMS equipment vendors have valuable resource materials available. Agencies such as the American Academy of Pediatrics, Poison Control Center, American Red Cross, and others also provide useful posters and brochures, often free of charge, for educational purposes.

A particularly useful resource is *Medical 911: The EMS Information Sourcebook* published by Jems Communications. This book offers complete and comprehensive listings of resources available specifically for EMS, from consultants, to publications and multimedia options, to abstracts and state EMS organizations.

Additional materials can be located through a local public or university library. Computer locating services such as Prodigy, Interlink, and other programs make locating available resources easier. Once located, audiovisual materials can often be ordered for use through the interlibrary loan program. Even if information specific for EMS is not available, other material geared toward health professionals could be modified or adapted as appropriate.

Commercially developed audiovisual materials are available from numerous publishers and other organizations. Publishers of textbooks for

Many training centers and other educational institutions have a central resource center available to instructors.

Even if information specific for EMS is not available, other material geared toward health professionals could be modified or adapted as appropriate.

EMS training programs usually offer supplemental materials as well, including slides, transparencies, and videos.

In addition to publishers, other organizations produce monthly or quarterly "magazine like" video series with four or five topics on each tape. These include items such as medical emergencies, physical assessments, physicians notes, and other features.

Should prepared media not be available or prove to be too costly, instructors can easily create alternative materials. Universities and EMS organizations may allow instructors to use their equipment to develop specific audiovisual material.

KEY POINTS

1. Instructional media is an essential part of the learning process and greatly affects how information is perceived and processed.
2. Audiovisual materials improve student motivation as well as the quality of instruction. They also provide a source for standardization, review, and remediation of information.
3. There are two channels for communicating information: single-channel and multichannel. The most beneficial forms of media are generally achieved when multiple senses are used during the presentation of information.
4. Learning objectives should be identified prior to the selection of audiovisual media to ensure appropriate use of instructional materials. Psychomotor objectives are best presented through the use of equipment and simulations; cognitive objectives are best presented with diagrams, videos, slides, and transparencies; and affective objectives are best presented with videos and multiscreen slide or tape presentations.
5. When inserting slides into a carousel, they should be placed upside down and backwards so that projection is correct.
6. When placing a transparency on an overhead projector, the instructor should be able to face the audience and read from the film, once placed on the projector.
7. The instructor should always be prepared with an alternative from of media in case of unforseen problems with audiovisual equipment.

REFERENCES

1. Malamed C. Tapping into the mind: how to design graphics to be remembered. *AV Video*. 1991; September:60–63.
2. Strauss R. Multimedia for the masses: designing for the TV screen. *AV Video*. 1992; February:48–58.
3. Faulkner L. *Invincible Visual Job Aids*. Huntsville, AL: Faulkner Consulting Services; 1991.
4. Bergeron R. The uses of colors to enhance training communications. *Performance and Instruction*. 1990; August:34–37.
5. Borsook T, Higginbotham-Wheat N. Interactivity: What is it and what can it do for computer-based instruction? *Educational Technology*. 1991; October:11–17.
6. Courseware GP. *Principles of Instructional Design*. Columbia, MD: General Physics Corporation; 1983.
7. Gustafson C. Increased stimulation with audiovisual aids in training. *JEMS*. 1985; June:59–62.

7 Alternative Teaching Methods Making Learning Fun

OBJECTIVES

Upon completion of this chapter, the reader will have sufficient information to:
1. Define game.
2. List four reasons for using games.
3. Relate the laws of learning to the use of games.
4. List four types of games.
5. Identify specific procedures for selected games.
6. Identify advantages and disadvantages of selected games.

KEY TERMS

Fun An enjoyable or pleasurable experience; a source of amusement or merriment

Game Any form of play, amusement, or recreation involving physical or mental competition under a specific set of rules

Puzzle A question or problem that exercises one's mind to test cleverness, skill, or knowledge

INTRODUCTION

Whoever said learning cannot be fun? In education, adding a little spice into a program can be all that is needed to make learning tolerable. In fact, it may even make learning fun, and although some educators may flinch at the thought of their students having fun in the classroom, students learn more in an interactive environment.

This chapter provides guidelines for games that can be used during any training session. An overview of each game is described along with procedures to follow in order to play the game. Specific questions for these games can be found in Appendix A.

WHY GAMES?

Participants of game play benefit in various ways including cognitive enhancement, attitude adjustment, and increased motivation. On a cognitive level, participants gain knowledge of facts and principles as well as improved decision-making skills[1]. People get very emotional about

articipants of game play benefit in various ways including cognitive enhancement, attitude adjustment, and increased motivation.

games. Since information related to strong emotions is more easily remembered, knowledge is increased through the use of games.

On a motivational level, participants exhibit increased interest and enthusiasm toward learning when games are used in the classroom. They tend to put more effort into the game than they would in an ordinary classroom session. On the attitudinal level, students gain more self-confidence with personal capabilities as well as a positive attitude toward the course in general. This might eliminate negative feelings over some other aspect of the program (*eg*, the number of hours, test anxiety).

One additional advantage regardless of the type of game used in training is excellence through competition. While students like to play, they strive to be better than their peers and will prepare harder for a game in which they do not want their peers to think they do not know the information. The fact is, students like competition.

DANGER WITH GAMES

It is important to spend time developing useful games. Games need to be designed at the right level for students. Games are only fun if they are challenging—note *challenging*, not frustrating or impossible. If a game is too easy, it won't be fun; if it is too difficult it will generate negative rather then positive feelings. This may be a difficult task to achieve since what is easy for one student may be hard for another. Therefore, when developing games format the design for the average student.

Do not make the instructions too confusing or complex. If the students are expected to play a game based on directions, be sure the directions are easy to follow or the students may become discouraged before the game begins.

In addition, it is important that games be related directly to course material. Students should be learning as they play. They need to feel the game is an important part of the course. Game play should not be used as a means to pass time, but as a necessary instructional tool.

Finally, when using games, always have a final score or some performance measure. Students prefer to have a game score to rate their overall performance. A score also helps justify the game as a instructional tool rather than a waste of time.

Students should be learning as they play. They need to feel the game is an important part of the course.

TYPES OF GAMES

There are various types of games, each designed for a specific purpose, including games for introductions, games to increase vocabulary, and general information games.

Introduction Games
Introduction games are designed to make the class feel at ease and become familiar with the rest of the group, either on the first night of class or at the beginning of a training session. Two games that provide this benefit have already been described in Chapter 3: The Name Game and The Scavenger Name Hunt.

Vocabulary Games
Vocabulary games are designed to increase the ease of learning terms, illnesses, anatomy, and other words that are important but difficult to remember. There are multiple methods to learning vocabulary and

Vocabulary games are designed to increase the ease of learning terms, illnesses, anatomy, and other words that are important but difficult to remember.

other specific information. One game, Professionals Use the Right Words, is an effective way to reinforce terminology. Puzzles and word finds can also improve retention of terminology and key points.

Puzzle Games

Puzzle games involve solving a puzzle and/or answering questions to win. A wide variety of puzzle games can be used to cover various topics throughout any course. For example, a crossword puzzle or word find can be related to specific course content. EMS Scrabble is a word puzzle in which clues for one word lead to the hidden term.

In addition, problem-solving word puzzles prove very beneficial in helping students work through the identification and/or treatment of various illnesses and injuries. Any theme can be used for these puzzles; Appendix A offers sample word puzzles including: "Illin' Dwarfs"[3], "The Shock of Her Life", and "A Traumatic Event." These word games can be modified to incorporate any illness or injury.

Puzzles can range from very simple to extremely complex. Complex puzzles can maintain student attention and motivation over long, tedious training programs. It is important, however, that puzzles relate directly to course objectives.

> Complex puzzles can maintain student attention and motivation over long, tedious training programs.

Quiz Games

Quiz games can be incorporated into any type question-and-answer session. Although most students have test anxiety, they enjoy quiz games. Traditional games such as Tic-Tac-Toe and War, as well as modifications for popular television game shows such as Jeopardy, Family Feud, Trivial Pursuit, and Win, Lose, or Draw can be used to achieve optimal training.

Even though questions used in quiz games may be the same as those included in an exam, students respond differently in a testing situation. If students think it is a game, they have fun answering questions; if they think it is a test, they approach the same questions with fear and anxiety.

Variations on quiz games can be found in Appendix A and include EMS Tic-Tac-Toe, EMS Jeopardy, EMS Family Feud, EMS Trivia Mania, EMS Feud, EMS Win, Lose, or Draw, and EMS Anybody's Guess.

Role Play Games

Role play games are designed to provide learners with a variety of choices within a storyline and ask participants to help create the story itself. There are endless role play games that can be incorporated into EMS training. "Beat the Reaper" is an example of a role play game and can also be found in Appendix A.

"Beat the Clock" is a simulation strategy role play game in which teams are timed on their speed and ability to assess and treat patients during various scenarios. Points are then awarded to the quickest, safest, most accurate, and most appropriate team.

> Role play games are designed to provide learners with a variety of choices within a storyline and ask participants to help create the story itself.

SPECIFIC GAMES FOR EMS EDUCATION PROGRAMS

The following pages provide a description of various EMS training games. Appendix A provides game cards and questions. The game format can be modified to meet specific training needs, and additional game cards created as necessary.

When developing additional games and questions, dare to be creative, and most importantly, have fun!

When playing games in a classroom setting, it is best to use small groups (not more than six participants) to allow for increased involvement and retention of information. Make certain to allow everyone equal turns. Be cautious of the rowdy student trying to dominate play by answering all the questions. When developing additional games and questions, dare to be creative, and most importantly, have fun!

Professionals Use The Right Words
When To Use:
During sessions that cover a large amount of terminology or for review sessions. This is an easy way to reinforce terminology for the lesson being covered.

Method:
1) As students enter the room, they are given a 3 × 5 card with a term on it. Students must match that term with its definition prior to the beginning of the class session. Definitions are on 4 × 6 cards secured to poster boards.
2) One of the first activities of the evening is for the instructor to review the terminology to ensure that students matched definitions correctly.
3) If one student has already placed a term with a definition, and another student feels his term matches the definition, the instructor intercedes to ensure that the correct term is matched with the appropriate definition.
4) Posterboards should be left in place for the entire session in order to allow students the opportunity to review them during breaks.

Purpose:
To motivate students to read prior to class and to test recall ability.

Materials:
3 × 5 cards with definitions.
4 × 6 cards with terms on posterboards (Figure 7.1).

Advantages:
☑ Provides an incentive for students to read assigned chapters prior to attending class.
☑ Quizzes students on information learned.
☑ Uses up time prior to the start of class, in a productive way.

Disadvantages:
☒ Takes time to create game cards and boards.

Word Puzzles
When to Use:
Whenever puzzles are available for a specific lesson.

Method:
Word puzzles can be created by computer-generated boxes, or by using graph paper to space letters and boxes appropriately. Word puzzles can be designed for any topic.

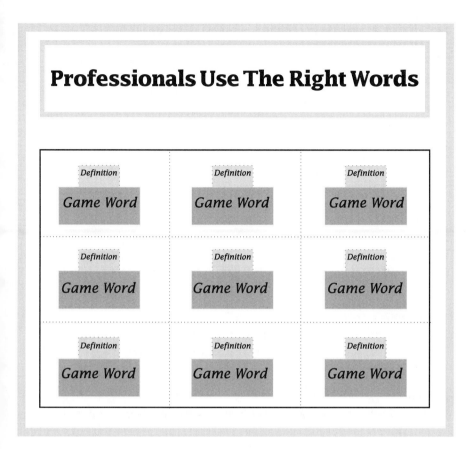

FIGURE 7.1 Professionals Use the Right Words Game Board

Purpose:
To improve and review vocabulary, promote incidental learning, and encourage completion of assigned reading.

Materials:
Prepared puzzles and answer keys to be distributed to learners.

Advantages:
☑ Help learners review key material and think through concepts.
☑ Help learners differentiate between different illnesses and injuries.
☑ Word finds and crossword puzzles help learners with the identification and spelling of key words.

Disadvantages:
✖ Takes time to create puzzles.
✖ Costs money for duplication of puzzles.

EMS Tic-Tac-Toe[2]
When to Use:
During review of any information, or to use up time at the end of a session.

Method:
1) Before the game session, assign appropriate reading and study material.
2) Divide the class into two teams and have teams select a team name and captain.

3) By way of a coin toss, decide who is "X" and who is "O" and which team goes first.

4) The team winning the toss selects a Tic-Tac-Toe square for strategic reasons.

5) Cards may be positioned in pockets on a poster board, as shown in Figure 7.2, with more difficult questions in more popular squares and/or toward the back of the stack.

6) The game host reads the question from the square chosen by the first team.

7) Both teams should be instructed to listen. The second team will have to evaluate the first team's answer and offer an alternative answer if the answer provided is not correct.

8) If team 1 is correct, they get 2 points and their mark (X or O) in the appropriate square.

9) If team 1 is incorrect, team 2 is provided the opportunity to answer. If team 2 is correct, they get 1 point and play moves to them.

10) If neither team is correct, the correct answer is discussed, and play moves to team 2.

11) Play proceeds until someone gets "Tic-Tac-Toe" or until all squares are used. An extra 5 points are awarded to the team that wins a Tic-Tac-Toe.

Purpose:
To reinforce key material and practice answering test type questions.

Materials:
Tic-Tac-Toe board. A piece of poster board, appropriately titled, with envelopes affixed and labeled in a Tic-Tac-Toe pattern (Figure 7.2).
Chalkboard or flipchart on which to keep score.
Question cards (at least six per square).

Advantages:
- ✓ Promotes excellence through competition.
- ✓ It is easy to create these types of questions since they are test-type multiple choice questions.
- ✓ Questions can cover any topic.
- ✓ The game provides an incentive for students to study and read material prior to attending class.

Disadvantages:
- ✗ The game takes time to play.

EMS Scrabble[2]
When to Use:
Whenever a review of content is needed, or as a break from traditional lecture sessions.

Method:
1) Divide the class into two teams and have teams select a team name and captain. Determine the starting team by way of a coin toss.
2) One member from each team comes to the front of the room.
3) The starting team picks a clue number.
4) The clue is read by the host and the first player to raise his or her hand attempts to answer.

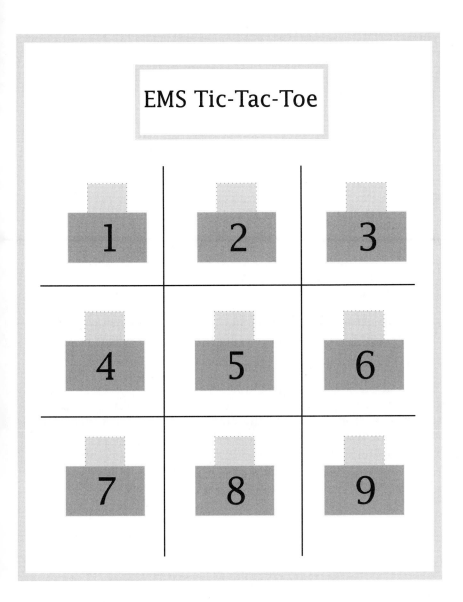

FIGURE 7.2 EMS Tic-Tac-Toe Game Board

5) If unsuccessful, the other team may try.
6) A score of two points is given to the team that answers the question on the first try.
7) The team to guess the key word is given a 10-point bonus.

Purpose:
To quiz students on key material and provide a review of content.

Materials:
A white- or chalkboard with the game pieces marked. An overhead transparency with nonpermanent markers can also be used.

Advantages:
☑ Promotes excellence through competition.
☑ Provides a good review at the end of a session.
☑ Acts as a good "filler" if class session ends early.

Disadvantages:
- ✖ Takes time to create initial game pieces.
- ✖ Takes time to play.

Beat the Reaper[2]
When to Use:
Whenever a review of content is needed to help students learn and sift through critical information for patient assessment and emergency care techniques.

Method:
1) Divide the class into small teams and have them select a team spokesperson.
2) Assign each group a topic, using 3×5 cards with a category or topic (*eg*, spontaneous pneumothorax).
3) Each group is given the following instructions:
   a. Develop a complete scenario with all details necessary for the identification of a patient problem or condition
   b. Include all information necessary to answer other learner's questions regarding patient history and physical examination
   c. Include all scene-related information whether pertinent to the patient's condition or not
4) The first group moves to the front of the class and gives the dispatch information that "gets the class to the call" (*eg*, dispatched to a man down at the Duck Pond Motor Lodge).
5) The remaining groups are then given the opportunity to gather information one team at a time (*eg*, "Is the dispatcher able to get any further information?" "What is the patient's chief complaint?" "What is the patient's blood pressure?" "What does the patient's skull feel like?").
6) Information is only given when asked for by the audience.
7) Once a team is able to correctly identify the condition or illness, they should state so. If they are correct in their response, they are given 10 points; if they are incorrect, they are penalized 5 points.
8) The game ends when all scenarios have been played, and the team with the highest score wins.

Purpose:
If participants put data together quickly and accurately enough, they may be able to "Beat the Reaper."

Materials:
3×5 cards with patient conditions / illnesses.
A board (paper or blackboard) for keeping score.

Advantages:
- ☑ Lets students do the studying and presentation of information.
- ☑ Students learn one illness or condition well.
- ☑ Promotes a cooperative effort with classmates working together; building teams is a useful tool in the EMS field.

Disadvantages:
- ✖ If students do not cover all key material, or if they provide inaccurate information, instructors must be prepared to fill in.

✖ Students only learn one illness well, and then rely on their peers for the rest of the information.

EMS Jeopardy
When to Use:
Whenever a review of content is needed, or as a break from traditional lecture sessions.

Method:
1) Divide the class into teams and have each team select a team name and captain. The captain will choose categories and give answers after conferring with the rest of his team.
2) The answers the captain gives should always be based on the team's direction.
3) Toss a coin to determine which team goes first.
4) Team A chooses a category and dollar amount.
5) If team A answers correctly, they get that amount; if they answer incorrectly, they are penalized that amount. If team A answers incorrectly, then team B gets an opportunity to answer. If team B answers correctly, they get the amount; if team B answers incorrectly they are not penalized.
6) The next questions goes to team B. If team B answers correctly, they get that amount; if they answer incorrectly, they are penalized that amount. If team B answers incorrectly, then team A gets an opportunity to answer. If team A answers correctly, they get that amount; if they answer incorrectly they are not penalized.
7) Each team has 15 seconds in which to answer the questions.
8) The game ends when all questions have been asked, and the team with the highest score wins.

Purpose:
To provide a mechanism for the review of important information and practice answering questions.

Materials:
A Jeopardy board with five or six categories, *eg*, Basic Life Support, Medical Emergencies, Fractures, Soft Tissue Injuries, General Knowledge, and Pediatric Emergencies. For each category identify dollar amounts and identify one "daily double." If a team selects a category with a secret "daily double" and answers the question correctly, they are awarded two times the dollar amount in points. Figure 7.3 provides an example game board.

A board (paper or black board) for keeping score.

Advantages:
☑ Students enjoy the game.
☑ Promotes excellence through competition.
☑ Allows for informal evaluation of class progress.

Disadvantages:
✖ Takes time to create initial game pieces.
✖ Takes time to play.

EMS Jeopardy

$ Amount	Fractures	Patient Assessment	Medical Emergencies	Trauma	Basic Life Support
$ 100					
$ 200					
$ 300					
$ 400					
$ 500					

FIGURE 7.3 EMS Jeopardy Game Board

EMS Family Feud
When to Use:
Whenever a review of content is needed, or as a break from traditional lecture sessions.

Method:
1) Divide the class into two teams (four to six members on a team is preferable; an extra person can be scorekeeper). Each team should select a team name and captain.
2) The first player from each team is asked a question to determine who gains control of play. The first player to identify a correct response will have control.
3) Each of the remaining team members are asked to identify items remaining on the response list. Points are awarded for each correct response according to the popularity of responses, with the most common answers resulting in higher scores. Each team is allowed only three incorrect responses before the opposing team is given the opportunity to "steal the pot." If the first team gets three strikes (incorrect responses) and the opposing team provides one of the remaining responses, the opposing team is awarded the points accrued during that question, and the first team receives no points.
4) The game ends when all questions have been played, and the team with the highest score wins.

Purpose:
To quiz students on key material and provide a review of content.

Materials:
Game question cards (at least 20 questions).
A board (paper or blackboard) for keeping score.

Advantages:
- Good for regurgitation of facts and information.
- Promotes excellence through competition.

Disadvantages:
- Can only be used effectively for lists of information such as types of devices or treatment modalities.

EMS Trivia Mania
When to Use:
Whenever a review of important material is necessary, as a means to practice answering test questions, or as a break from traditional lecture sessions.

Method:
1) Divide the class into teams and have each team select a team name and captain. The captain will choose categories and give responses after conferring with the rest of the team.
2) The answers the captain gives should always be based upon the team's direction.
3) Give each team a playing card.
4) Toss a coin to determine which team goes first.
5) The first team is asked to pick a category. The moderator asks the question and allows the team captain 15 seconds to provide an answer. If they provide a correct response, they are given a game piece for that category. If they are incorrect, the opposing team is given the opportunity to answer the question. If the opposing team is correct, they are given the game piece. Play then moves to the opposing team.
6) Play ends with the first team to collect enough category game pieces to fill the entire play card.

Purpose:
To provide a mechanism for the review of key information and provide practice in answering test questions.

Materials:
Game cards (at least 20 sets of questions). Playing cards (gameboard) and game pieces. Figures 7.4 and 7.5 provide an example game board and game categories.

Advantages:
- Can be used anytime. If there is not enough time in class for a formal game, game cards can be used to quiz students during available time or while waiting for class to begin.
- Includes a variety of topics.

Disadvantages:
- Takes time to create game pieces and game cards.
- Takes time to play.

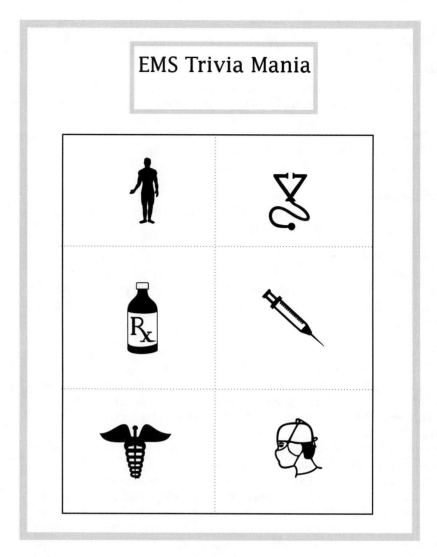

FIGURE 7.4 EMS Trivia Mania Game Board

EMS Feud

When to Use:
Whenever a review of content is needed, or as a break from traditional lecture sessions.

Method:
1) Divide the class into two teams (four to six members on a team is preferable; an extra person can be the scorekeeper). Toss a coin to identify the starting team.
2) Each team selects a team name and captain.
3) The first team is asked a question. The team has 15 seconds to decide on an answer, which is relayed through the team captain. If more than one answer is voiced, only the captain's will count.
4) The opposing team then evaluates the first team's answer and agrees or supplies what they think is the correct response.
5) Two points are awarded to the team for each correct answer

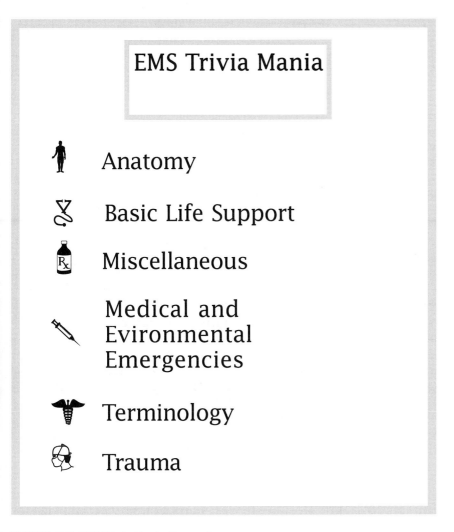

FIGURE 7.5 EMS Trivia Mania Categories

given on the first attempt. If the opposing team was also correct, they receive one point. No points are given for wrong answers.
6) The game ends when all questions have been played, and the team with the highest score wins.

Purpose:
To quiz students on key material and provide a review of content.

Materials:
Game question cards (at least 20 questions).
A board (paper or blackboard) for keeping score.

Advantages:
☑ Questions can be used any time; it does not need to be a structured game.
☑ Old test questions can be used as game cards.

Disadvantages:
☒ Takes time to create initial game cards.

EMS Win, Lose, or Draw
When to Use:
Whenever a review of the identification of anatomy or signs and symptoms of specific illnesses are needed, or as a break from traditional lecture sessions.

Method:
1) Divide the class into teams and have each team select a team name.
2) Toss a coin to determine which team goes first.
3) The first player from team one stands in front of the class with a marker and large pad. The moderator holds the first playing card (with a descriptor), and the player draws clues that should lead team members to the identification of the word. Team members have 30 seconds to guess what the word is. If team members guess the word, they receive one point. If, at the end of 30 seconds, team members have not successfully identified the descriptor, the opposing team has the chance to guess. If the opposing team is correct, they receive one point.
4) Each team takes turns playing, rotating through each player so everyone is given the opportunity to draw clues.
5) At the end of 15 minutes of play, the super-round begins. The team with the least points begins. The first team has 90 seconds to guess as many words as possible. The opposing team then has 90 seconds to guess as many words as possible to beat the first team's score (again, giving one point for each correct answer).
6) The game ends at the conclusion of the super-round. The team with the highest score wins the game.

Purpose:
To provide a mechanism for the review of key words, terms, and anatomy, as well as practice identifying signs of illnesses, injuries, or conditions.

Materials:
Game cards (at least 30).
A board (paper or blackboard) or easel.
Markers.

Advantages:
☑ Helps student work through words through descriptions, signs, and symptoms or other key concepts.
☑ Assists with the assessment of injuries and illnesses by putting "clues" together.
☑ Builds team spirit.

Disadvantages:
☒ Takes time to play.
☒ Need small groups to make the experience worthwhile.

EMS Anybody's Guess
When to Use:
Whenever a review of the identification of specific illnesses or injuries are needed, or as a break from traditional lecture sessions.

Method:
1) Divide the class into teams and have each team select a team name and captain.

2) Toss a coin to determine which team goes first.
3) The first player from team one reveals the first slot from the game card. He is then given the opportunity to guess the illness or injury the card is describing. If he answers correctly, the player's team is given 10 points. If the player cannot provide a correct response, the next clue is revealed and the second player from team one is given the opportunity to guess. If he is correct, the team receives 7 points. If he cannot provide a correct response, the third slot is revealed and the third player from team one is given a chance. If he provides the correct response, his team receives 5 points. If after the forth clue, the team provides a correct response, the team receives three points. If after the forth clue, team one is still incorrect, the opposing team has the opportunity to identify the term. If they are correct, their team receives 3 points.
4) The game ends when all game cards have been exhausted. The team with the highest score wins the game.

Purpose:
To provide a mechanism for the review of identifying key illnesses, injuries, and conditions.

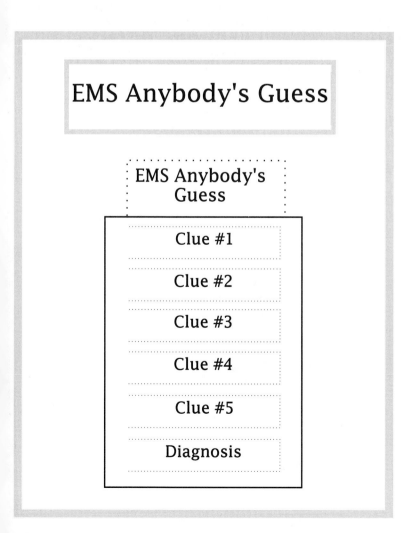

FIGURE 7.6 EMS Anybody's Guess Game Board

Materials:
Game cards (at least 30).
An Anybody's Guess game board with reveal slots (Figure 7.6).
A board or paper for keeping score.

Advantages:
☑ Works well as a test for identifying illnesses, injuries, and conditions.

Disadvantages:
☒ Is only effective with assessment of injuries, illnesses, and conditions.
☒ Works best in small groups.

KEY POINTS

1. Any topic can be turned into a game to make learning an enjoyable process. The use of games is extremely beneficial in EMS education; when students enjoy learning, the retention of important information is increased.

2. One of the advantages, regardless of the type of game played, is excellence through competition. Most students strive to do better than their peers because of an inherent competitive instinct. While students like to play, they strive to be better and will prepare harder for a game in which they do not want their peers to think they do not know the information. Instructors who tap into that competitive state help students help themselves learn important information.

3. The games included in this chapter are just a few of those available to EMS educators. Others can be developed as needed. The primary disadvantage consistent through all these games is *time*; the initial time to create game pieces and time to actually play the game.

4. While games are not intended to replace traditional classroom activities and lectures, they can be used to augment them and liven up a session. Some games can be used as "fillers" to use up extra time at the end of a class or before the session begins. Other games can be used to present information in a more effective manner than the traditional lecture. Other games can also be used as an evaluation too.

REFERENCES

1. Magney J. Game-based teaching. *The Education Digest*. January 55(5):54–57.
2. Head J. *Instructor's Resource Manual: Emergency Care*. Englewood Cliffs: NJ: The Brady Company; 1990.
3. Caroline N. *Workbook in Emergency Medical Treatment: Review Problems for EMTs*. Boston: Little Brown and Company; 1982.

8 EVALUATING STUDENT PERFORMANCE

Upon completion of this chapter, the reader will have sufficient information to:
1. Describe the purpose of exams.
2. List five question format types and a purpose for each type.
3. Provide seven guidelines for creating effective true-false questions.
4. Analyze multiple-choice questions to determine their effectiveness and make modifications as necessary.
5. List eight guidelines for developing effective multiple-choice questions.
6. Identify appropriate uses for matching questions.
7. Use five guidelines to develop effective matching items.
8. Describe two variations of short-answer questions.
9. Use three guidelines to develop effective short-answer questions.
10. Develop effective essay questions to test higher learning objectives.
11. List seven strategies to increase the accuracy of scoring essay questions.
12. Analyze exams to determine their effectiveness, and make modifications as necessary.
13. Calculate difficulty and discrimination indices for test questions.
14. Define statistical terms relative to analyzing exam scores.
15. Identify the mean, mode, and median of a set of exam scores.

KEY TERMS

Content validity The extent to which a test is representative of a defined body of knowledge

Criterion-referenced assessment Measurement in which a student's score is interpreted against a defined body of student behavior or to some specified level of performance

Diagnostic test A test used to measure student strengths and weaknesses in a given area

Distractor An incorrect option or possible response on a multiple-choice item

Essay item A test format that requires students to structure long written responses

Evaluation The process of making a value judgement based on information from one or more sources

Grammatical clue A flaw in wording or punctuation that directs the examinee to the correct answer

Guessing A conjecture, often at random, made when the correct answer to a question is not known

Halo effect An effect that can enter into the scoring of essay items, whereby there is a tendency to give higher scores to those individuals known to be good students and lower scores to those known to be poor students, independent of the quality of responses

Intelligence The capacity for reasoning and understanding

Intelligence quotient (IQ) The ratio of mental age (MA) to chronologic age (CA), multiplied by 100 ($100 \times [MA/CA]$)

Matching format A test item consisting of a two-column format (item and response) that requires students to make a correspondence between the two

Mean The arithmetic average of a set of scores

Median   The midpoint in a distribution; the 50th percentile

Mode   The score that occurs most frequently in a set of scores

Multiple-choice format   A test format in which the examinee selects the correct answer from a list of possible options

Negative skewness   Asymmetry of test scores in which most scores in a distribution are high

Normal distribution   A bell-shaped, symmetric distribution of scores, normally found in test results

Oral tests   Exams in which both questions an answers are given out loud

Performance test   A nonpaper, nonpencil test that requires students to engage in some type of process or skill performance

Positive skewness   Asymmetry of test scores in which most scores in a distribution are low

Range   The area between the highest and lowest scores in a distribution

Reading difficulty   The level of reading ability required to understand test questions

Relevance   The correlation between test items and the content area to be assessed

Reliability   The extent to which a test is consistent in measuring student performance

Short-answer format   A test item for which the student must provide a brief response to stem questions, usually consisting of a word or phrase

Stem   The portion of a multiple-choice test item that consists of an incomplete statement or question and is followed by a list of options

Test anxiety   A psychological state of stress caused by a testing situation

Test bank   A set of test questions from which exams can be created to match course objectives

True-false format   A test format in which examinees indicate whether a statement is correct (true) or incorrect (false)

Validity   The extent to which a test measures what it is intended to measure

ASSESSING OUTCOMES

While tests may not be perfect, they serve as a valuable tool in identifying the extent to which students have met course objectives.

There are many reasons for administering tests. Generally, they are used to provide information regarding student performance and progress. There is considerable controversy regarding the use and types of examinations in education, and EMS education is no exception. While tests may not be perfect, they serve as a valuable tool in identifying the extent to which students have met course objectives.

TYPES OF EVALUATION TOOLS

Test questions can be written in a variety of formats. There are two primary classifications, objective items including true-false, multiple-choice, and matching questions, and essay-type items including short-answer and essay questions. Such formats are useful in different circumstances; and, since there are various reasons for instruction, there is no one format best for all situations.

Objective questions are more easily and reliably scored, but, they usually take more time to construct.

In general, objective questions are more easily and reliably scored, but usually take more time to construct. Essay questions, on the other hand, are easier to develop but take more time to correct. In addition, essay test items often require subjective scoring from the instructor.

True-False Items

True-false test questions require the examinee to determine whether a given statement is true or not. To increase the difficulty of such questions, examinees could be required to explain why false statements are false or to identify and correct false areas of a statement.

A good true-false item is often difficult to construct. In addition, because they measure only what is absolutely true or false, they do not provide information about why a student responds incorrectly. Finally, since there are only two options to true-false questions, students have a fifty-fifty chance of answering correctly, even when guessing.

A good true-false item is often difficult to construct.

To ensure the validity of test questions, it is important to keep in mind the following tips when creating true-false questions:

- **Use true-false questions only when there is a clear-cut true or false answer.** For example:

> The most common cause of cardiac arrest is respiratory arrest.
> True or False

This statement is true when talking about infants and children, but not for adult victims of cardiac arrest. A better statement would be as follows:

> The most common cause of cardiac arrest in children is respiratory arrest.
> * True or False

- **Construct the statement as entirely true or entirely false.** Ambiguous statements should be avoided. For example:

> Biological death, which occurs when breathing and circulation cease, is irreversible.
> True or False

This statement is poor because clinical death occurs when breathing and circulation cease. A better question would be one of the following:

> Biological death occurs when breathing and circulation cease.
> True or False *

> Biological death is irreversible.
> * True or False

- **Avoid lifting statements directly from a textbook.** Textbooks are written so that sentences fit into paragraphs and do not necessarily stand alone. In addition, if students identify that questions simply follow the text, they may begin memorizing the text rather than understanding concepts and information. For example:

> Gamma rays and x-rays can be considered the same thing. Gamma radiation is extremely dangerous, carrying high levels of energy able to penetrate thick shielding.
> * True or False

While this statement is true, it is taken directly from the textbook and is somewhat complex. A better statement would be as follows:

> Gamma radiation can be stopped by a layer of clothing.
> True or False *

🍎 **Avoid specific determiners such as all, none, always, and never.** Students know such questions are usually false since at least one exception to a statement can usually be found. For example:

> Closed fractures always produce minor soft tissue damage.
> True or False

While closed fractures can produce minor soft tissue damage, sometimes it causes no damage to surrounding tissue, and other times it causes great damage. A better statement would be as follows:

> Closed fractures often causes minor soft tissue damage.
> * True or False

🍎 **Construct approximately the same number of true and false statements, and make such questions of equal length.** If most true statements are longer, students may guess answers based on question length rather than content.

🍎 **Avoid setting a pattern of answers (ie, two true, two false, two true, etc.).** When students become aware of patterns, they tend to guess based on them.

🍎 **Avoid trick questions consisting of minor adjustments to true statements in order to create a false response.** Such changes are usually trivial and have little bearing on the question at hand. For example:

> When rewarming a frostbitten body part, water heated to 100°F should be used.
> True or False

While this statement could be technically correct, students could answer it true or false. A better statement would be as follows:

> When rewarming a frostbitten body part, water heated to 100° to 105°F should be used.
> * True or False

Multiple-Choice Items

Multiple-choice questions require the examinee to select one or more correct responses to a question. A multiple-choice item consists of two parts, the stem or the incomplete statement or question, and the options. Options usually consist of one correct answer and three or four distractors.

In EMS training programs, multiple-choice tests are the most common form of written examinations. Most states, as well as other agencies, use multiple-choice tests to assess student competency. Properly written multiple-choice questions can prevent the likelihood of students passing a test simply by guessing. In addition, this type of test format is easily scored and validated.

The following guidelines will help with the development of effective multiple-choice questions:

🍎 **Do not give away answers by grammatical clues.** The wording of questions and options could provide clues leading to the

In EMS training programs, multiple-choice tests are the most common form of written examinations.

correct response, even if students do not know the answer. The most common grammatical clues include plurals, articles, and tenses. For example:

An injury in which the skin is bruised is referred to as a:
   (a) abrasion
   (b) avulsion
   (c) ecchymosis
* (d) contusion

The student can identify the correct answer as (d) even if he is unsure of the term, providing he knows grammatical skills. Since responses (a), (b), and (c) all require the antecedent *an* rather than *a*, the only grammatically correct response is (d). An improved question would be as follows:

An injury in which the skin is bruised is referred to as a(n):
   (a) abrasion
   (b) avulsion
   (c) ecchymosis
* (d) contusion

🍎 **Make all distractors the same length.** For example:

The best way to care for a pediatric patient with abdominal pain is by:
   (a) thoroughly assessing for the location of pain.
* (b) allowing the child to seek a position of comfort and transporting the patient quickly and carefully with oxygen delivered as tolerated.
   (c) allowing the parents to transport the child on their own.
   (d) rapidly transporting the patient.

Most examinees would select choice (b) simply because it is the most complex answer. A better question would be:

The best way to care for a pediatric patient with abdominal pain is by:
   (a) thoroughly assessing for the location of pain.
* (b) allowing the child to seek a position of comfort.
   (c) allowing the parents to transport the child on their own.
   (d) rapidly transporting the patient.

🍎 **Place all key words in the stem rather than the options.** For example:

Manual stabilization is begun prior to application of a cervical collar and may be discontinued:
   (a) after the cervical collar is completely secured.
   (b) after a short board has been applied.
* (c) after the patient is secured to a long spine board.
   (d) after the patient's head is secured to the short spine board.

Repeating "after" in all four options tends to de-emphasize the key information presented in each option. It is more effective to include key information in the stem only, as identified below:

Manual stabilization is begun prior to application of a cervical collar and may be discontinued after:
  (a) the cervical collar is completely secured.
  (b) a short board has been applied.
* (c) the patient is secured to a long spine board.
  (d) the patient's head is secured to the short spine board.

🍎 **Phrase stems positively unless it is important to emphasize an exception.** For example:

Which of the following is not a sign or symptom of shock?
  (a) diaphoresis
* (b) paralysis
  (c) increased pulse
  (d) decreased blood pressure

In cases in which an exception is key, underline or capitalize the exception to point it out to the examinee so as to decrease the likelihood of misreading the question. Either of the following two examples would be appropriate:

Which of the following is *not* a sign or symptom of shock?
  (a) diaphoresis
* (b) paralysis
  (c) increased pulse
  (d) decreased blood pressure

All of the following are sign or symptoms of shock EXCEPT:
  (a) diaphoresis
* (b) paralysis
  (c) increased pulse
  (d) decreased blood pressure

🍎 **Construct test items with a single correct answer.** For example:

The liver is located in which abdominal quadrant?
* (a) RUQ
* (b) LUQ
  (c) LLQ
  (d) RLQ

Since the liver extends into the left upper quadrant, examinees may find this question confusing. A better question would be:

The liver is primarily located in which abdominal quadrant?
* (a) RUQ
  (b) LUQ
  (c) LLQ
  (d) RLQ

🍎 **Include a minimum of four and maximum of five options.**
Using less than four options increases the examinee's chance of
guessing at the correct response, and it is often difficult to create more than four good distractors.

🍎 **Use plausible distractors.** For example:

> The primary life-threatening consequence of anaphylactic shock is
> a(n):
> * (a) airway obstruction
>   (b) sprained airway
>   (c) punctured lung
>   (d) headache

The only possible answer to the above question is (a). As such, even
if examinees do not know what anaphylactic shock is, they would still
most likely choose answer (a). A better question would be:

> The primary life-threatening consequence of anaphylactic shock is:
> * (a) an airway obstruction
>   (b) cardiac arrest
>   (c) brain damage
>   (d) dehydration

🍎 **Arrange options in a logical sequence.** For example:

> What percentage of body surface is affected if an adult is burned on
> the back of both legs?
> * (a) 18%
>   (b) 36%
>   (c) 9%
>   (d) 27%

Be certain to vary the placement of responses. Most examinees
will guess by selecting the middle number. A better sequence of responses follows:

> What percentage of body surface is affected if an adult is burned on
> the back of both legs?
>   (a) 9%
> * (b) 18%
>   (c) 27%
>   (d) 36%

🍎 **Alternate the order of correct responses randomly among
all options.** As with true-false questions, if examinees can identify a pattern of responses, they are more likely to guess such.
For example, if choice (c) is used excessively, when a student
does not know the answer, he will most likely choose (c).

🍎 **Refrain from using the choices "all of the above" or "none
of the above."** Most students know that if "all of the above" is
an option, it is usually the correct choice.

Matching Items

Another objective format of test questions involves the examinee
matching two columns, using some form of association criterion. The

two columns are termed the *premises*, consisting of the item stem, and the *responses,* which consist of possible responses.

Matching questions are useful for testing student knowledge of definitions or relationships to ideas, concepts, principles, or items. Matching items are generally easier to develop since they do not require the construction of plausible distractors. In addition, since a relatively large amount of material can be covered into matching stems, a large amount of material can be tested in a short period of time, with answers scored quickly and reliably.

Entire exams are rarely comprised solely of matching items, but, a combination of multiple-choice, true-false and matching items may provide the best method for accurately testing student knowledge. In such exams, matching items are most often confined to a section of associated terms or definitions.

The following guidelines will help with the development of effective matching items:

> **Keep the list of items to a short but challenging length.** Include, generally 10 to 15 items in each matching group.
> **Construct lists that are homogeneous in content** (*ie*, all relative to the same item). Including heterogenous content enables the examinee to eliminate certain choices simply because they lack similarity between the premise and response. When this occurs, the chances of an examinee guessing at the correct response increases. Consider the following example:

_____	1. a sign of arterial bleeding	a. 15:2
_____	2. a mechanical immobilization device	b. slurred speech
_____	3. a sign of stroke	c. bright spurting blood
_____	4. the definition of lateral	d. traction splint
_____	5. the ratio of compression to ventilation for 1 person adult CPR.	e. to the side of the body

The examinee who knew nothing about the information contained on the test would be able to answer these questions without error, simply because there is only one plausible answer for each item. Likewise, the following example adds a few test items to increase the need to choose between plausible responses, but there is still only two potential correct responses. As such, the examinee's chance of guessing the correct answer is still 50%.

_____	1. a sign of arterial bleeding	a. 15:2
_____	2. a sign of venous bleeding	b. KED
_____	3. a mechanical immobilization device	c. chest pain
_____	4. an alternative to the short board	d. toward the center of body
_____	5. a sign of stroke	e. slurred speech
_____	6. a sign of a myocardial infarction	f. bright spurting blood
_____	7. the definition of lateral	g. 5:1
		h. traction splint

_____	8. the definition of medial
_____	9. the ratio of compressions to ventilations for 1 person adult CPR.
_____	10. the ratio of compressions to ventilations for 2 person adult CPR.

i. steady flow of dark blood
j. to the side of the body

A more effective type of matching item would include stems from a homogeneous content, such as a single concept or basis for classification. The following is an example:

_____	1. anaphylactic shock
_____	2. cardiogenic shock
_____	3. hypovolemic shock
_____	4. metabolic shock
_____	5. neurogenic shock
_____	6. psychogenic shock
_____	7. septic shock

a. a life threatening reaction to an allergen
b. failure of the heart to pump adequately
c. loss of body fluids causing a change in chemical balance
d. caused by the inability to control the diameter of blood vessels
e. a sudden dilation of blood vessels causing the patient to faint
f. caused by severe infection
g. caused by the loss of blood, plasma or other body fluids

- **Provide more responses than needed to prevent students matching items by a process of elimination.** This practice also protects students from automatically answering a second question wrong when an equal number of premises and responses are provided.
- **Provide directions as to whether examinees are permitted to use a response more than once.**
- **Make certain responses are plausible.**

Short-Answer Items

Short-answer questions require the examinee to provide the correct response, rather than selecting from a variety of options. As such, these questions do not require the development of plausible distractors.

Short-answer questions take on two main formats: questions and completion items. The question format requires the examinee to provide the answer to a question. For example:

What is the compression to ventilation ratio for one rescuer adult CPR?
Answer: _____

Completion items provide a statement with one or more missing words, and require the examinee to fill in the blanks. A common problem with this type of question is ambiguous wording, which could lead to multiple possible answers. An example of a completion type question follows:

Short-answer questions take on two main formats: questions and completion items.

When necessary, the _____ pressure point can be used to help control facial bleeding.

The following guidelines should be followed in order to increase the validity of short answer questions:

🍎 **Ensure that questions are worded so there is only one correct answer.** For example:

Diaphoresis, a rapid pulse and low blood pressure are signs and symptoms of what illness? _____

These symptoms could be present with numerous illnesses. As such, a better question would be as follow:

What are three signs or symptoms of a patient in shock?

_____

_____

_____

🍎 **Place the blank toward the end of the statement** to avoid making students read the question twice. For example:

_____ is a true emergency resulting from a patient experiencing multiple seizures without regaining consciousness.

A better statement would be as follows:

The syndrome which occurs as a result of a patient experiencing multiple seizures without regaining consciousness is known as _____ (Status Epilepticus) _____.

🍎 **Limit the number of blanks to one or two.** For example:

_____ is a medical condition which occurs due to the _____ not receiving enough oxygen. Patients with this condition often take_____.

When too many words are missing from a statement, examinees will have difficulty identifying the intent of the question. It is important that short-answer test items retain structure with blanks so that examinees can understand adequately and respond appropriately. A better question would be as follows:

The medical condition that occurs as a result of insufficient blood supply to the heart, often brought on during physical or emotional stress, is known as _____. Patients with this condition often take what medication? _____

Another form of completion questions involves placing labels on a diagram. For example, Figure 8.1 provides a diagram of the human body. Examinees can be given diagrams with directions to label each blank with the appropriate name of the bone to which it is pointing. Another variation would be a matching diagram in which a list of options (names

ANATOMY & PHYSIOLOGY QUIZ
Pressure Points

NAME: _____   DATE: _____

DIRECTIONS: Fill in all blanks with the complete name of the pressure point to which it points.

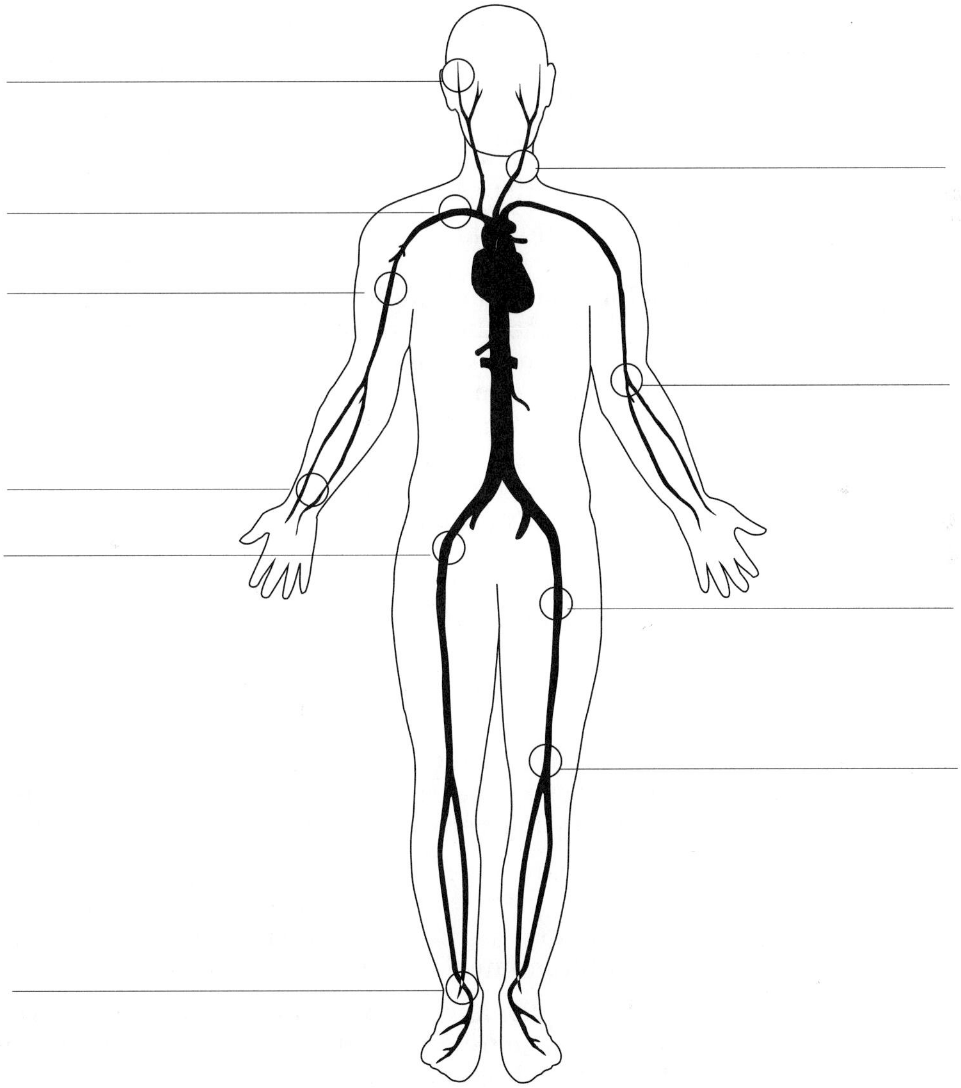

FIGURE 8.1 Sample Diagram Completion Quiz

of various bones) is provided, with directions that the examinee must match the name of the bone to the correct location on the body.

Essay Items

Essay-type questions are often used in college–level courses in order to elicit student responses such as organizing ideas, analyzing information, comparing and contrasting ideas or opinions, or solving problems. These questions require the examinee to understand concepts and processes rather than memorize isolated facts.

> Essay questions are used effectively to measure higher-level objectives such as analysis, synthesis, and evaluation.

Essay questions are used effectively to measure higher-level objectives such as analysis, synthesis, and evaluation. They are not effective, however, as a means of measuring lower-level objectives. Examples of higher-level skills that can be measured by essay questions include the following[1]:

- Organizing information to defend a position.
- Developing a plan to solve a potential problem.
- Comparing and contrasting positions or issues.
- Formulating conclusions based on data provided.
- Explaining the application of certain principles.
- Describing the cause-and-effect relationship between items.

Essay questions are easy to construct, but are quite time-consuming to grade. In addition, grading essay questions is often subjective, and instructors may mark students off for poor writing skills and not necessarily because they did not know the material. In addition, essay questions often take time for examinees to complete and, although they prevent the opportunity for cheating, they tend to encourage examinees to bluff or exaggerate the response.

In essence, essay questions provide the opportunity for the instructor to determine exactly what the examinee knows about a particular topic. For example:

> Compare and contrast diabetic coma and insulin shock, including pathophysiology, signs and symptoms, and treatment.

When creating essay questions, it is important to follow some guidelines:

- 🍎 **Incorporate specific phrases within the question that elicit the exact response needed.** As with performance behaviors, the following verbs are best:

  - Compare
  - Justify
  - Explain
  - Differentiate
  - Contrast
  - Describe
  - Illustrate
  - Rationalize

- 🍎 **State specifically what information the examinee is expected to provide, including the length and detail expected.** Without such guidelines, it is difficult for the instructor to judge a response and the student to know when enough information has been provided.

- 🍎 **Judge the examinee based on the response provided rather than on personality or previous work.** In order to minimize instructor bias:
  - Score essay questions without knowing the identity of the examinee. Substituting social security numbers or other identi-

fiers for names causes the instructor to score questions based solely on the response provided.

- Prior to scoring any exam, read a sample of responses in order to establish a range for judging how the overall group performed.
- Disregard neatness, spelling, grammar, punctuation, and handwriting unless such criteria were previously established within the directions. If such criteria are necessary, a separate score should be given for grammar and content.
- Compare examinee responses to a model answer prepared by the instructor in advance. The model should include items the examinee is expected to provide.
- Use essay items to measure the examinee's ability to apply, evaluate, or analyze the information learned.
- Since essay questions require a different approach to studying, it is important to advise students that such questions will be on the exam.
- Use essay questions in combination with other types of questions.

DEVELOPING EXAMS

Developing effective exams that accurately measure student performance requires careful planning and design. When doing so, adhere to the following guidelines[2]:

- 🍎 **Organize the exam in a logical manner.**
  - Group like items together, such as multiple-choice items, true-false questions, or matching items, as well as content-specific items such as all questions relative to a specific objective.
  - Place easier questions at the beginning of the exam to allow students to breeze through the beginning and concentrate on the latter, more difficult questions. This prevents students from becoming discouraged from the inability to answer the first few difficult questions.
- 🍎 **Make certain the exam tests the items intended.** Each question should be referenced to a specific lesson objective in order to be determined valid.
- 🍎 **Organize the test format for ease of scoring.** If the student is to write directly on the exam, place all answer blanks of equal length on one side of the paper. Using a separate answer sheet will allow instructors to score exams easily and allows for exams to be reused, thereby minimizing duplication costs.
- 🍎 **Write clear, complete directions that define exactly how and where the examinee is to respond to questions.** When appropriate, include information regarding how much each question is worth, and any time limits being placed on the examinee to complete the test.
- 🍎 **Be sure to include proper identification of the exam title on both the exam and answer sheet.** Also include an area for the date and examinee's name or other identification code (such as social security number) on the answer sheet.
- 🍎 **Be sure numbering and format of the exam questions match those of the answer sheet.** For example if the exam has response options a, b, c, and d, do not use A, B, C, or D or 1, 2, 3, or 4 on the answer sheet.

- **Be sure the exam is of adequate length and give the time allotted.**
- **After development, field test the exam by administering it to peers or recent graduates.** Allow these students the opportunity to write comments directly on the exam for items that are inaccurate or difficult to understand. Compile results of the field test and revise the examination accordingly.
- **Prepare legible copies of the exam that are free of all typographical, grammatical, and content errors.** Keep examinations in a locked storage area and number each one to assure security. Once security has been violated, the validity of an exam is compromised.
- **Make an accurate answer key, validating it to make certain it is correct.**

ANALYZING EXAMS

In order to determine the effectiveness of an exam, it is necessary to analyze results. One method requires student participation. Once the exam is scored, return it to the class and discuss test items. This provides useful information regarding why students chose an incorrect response, misleading questions or typographical errors on the exam, or other problems such as lack of time to complete all answers, poor sentence structure, discrepancies between the content covered within a course and the material presented on the exam, as well as other valuable information that can be used to modify future tests.

It is important that instructors not be defensive when discussing exams with students. It is normal to believe that an exam is perfectly constructed; however, there are times when exams can be improved. The goal of a test is to measure student competency; if this requires a rewrite, do not take it personally.

The second method for determining the effectiveness of an exam involves an item analysis. This will provide valuable information regarding which items were most often answered incorrectly and which distractors were most effective. Finally, an item analysis will provide information regarding how high-scoring and low-scoring students answered specific questions, thereby validating certain questions and suggesting elimination of other questions[2].

Complete the following steps in order to calculate item difficulty:

1) Score the exams and rank the scores in order from highest to lowest number of correct responses.
2) Select the exams for approximately the top 25% and bottom 25% of scores and add the number of correct responses in each group (high scorers and low scorers) for each question on the exam.
3) Calculate the item difficulty index for each question by:
   - Adding the number of correct responses in the high group (H) with those of the low group (L),
   - Divide the number of responses by the total number of examinees in both groups (T); and
   - Multiply by 100.
4) Express the difficulty index as a percentage. Items with a difficulty index above 70% are considered relatively easy, and those below 30% are classified as difficult.

> *Once the exam is scored, return it to the class and discuss test items.*

Example: $\dfrac{H+L}{T} \times 100 = $ Item Difficulty

$H = 8$
$L = 4$
$T = 20$

$\dfrac{8+4}{20} \times 100 = 60\%$

With the above example, there were 20 scores selected for analysis. Of those 20, eight from the group of high scorers and four from the group of low scorers answered this question correctly, thereby resulting in an item difficulty index of 60% for this test question.

To determine how an item was responded to by both high and low achievers, complete the following:

1) Score the exams and rank the scores in order from highest to lowest number of correct responses.
2) Select the exams for approximately the top 25% and bottom 25% of scores and add the number of correct responses in each group (high scorers and low scorers) for each question on the exam.
3) Subtract the number of correct responses of the low scoring group (L) from that of the high scoring group (H), and divide by half the total number in the sample groups (.5T).
4) Express the difficulty index as a decimal.

Example: $\dfrac{H-L}{0.5T} = $ Item Discrimination

$H = 8$
$L = 4$
$T = 20$

$\dfrac{8-4}{0.5(20)} = +0.40$

With the above example, there were again 20 scores selected for analysis. Of those 20, eight from the group of high scorers and four from the group of low scorers answered this question correctly, thereby resulting in a discrimination index of +0.40 for this test question.

Difficulty indices will range from -1.00 to $+1.00$. Those items that discriminate effectively between high and low scorers have a discrimination index of $+0.40$ or better. These items are answered correctly more often by high scorers than low scorers and are valid test questions. Items that are answered correctly equally between high scorers and low scorers have a discrimination index of 0.00. A negative discrimination index identifies that more low scoring students answered a question correctly than did high scorers and these questions should be reviewed for validity.

Once the difficulty and discrimination indices have been calculated, the information should be charted and analyzed. Figure 8.2 provides a chart of sample item analysis data. When analyzing these results, it is important to adhere to the following guidelines:

• Items with a high difficulty index are usually too easy and should be modified to make them more difficult by rephrasing the statement or providing more plausible distractors.

Test: Medical Emergencies		EMT-Basic Course #2		Date: 12/5/94

		Number students taking the exam	40	
		Number students scoring in upper 25% of class	10	
		Number students scoring in lower 25% of class	10	

	Totals		Difficulty Index	Discrimination Index
Item #	High (H)	Low (L)	$\dfrac{H + L}{T} \times 100$	$\dfrac{H - L}{.5T}$
1	10	10	100%	0.00
2	10	5	75%	+0.50
3	8	10	90%	-0.20
4	0	2	10%	-0.20
5	7	3	50%	+0.40
6	4	4	40%	0.00
7	10	0	50%	+1.00
8	9	3	60%	+0.60
9	6	2	40%	+0.40
10	10	3	65%	+0.70

FIGURE 8.2 Sample Item Analysis Report (*adapted from TIPS[2]*).

- Items with a discrimination index below +0.19 or with negative indices should be revised.
- Items with discrimination indices between +0.20 and +0.39 should be examined for errors.
- Most items on an exam should be targeted at the 50% difficulty level. Extremely easy or difficult questions should be modified accordingly.
- Select a few items that are relatively easy (80% to 90%) and a few that are relatively difficult (10% to 20%).
- Use items with a discrimination power of +0.40 or higher.

These guidelines should produce exams that result in a wider range of scores, with most scores occurring in the middle as identified in a normal bell curve. For the scores presented in Figure 8.2 items should be revised as follows:

Item #	Revision
1	Revise to increase difficulty
2	No revision necessary
3	Review and revise wording
4	Review and revise wording
5	No revision necessary
6	Revise to increase difficulty
7	No revision necessary

Item #	Revision
8	No revision necessary
9	No revision necessary
10	No revision necessary

STATISTICAL CONCEPTS OF TESTING

In order for test scores to describe student progress adequately, they must be analyzed and judged against certain criteria. To do this, test results must be placed into arithmetic measurements.

A *frequency distribution* describes a set of test scores by listing all possible scores and the number of students achieving each score, as shown in Boxes 8.1 through 8.3.

The *mean* of a set of scores is simply the average of scores, and can be identified by summing all scores and dividing the total by the number of scores. The mean is the most commonly used standard of determining how well a class performed on an exam. For the scores identified in Box 8.1, the mean score is 84.43.

The mean is the most commonly used standard of determining how well a class performed on an exam.

BOX 8.1 Test Scores of 30 Students

Student	Score	Student	Score	Student	Score
1	98	11	85	21	84
2	76	12	92	22	78
3	83	13	100	23	82
4	86	14	76	24	96
5	85	15	75	25	79
6	92	16	92	26	82
7	86	17	83	27	73
8	94	18	83	28	83
9	83	19	86	29	87
10	79	20	68	30	88

Test scores of 30 students.

BOX 8.2 Frequency Distribution for 30 Scores

Score	Frequency	Score	Frequency	Score	Frequency
100	1	89	0	78	1
99	0	88	1	77	0
98	1	87	1	76	2
97	0	86	3	75	0
96	1	85	2	74	1
95	0	84	1	73	1
94	1	83	5	72	0
93	0	82	2	71	0
92	3	81	0	70	0
91	0	80	0	69	0
90	0	79	2	68	1

Frequency distribution for 30 scores.

BOX 8.3 Grouped Frequency Distribution

Score	Frequency
95–100	3
90–94	4
85–89	7
80–84	8
75–79	5
70–74	2
65–69	1
60–64	0

Grouped frequency distribution.

The *median* is the score that divides the distribution in half, whereby 50% of scores fall above and 50% fall below the median. For the scores identified in Box 8.1, the median score is the middle score, in this case 85. In this example, 15 scores fell at or above 85 and 15 scores fell below 85. If there were only 25 student scores in a distribution, the 13th score would be the median.

The *mode* is the score that occurs most frequently in a distribution. The mode of the scores in Box 8.2 is 83 since five students scored an 83 and no other score occurred more often.

TEST VALIDITY AND RELIABILITY

Validity refers to the extent to which a test measures what it is intended to measure. Without validity, exams cannot accurately reflect student progress and performance. Test validity incorporates three areas: content, criterion, and construction[1].

Validity

Content validity is extremely important to measure student academic and performance skill levels accurately. To establish content validity, it is necessary to determine if the test assesses the skills and knowledge intended by the instructional objectives. In order to be valid, the test must be representative of the material presented during the course.

Consequences of administering a test that is not representative of the skills and knowledge taught are threefold. First, students cannot demonstrate skills they possess if the skills are not tested. Second, students may answer questions incorrectly when information was not taught or is considered irrelevant.

Lastly, irrelevant questions will result in poor test scores, leading to bad feelings of students. They may begin to question the competency of instructors or their own ability to learn material. Administering tests that cannot measure student performance adequately relative to course content presented may have a significant effect on student's self-confidence and self-esteem.

To ensure test validity, it is essential that test items be developed from course established objectives. Each test question should be referenced to at least one course objective. If a question cannot be so referenced, provided objectives were appropriately written and instruction was provided to meet such objectives, the question should not be used.

In order to be valid, the test must be representative of the material presented during the course.

Each test question should be referenced to at least one course objective.

Reliability

Criterion validity refers to the relationship between test scores and scores representing some type of norm. For example, state EMS written exams are often validated by providing statistical information for a specific class as well as information for other classes testing around the same time.

Reliability is the measurement of consistency for a test. For example, if one version of a test is administered to a student, and a second version of the same test given to the same student, scores should be the same or the test would not be considered reliable.

> *Reliability* is the measurement of consistency for a test.

KEY POINTS

1. There are five basic question types that can be used effectively to assess students' progress, including true-false, multiple-choice, matching, short-answer, and essay questions.
2. Review true-false questions to ensure they are written with a clear-cut true or false answer; avoid using specific determiners such as all, none, always, and never; and avoid developing trick questions.
3. When creating multiple-choice questions, use between three and four plausible distractors of equal length; place all key words in the stem of the question rather than in the options, avoid providing grammatical clues; and make certain there is a single correct answer.
4. When developing matching sections, construct items that are homogenous in content; provide 10 to 15 items for each section; provide more options than necessary; and make certain responses are plausible.
5. Short-answer questions take on two formats: questions and completion items. When developing such questions ensure that they are worded so there is only one correct answer; create blanks of equal length with a limit of two blanks per question; and place blanks toward the end of the statement.
6. Use essay-type questions to assess higher-level skills such as organizing information, developing a plan, comparing and contrasting positions or issues, formulating conclusions, explaining the application of certain principles, or describing the cause-and-effect relationship between items.
7. When scoring essay-type questions, refrain from looking at the examinee's name prior to reading responses; read a sample of responses in order to establish a range for judging group overall performance; disregard grammar and writing skills unless such criteria were previously established; and develop a model answer with which to evaluate examinee responses.
8. After scoring examinations, perform an item analysis to calculate item difficulty and discrimination indices. Use the results to modify test questions in order to increase the effectiveness and validity of such exams.

FOLLOW-UP ACTIVITIES

1. Develop a 10-question true-false quiz using the guidelines presented in this chapter.
2. Develop two essay questions complete with directions and guidelines as presented in this chapter.
3. Develop a 10-question completion quiz using the guidelines presented in this chapter.
4. Develop a 10-question multiple-choice quiz using the guidelines presented in this chapter.
5. Develop two matching sections, consisting of at least 10 items per section, using the guidelines presented in this chapter.
6. Develop a diagram that requires examinees to either match items or complete statements.
7. Administer the above exams to a group of students and provide the following statistical information based on their scores:
   - Mean
   - Mode
   - Median
   - Difficulty index of each question
   - Discrimination index for each question

REFERENCES

1. Wiersma W, Jurs S. *Educational Measurement and Testing.* Boston MA: Allyn and Bacon, Inc.; 1985.
2. *Teaching Improvement Project Systems For Health Care Educators (TIPS).* Lexington, KY: Center for Learning Resources, College of Allied Health Professions, University of Kentucky.

9 Course Coordination

Upon completion of this chapter, the reader will have sufficient information to:

1. List three roles and responsibilities for key training personnel, and qualifications for each.
2. Develop a budget for training programs.
3. Describe five factors to consider when scheduling and using instructional staff including primary instructors, assistant instructors, and guest lecturers.
4. State the role of clinical and field affiliations in EMS training.
5. Identify five factors to consider when affiliating with clinical facilities.
6. List class materials that should be provided the first night of class.
7. Describe key information that should be included in a student course overview.
8. Describe the process and need for conducting student counseling sessions.
9. Develop effective course evaluation forms for instructors, students, and administrative personnel to use while analyzing the effectiveness of training programs.
10. Identify key elements of documentation for training programs.
11. List 10 types of class records that should be maintained.
12. Identify three areas of legal liability for training programs.
13. Describe principle elements of the professional code of ethics for educators.
14. Define and provide three examples of discrimination and sexual harassment.
15. Describe elements of legal issues regarding the use of copyrighted materials.

KEY TERMS

Administrative director The individual responsible for the overall administration of a training program; sometimes referred to as the program director

Assistant instructor An individual who assists a primary instructor with skills instruction; also referred to as practical skills instructor or lab instructor

Clinical facility An institution or agency that, in coordination with an accredited training institute, provides medical direction and continual assessment of student performance for in-hospital observation and skill performance

Defamation The act of attacking or injuring the reputation or honor of an individual by false and malicious statements

Discrimination The showing of partiality or prejudice in treatment generally directed against a minority group

Field affiliation A licensed ambulance service that, in coordination with an accredited training institute, provides continual assessment of student performance of prehospital observation and skill performance

Field internship The portion of required training during which a student obtains a supervised learning experience on a licensed prehospital emergency care unit

Harassment The act of troubling, worrying, or tormenting an individual by repeated attacks or actions

Libel A false and malicious written or printed statement, or any sign or picture that accuses another of immoral or unlawful conduct, thereby exposing the individual to public ridicule or injuring the individual's reputation in any way

Malpractice Unprofessional treatment or neglect, misconduct, or improper practice in any professional or official position

National Standard Curriculum The current edition of a specific national training program adopted by the Department of Transportation, and amendments or revision thereto

Negligence Failure to use a reasonable amount of care resulting in injury or damage to another

Preceptor An individual who evaluates a student's performance in a prehospital or in-hospital clinical setting

Standard of care The level of conduct expected of similarly trained professionals in a given field

Training institute An educational institution approved by state or other regulatory authorities to provide EMS training

INTRODUCTION

Course coordination is the basis for EMS training success. A poorly coordinated program will most likely result in poorly trained, frustrated students. On the other hand, a well planned, coordinated, and executed program, should result in a highly effective training program producing well-prepared, highly skilled, qualified EMS providers.

Many individuals, with various skills and responsibilities, comprise the training staff. The abilities and enthusiasm of such personnel ultimately dictate how successful a training program will be. Effective coordination of a training program requires extensive organizational skills and the implementation of policies and procedures that place emphasis on students and the learning process, and on ways to improve these.

Course coordination involves multiple tasks including securing facilities and training equipment, selecting and preparing instructional staff, scheduling and announcing programs, affiliating and scheduling with clinical sites, preparing necessary course materials, and other necessary tasks. The manner in which these tasks are completed will influence the effectiveness and ease with which a training program proceeds.

In addition to specific coordination tasks, a quality training program requires forethought into legal and ethical liability factors that may influence the outcome of training, and implementation of policies and procedures to protect all individuals involved.

> *A well planned, coordinated, and executed program, should result in a highly effective training program producing well-prepared, highly skilled, qualified EMS providers.*

TRAINING ORGANIZATION KEY PERSONNEL

The administration of EMS training programs requires significant coordination, planning, and preparation. Key personnel required to successfully implement a training program include a program manager or administrative director, course coordinator, instructional staff, an equipment maintenance person, a counselor, a medical director, and a fiscal analyst.

Qualifications for each job vary and may be determined by each state and one individual could perform multiple responsibilities. General recommended qualifications along with job responsibilities for each staff position are provided below.

Administrative Director

The administrative director, or program director, is ultimately responsible for all aspects of a training program, including course planning, operation, and evaluation. Specific duties include but are not limited to:

> *The administrative director, or program director, is ultimately responsible for all aspects of a training program.*

- Scheduling courses and assigning course coordinators and/or instructors
- Preparing and distributing course announcements
- Processing course registration forms and supervising the student selection process
- Preparing, maintaining, procuring, and taking inventory of all necessary training equipment
- Preparing exposure control plans
- Evaluating training programs including all course written and practical skills examination results and course evaluation forms
- Maintaining all training files and student records
- Serving as a student/faculty liaison
- Maintaining the quality of classes
- Overseeing the handling of financial matters
- Grant writing and research
- Coordinating with community colleges and universities as appropriate
- Serving as liaison and coordinating with community colleges as necessary

Qualifications
The administrative director of a training program may have additional responsibilities depending on the organization itself, but in general, the recommended qualifications for this individual would include:

- A degree in education
- Management experience (*eg,* personnel issues, discipline and conflict resolution, budgets, planning)
- Minimum certification as an EMT
- Current state certification as an EMT and CPR instructor

Course Coordinator
The course coordinator is responsible for overseeing and coordinating individual class sessions of emergency care training programs. Such responsibilities might include:

- Scheduling qualified primary and assistant instructors and ensuring that an instructor/student ratio of 1:6 is maintained for practical work
- Scheduling qualified evaluators and victims for course exams
- Preparing and assisting guest lecturers with audiovisual material
- Reviewing with all instructors and assistant instructors their responsibilities during each class session
- Ensuring that all training and visual aids are at the disposal of a designated instructor as necessary
- Assuming responsibility for classroom facilities by ensuring that rooms are kept neat and orderly and making certain local policies are enforced
- Being accountable for all training aids, equipment, and course materials and ensuring their proper use and storage while at a training site
- Maintaining a safe and effective learning environment for students
- Providing appropriate feedback by identifying and reporting any student or instructor problem or weakness
- Providing counseling services to students and instructors as necessary

The course coordinator is responsible for overseeing and coordinating individual class sessions of emergency care training programs.

- Scheduling student clinical observation and internship rotations
- Acting as liaison between the training institutes, students, and clinical facilities
- Ensuring that Department of Transportation lesson plans and skill sheets are adhered to by all instructors, and reporting any discrepancies to the administrative director
- Ensuring that course goals and objectives are met
- Supplementing lecture material as needed to meet lesson plan requirements
- Organizing and supervising all practical exercise activities including coordinating the use of assistant instructors and maintaining high performance standards
- Evaluating instructor performance with regard to information presented as well as instructional methods and teaching activities
- Being prepared to assume the role of primary instructor when a scheduled instructor cancels on short notice
- Maintaining appropriate student and class records
- Maintaining instructor attendance/participation records as required
- Protecting the privacy of students and the confidentiality of course records as required
- Serving as a positive role model by maintaining appropriate personal hygiene and appearance; recognizing personal limitation by seeking assistance when appropriate; and displaying personal mental and physical health

Qualifications

The course coordinator should be knowledgeable in all aspects of EMS training including state reporting requirements. Qualifications for this individual include:

- Some management or coordination experience
- Knowledge of educational principles and instructional design
- Knowledge of patient care protocols and state regulatory agency requirements (if applicable)
- Current state certification as an EMT instructor
- Current certification as a CPR instructor
- Minimum of 3 years experience as an EMT-Basic (or higher)

The course coordinator should be knowledgeable in all aspects of EMS training including state reporting requirements.

Instructional Staff

Instructional staff consists of primary and assistant instructors. While it is optimal to use the same instructors for an entire training program, unless a training institute has full-time faculty devoted to such training, it is often difficult to do so. Most EMS instructors are part-time contracted employees with other full-time responsibilities. As such, they may not be available to teach multiple sessions. This problem may lead to inconsistencies in training and a fragmented program.

Primary Instructors

Primary instructors are usually responsible for teaching individual class sessions. They generally present a lecture, facilitate discussions, and orchestrate practical skill sessions. Primary instructors usually receive some type of certification or recognition from a state governing agency by participating in an approved instructional methodology course, or by possessing other credentials such as a degree in education or teaching certificate.

Primary instructors are usually responsible for teaching individual class sessions.

Specific responsibilities of primary instructors might include:

- Providing a safe and effective learning environment
- Providing appropriate feedback to students and course coordinators as necessary
- Completing appropriate student and course records as required by regulatory agencies
- Presenting course material following the National Standard Curriculum
- Consistently monitoring student performance and evaluating for safe and effective performance in accordance with established state and national standards
- Ensuring that training equipment is maintained in a safe and acceptable working condition
- Protecting the privacy of students and the confidentiality of training records as required
- Orienting and supervising assistant instructors
- Serving as a positive role model by exhibiting personal mental and physical health, maintaining appropriate personal hygiene and appearance, and recognizing personal limitations by seeking assistance when appropriate

Qualifications
- Current state certification as an EMT instructor
- Current certification as a CPR instructor (recommended)
- Minimum of 1 year experience as an EMT-Basic (3 years recommended)
- Knowledge of all aspects of prehospital emergency care and techniques
- Knowledge of principles of adult education
- Demonstration of competence in teaching both didactic and practical skills portions of the curriculum by serving as an assistant instructor for a minimum of one EMT course in order to prove teaching abilities

Assistant Instructors
Assistant instructors teach hands-on skills training. Most EMS training programs require an instructor:student ratio of 1:6 for skills practice. When classes are divided into practice groups, they are usually led by assistant instructors.

Assistant instructors often have not participated in an instructional methodology course but hopefully have attended at least a 6-hour assistant instructor course, which teaches them basic principles of learning and how to teach practical skills, as well as administrative aspects of a particular training institute.

> Most EMS training programs require an instructor:student ratio of 1:6 for skills practice.

Qualifications
- Participation in an assistant instructor course
- Current certification as a CPR instructor (recommended)
- Minimum 1 year experience as an EMT-Basic (recommended)

Guest Lecturers
Guest lecturers are not certified "EMT instructors" but possess advanced education in a specialty field. Emergency department physicians and nurses are often used as guest lecturers as are some EMT paramedics and respiratory technicians.

Evaluators

Evaluators are those individuals responsible for ensuring student proficiency at skill performance stations. It is recommended that evaluators not evaluate those students whom they have taught previously, are related to, or are members of the same EMS service.

Specific responsibilities of evaluators include:

- Evaluating student performance during practical skills evaluation testing
- Documenting unsatisfactory skill performance using state-approved evaluation forms
- Using only scenarios approved by regulatory agencies
- Putting students at ease by providing a calm testing environment
- Exhibiting good personal hygiene, a neat and well-groomed appearance, and refraining from smoking, eating, and drinking while evaluating students
- Protecting the privacy of students and the confidentiality of training records as required

Qualifications
- Participation in an evaluator course
- Current certification as a CPR instructor (recommended for all, required for those evaluating CPR skills)
- Minimum 1 year experience as an EMT-Basic (3 years recommended)

Victims

Programmed victims are used for course practical skills exams and practice sessions to provide realism in the training environment. Some state regulatory agencies may have minimum age requirements for victims in order to decrease the risk of liability.

It is recommended that victims not be used when evaluating fellow class members, members of the same service, or those to whom they are related. To increase the realism of practice emergency situations, victims should be oriented to the role playing scenarios and be moulaged appropriately.

Preceptors

Preceptors are responsible for evaluating and ensuring student proficiency during clinical and field affiliation rotations. Specific responsibilities of evaluators include:

- Providing the opportunity for students to practice skills in order to obtain proficiency
- Serving as a positive role model
- Evaluating student performance of skills
- Providing feedback to students regarding their ability to meet program objectives successfully as they relate to skill performance
- Providing remedial training in specific skills, as necessary
- Accurately documenting student performance of skills in the hospital or field setting

Qualifications
- Current state certification at the level for which they are precepting
- Current certification as an EMT instructor (recommended)

Evaluators are those individuals responsible for ensuring student proficiency at skill performance stations.

Preceptors are responsible for evaluating and ensuring student proficiency during clinical and field affiliation rotations.

- Minimum of 1 year experience at current level of training (3 years recommended)
- Attendance at a training program designed to teach individuals how to be an effective preceptor (recommended)
- Approval by the medical director
- Knowledge of all aspects of prehospital emergency care and skill performance
- Knowledge of all aspects of evaluation, documentation, and reporting requirements as identified by the sponsoring agency
- Knowledge of principles of adult education
- Demonstration of competence in performing and teaching practical skills included in the National Standard Curriculum

Equipment Maintenance Person

The equipment person is responsible for all aspects of EMS training equipment. Such responsibilities include:

- Maintaining a complete EMS training equipment and audiovisual aids inventory
- Ensuring the working order of all equipment, and repairing items as necessary
- Being knowledgeable of proper infection control procedures and following appropriate guidelines
- Notifying a supervisor when items are in need of additional repair or when parts need to be ordered
- Ensuring that equipment is available when needed
- Transporting equipment to appropriate facilities as necessary

Counselor

The counselor is responsible for making counseling sessions available upon student request in order to address academic deficiencies or personality conflicts. Responsibilities include:

> The counselor is responsible for making counseling sessions available upon student request in order to address academic deficiencies or personality conflicts.

- Making counseling sessions available upon student request, or at the course coordinator's discretion, to discuss educational difficulties, skill performance deficiencies, or personality conflicts
- Maintaining appropriate documentation regarding counseling sessions
- Educating students about the grievance process

Qualifications

The administrative director or course coordinator often serves as the counselor for students with problems interfering with learning. The individual serving as the counselor should be knowledgeable in how to deal with people and conflict resolution strategies. Additional qualification for this individual would include:

- Some counseling experience
- Knowledge of state regulatory agency requirements (if applicable)
- Current state certification as an EMT instructor
- The ability to communicate effectively with individuals

Medical Director

The medical director is responsible for providing oversight, ensuring the quality of educational experiences for all training programs, and providing assistance to the administrative director and course coordinator as needed.

The medical director has ultimate authority regarding course con-

The medical director has ultimate authority regarding course content and emergency procedures and protocols.

tent and emergency procedures and protocols within the confines of the National Standard Curriculum. Additional responsibilities might include:

- Providing oversight to ensure that course content complies with standards set forth in the National Standard Curriculum(s) or other approved courses
- Providing oversight to assist with the recruitment, selection, and orientation of instructional faculty
- Providing technical advice and assistance to instructional faculty and students
- Providing oversight to ensure the quality of educational experiences.

Qualifications

The medical director should provide technical advice and insight into medical aspects of EMS training, such as the proper method for applying a device. The individual should be knowledgeable in emergency medicine.

He should also be well versed in adult educational principles and EMS training. Preferably, this individual would have participated in an EMS training program in order to understand specific aspects of such training and in order to suggest methods to improve it. Qualifications include:

- A medical license (MD or DO) in the state in which he is serving as medical director (preferably board-certified by state EMS)
- Knowledge of state regulatory agency requirements (if applicable)
- Past experience in the delivery of training programs
- Current certification as a CPR or ACLS Instructor (preferred)

Fiscal Analyst

The fiscal analyst is responsible for all financial matters relative to training programs. Such responsibilities might include:

- Posting payments for student tuition
- Generating bills for outstanding balances
- Preparing purchase orders for books, equipment, and other instructional supplies and materials
- Ordering necessary equipment and supplies
- Preparing payments for outstanding bills
- Generating instructor payments (as appropriate)
- Maintaining account balance ledgers as necessary

Qualifications

The fiscal analyst should be knowledgeable in all aspects of accounts receivable and accounts payable. Recommended minimum qualifications for this individual would include:

- Coursework in accounting principles
- Knowledge of computer programs such as dBase and Lotus.

The fiscal analyst should be knowledgeable in all aspects of accounts receivable and accounts payable.

PLANNING AND IMPLEMENTING TRAINING PROGRAMS

The planning process is extremely important to the overall success of a training program. Through effective planning, the administrative di-

BOX 9.1　Preparation Checklist

Three Months Prior to a Course

- Select dates for the training program.
- Select and reserve an appropriate training site, (ensuring adequate size, lighting, ventilation, and accessibility).
- Mail a facility agreement.
- Create and distribute course announcements.
- Assign a course coordinator.
- Schedule primary and assistant instructors.
- Mail instructor agreements.
- Locate and reserve appropriate audiovisual aids.
- Order books, workbooks, skill sheets, and other course materials.
- Ensure that equipment is in working order.
- Order duplication of class materials (*eg,* handouts, course overviews, reading lists, syllabus).

Three Weeks Prior to a Course

- Determine number of participants registered for the program.
- Send confirmation letters and directions to classroom location (if appropriate).
- Make certain duplication material, books, and other supplies have been received.
- Make certain audiovisual aids have been reserved; review audiovisual materials prior to class session.
- Submit regulatory agency paperwork (if required).

Day of Training

- Arrive for class at least 30 minutes prior to start.
- Check that training equipment, including audiovisual equipment, is in working condition.
- Organize materials on a table or lectern.
- Make certain room arrangement meets the needs of the session. Move furniture as necessary.
- Tape audiovisual equipment electrical cords to floor (if appropriate).
- Check for spare bulbs for audiovisual equipment.
- Make certain chalk, pens, and markers are available

Course preparation checklist (adapted from Margolis and Bell, 1986[1]).

rector and course coordinator can anticipate problems and help a program run smoothly.

One of the most important components of effective EMS training is preparation. A task analysis can help with such preparation. It involves identifying all key steps required to conduct a training program effectively and efficiently. Once key elements of a program are identified, they must be prioritized and placed into a time line in order of what tasks must be completed first.

Checklists are an important part of a task analysis and course development. Box 9.1 identifies tasks that should be completed in order to improve chances of success with a training program. Requirements and time lines may vary from state to state.

One of the most important components of effective EMS training is preparation.

An appropriate facility promotes learning because it is free of distractions.

Facility

The facility itself is extremely important to the learning process. Every environment creates its own climate and mood. An appropriate facility promotes learning because it is free of distractions. The preferable location has adequate classroom space, secured storage for training equipment, and is of sufficient size to conduct didactic and skills instruction as well as performance evaluation sessions.

The facility should also be convenient and accessible. If the classroom is located on the third floor of a building with no elevators, and the equipment is on the first floor, students may be exhausted before the class starts, especially if they are asked to help move equipment. The room should also be easily accessible to students. If an individual has to go through three locked doors and a security guard to enter the classroom, he may become discouraged and annoyed prior to class, or may arrive late.

Finally, the room should be comfortable. It must have adequate lighting, a comfortable temperature, and be free from noise and distractions. Classrooms should be properly ventilated with comfortable chairs and adequate tables or other writing surfaces. The room should also have electrical outlets that are accessible for audiovisual equipment without bulky extension cords.

Scheduling

How and when a program is scheduled and announced may affect the number of attendees. Sufficient time should be allotted to allow for adequate distribution of course announcements. A yearly schedule is recommended, with individual course announcements distributed a minimum of 3 months prior to the start of a program.

When scheduling a training program, it is important to take into account the time of day, day of week, and time of the year the program is offered. Evening programs should allow students time to return from work and eat supper prior to the beginning of class. Training sessions should also accommodate students with religious obligations. Saturday evenings and Sunday mornings may be difficult times for many students to participate in training programs.

Announcing Courses

Training programs should be announced a minimum of 3 months prior to the start of a class, although additional time is recommended. The announcement should include a course description, course fee, location, class dates and times, and an application deadline date. A sample course announcement is provided in Appendix E.

Course announcements should be distributed to all potential students. This might include ambulance services, fire departments, police departments, government agencies, municipalities, colleges, and universities. Programs can also be announced in newspapers and community publications.

Budget Considerations

It is the administration's responsibility to ensure adequate funding to conduct training programs.

It is the administration's responsibility to ensure adequate funding to conduct training programs. Generally, a budget is developed for a training department and includes various training programs. It is important for course coordinators and instructors to understand the financial limitations that may exist. Figure 9.1 identifies a sample budget and Figure 9.2 shows a sample year-to-date expense versus revenue budget comparison format.

PDQ EMS Training Institute

	EMT Class (3 Classes)	EMT-Refresher (2 Classes)	First Responder (2 Classes)	FR-Refresher (2 Classes)	Other	Total
INCOME						
Tuition EMT Class	42000	0	0	0	0	42000
Tuition EMT-Refresher Class	0	9000	0	0	0	9000
Tuition FR Class	0	0	8000	0	0	8000
Tuition FR-Refresher Class	0	0	0	3000	0	3000
Tuition Continuing Education	0	0	0	0	6000	6000
Tuition Instructor Training	0	0	0	0	4000	4000
Tuition Other	0	0	0	0	3000	3000
Fees	0	0	0	0	2500	2500
Contributions	0	0	0	0	10000	10000
Interest	0	0	0	0	1200	1200
Miscellaneous	0	0	0	0	1796	1796
Total Income	42000	9000	8000	3000	28496	90496
EXPENDITURES						
Instructor Fees	16617	2820	4444	1740	1200	26821
CPR Certification Cards	480	240	240	160	1000	2120
Textbook Purchase	5760	1800	2880	1200	500	12140
Audiovisual Purchase	0	0	0	0	1200	1200
Training Equipment (Capital)	0	0	0	0	4000	4000
Training Supplies (Disposables)	5640	3150	2340	1560	2500	15190
Training Equipment Maintenance	100	100	100	100	100	500
Administration Supplies	6000	1000	1500	800	700	10000
Library Book Purchase	0	0	0	0	1500	1500
Periodical Subscriptions	0	0	0	0	300	300
Advertising Costs	0	0	0	0	200	200
Award Program	0	0	0	0	250	250
Staff Training	0	0	0	0	250	250
Legal Fees	0	0	0	0	500	500
Insurance	0	0	0	0	2500	2500
Accounting Fees	0	0	0	0	500	500
Travel Expenses	200	50	100	50	200	600
Duplicating Costs	1800	900	900	600	2000	6200
Postage	0	0	0	0	5000	5000
Tuition Refunds	150	100	100	75	50	475
Miscellaneous	50	50	50	50	50	250
Total Expenditures	36797	10210	12654	6335	24500	90496

FIGURE 9.1 Sample Training Budget

A budget includes income and expenditures. Income includes any projected income through tuition, donations, or book sales. Expenditures are any bills generated for which the organization is responsible.

When developing a course budget, administrators should also take into account facility costs such as electricity, phones, postage, duplicating, printing, travel expenses, and associated costs. Salaries for adjunct personnel such as administrative support personnel (*eg,* fiscal analyst, receptionist, clerical staff) should also be included. While these may not be directly related to a specific course, such costs may need to be covered by dividing it evenly throughout all training programs.

Training programs can be funded by a variety of sources. Some training institutes are private, nonprofit entities. Others are part of hospitals, universities, or government agencies.

The reason an institute chooses to conduct training programs may determine budgetary constraints. For example, if a hospital conducts programs as a "public relations" service, it may not be necessary for

```
┌─────────────────────────────────────────────────────┐
│              PDQ EMS Training Institute               │
│                                                       │
│                    Year To Date                       │
│                                                       │
│                 Actual        Budget                  │
│                                                       │
│  INCOME                                               │
│                                                       │
│  Tuition EMT Class                          42000     │
│  Tuition EMT-Refresher Class                 9000     │
│  Tuition FR Class                            8000     │
│  Tuition FR-Refresher Class                  3000     │
│  Tuition Continuing Education                6000     │
│  Tuition Instructor Training                 4000     │
│  Tuition Other                               3000     │
│  Fees                                        2500     │
│  Contributions                              10000     │
│  Interest                                    1200     │
│  Miscellaneous                               1796     │
│                                                       │
│  Total Income                               90496     │
│                                                       │
│                                                       │
│                                                       │
│  EXPENDITURES                                         │
│                                                       │
│  Instructor Fees                            26821     │
│  CPR Certification Cards                     2120     │
│  Textbook Purchase                          12140     │
│  Audiovisual Purchase                        1200     │
│  Training Equipment (Capital)                4000     │
│  Training Supplies (Disposables)            15190     │
│  Training Equipment Maintenance               500     │
│  Administration Supplies                    10000     │
│  Library Book Purchase                       1500     │
│  Periodical Subscriptions                     300     │
│  Advertising Costs                            200     │
│  Award Program                                250     │
│  Staff Training                               250     │
│  Legal Fees                                   500     │
│  Insurance                                   2500     │
│  Accounting Fees                              500     │
│  Travel Expenses                              600     │
│  Duplicating Costs                           6200     │
│  Postage                                     5000     │
│  Tuition Refunds                              475     │
│  Miscellaneous                                250     │
│                                                       │
│  Total Expenditures                         90496     │
└─────────────────────────────────────────────────────┘
```

FIGURE 9.2 Sample Expense/Revenue Budget Comparison

income to cover all expenses; the hospital may be willing to subsidize the program. Government agencies are often subsidized, at least in part, from an outside source and, therefore, may not be as concerned with covering all associated costs.

If an organization conducts training programs in order to train their own personnel, they will most likely cover the cost of all programs. Income from tuition will most likely not cover expenses, in which case funds must be generated from a different area within the organization.

Regardless of specific instances surrounding the development of a budget, the end result is a boundary for which monies can be spent. If equipment breaks, and there is no money allocated for repairs, it may not be possible to fix the equipment until the next fiscal year. Likewise, if too many instructors are scheduled for a particular session (more than had been allocated in the budget), fewer instructors may be scheduled for future sessions in order to balance the budget.

Assigning Instructors

It is usually the course coordinator's responsibility to assign instructional faculty. When doing so, it is important to ensure instructor qualifications. Copies of current credentials (*eg,* EMT paramedic, EMT instructor, CPR instructor) should be kept on file in the training institute office for review and audit as necessary.

Once a list of qualified instructors has been developed, the course coordinator should assign primary instructors and determine how many assistant instructors are necessary for each class session.

Primary Instructors

It is optimal to have the same primary instructor teach all sessions of a course, in order to ensure continuity within a training program. However, unless these individuals are full-time employees of a training institute, this is usually not possible. More often, a course is conducted by multiple primary instructors.

If it is not possible for one instructor to conduct an entire course, the use of team teaching may increase the continuity of a training program. With team teaching, a small group of primary and assistant instructors is used throughout an entire program. They learn to communicate with each other and become accustomed to the way information is presented and the accuracy with which it is taught. Instructor meetings are essential for maintaining the consistency throughout the course.

> It is optimal to have the same primary instructor teach all sessions of a course.

Assistant Instructors

Assistant instructors are routinely needed for those lessons requiring the demonstration and practice of skills. Lessons with a large number of psychomotor objectives will most likely require assistant instructors. These instructors also evaluate student competency during practical skill exams.

From a budgetary viewpoint, it is best to combine lecture-type lessons into one class session, and then have a separate class of combined practical sessions. For example, during patient assessment lessons, rather than requiring assistant instructors to attend 1 hour of three consecutive classes in order to demonstrate various patient assessment techniques, it would be more beneficial to combine the lecture/demonstration sessions into two 3-hour sessions and combine the last 3 hours into a full practice session.

While educators may argue in theory that it is best to teach a little and practice a little, budgetary constraints may prevent such in application. Likewise, the time it takes for equipment set up and clean up, 1-hour practice modules may waste too much class time.

It is estimated that approximately 36 to 40 hours of the 110 hour EMT-Basic curriculum require the use of assistant instructors. It is recommended, however, that one assistant instructor be assigned to attend the entire program to help the primary instructor with simple demonstrations, obtaining equipment and other tasks during a training session.

> Lessons with a large number of psychomotor objectives will most likely require assistant instructors.

Guest Lecturers

Guest lecturers can provide added expertise on certain topics. Emergency department physicians, Critical Incident Stress Debriefing (CISD) team members, nurses, and respiratory technicians may provide valuable information during EMS training programs as guest lecturers. When using these individuals, it is important to explain course objectives fully as well as what information is to be covered in a specific lesson.

In addition, it is helpful if guest lecturers understand the audience to whom they are teaching, so information can be provided at their level of knowledge and understanding. A common complaint when using guest lecturers is that students do not understand the jargon used. A physician in the emergency department needs to be able to communicate experiences using terminology that EMS students can understand and relate to.

Guest lecturers should also be informed on what tasks the group will be permitted to perform at the conclusion of a course. For example, it would be inappropriate for a respiratory therapist to provide information relevant to intubation if he is teaching an EMT-Basic class that may not be authorized to use such a skill.

Affiliating with Clinical Facilities

Clinical facilities such as ambulance services, hospitals, clinics, and physician's offices can be used at both Basic Life Support (BLS) and Advanced Life Support (ALS) training levels. For BLS programs, time requirements for a clinical facility are minimum; at present only 10 hours of clinical time per student is required for EMT programs.

When affiliating with clinical facilities, it is important to use one contact person for scheduling rotations and evaluating student progress.

For EMT-Intermediate and other advanced EMT modules, time requirements increase. In addition, with ALS training programs, including paramedic and prehospital nursing programs, time and liability requirements for clinical facilities increase dramatically. To decrease potential problems when affiliating with clinical facilities, it is important to use one contact person for scheduling rotations and evaluating student progress.

Facilities

There are primarily two types of clinical facilities that serve to provide clinical experience for EMS students in hospital and field facilities. Clinical affiliations are usually hospital critical care departments. In ALS training programs, students may be permitted to attend multiple clinical sites, often termed *primary* and *secondary sites.*

The primary site generally provides in-hospital experience within the emergency department, critical care units, maternity and pediatric departments, the operating room, and the morgue. The secondary clinical site is used primarily to provide the opportunity for additional field training experience to obtain proficiency in ALS skills.

CLINICAL (IN-HOSPITAL) AFFILIATIONS

The 1994 EMT-Basic National Standard Curriculum requires that students to assess and interview a minimum of five patients, and document their interaction using approved regulatory agency forms. The National Standard Curriculum also recommends that students be graded on clinical interactions and the competency of documentation on patient reports, and that feedback be given to individual students regarding their performance.

One problem that may be encountered when affiliating with a clinical site is that many hospitals now require proof that students have received hepatitis B vaccinations. If students have not received shots, who is responsible for payment of vaccines? Or if a student refuses such vaccinations, could it be deemed discrimination if he is not allowed to participate in training? These issues may require a legal opinion.

In addition, it is important that students found to have difficulty in successfully meeting the objectives of clinical rotations obtain remediation and redirection. These students should participate in additional clinical activities until they are deemed competent by the course coordinator or program director[6]. If such remediation proves unsuccessful, the student will most likely need to be dismissed from the program with adequate counseling and documentation provided.

FIELD (PREHOSPITAL) AFFILIATIONS

Field affiliations have been used primarily for ALS and advanced EMT training programs. Future training programs, however, may direct field evolutions during BLS training programs as well.

Field affiliations should be licensed ALS units (for ALS training programs) approved by a training institute's medical director and state regulatory agencies. They are affiliated with a training institute to provide prehospital field internship training. Such services should be staffed with qualified field preceptors to oversee field training experiences.

Field internships are designed to allow students the opportunity to become familiar with the prehospital environment and to become proficient at performing skills associated with the level of training they are obtaining. Paramedic students use field experience to practice and refine ALS skills such as intubation, intravenous insertion, defibrillation, cardioversion, medication administration, and other advanced techniques while under direct supervision.

Field internships also provide the opportunity for ALS and BLS students to gain additional practice at BLS skills such as CPR, patient assessment, documentation, and report writing in the prehospital environment. Clinical preceptors should be available during all clinical rotations to teach and evaluate students in order to promote proficiency of skills.

> Field affiliations have been used primarily for ALS and advanced EMT training programs.

> Field internships are designed to allow students the opportunity to become familiar with the prehospital environment.

GUIDELINES

When affiliating with either an in-hospital or field clinical facility, policies and procedures should be developed as guidelines to ensure quality and professionalism. In addition, the following items should be provided to each affiliation:

- A contract between the training institute and clinical facility
- Program guidelines, policies, and procedures including:
  - A dress code for students during clinical and field rotations
  - An attendance policy
  - A statement of what is expected of students
  - Preceptor guidelines for evaluating and grading students
  - Guidelines for completing skills verification and skill authorization forms
- Skill guidelines

CONTRACTS

It is advisable to have a yearly contract with each clinical facility associated with a training institute. Contracts should identify responsibilities of each party, names and credentials of each preceptor, a description of how much interaction students should have with patients, responsibilities of students during clinical rotations, and other important information.

POLICIES AND PROCEDURES

Preceptors need to understand policies and procedures implemented by a training institute. Items such as student dress codes, documen-

An itemized list of those skills that students are permitted to perform should be provided to preceptors.

It is important that all areas of learning be evaluated including the knowledge level (cognitive domain), level of professionalism (affective domain), and the competency of skill performance (psychomotor domain).

tation procedures, evaluation methods, and other information must be provided to preceptors to add professionalism and quality to an internship program.

Preceptors also need to be informed as to the attendance policy for students as well as information regarding what is expected of both students and preceptors. In addition, an itemized list of those skills that students are permitted to perform should be provided to preceptors.

It is advisable that a skills authorization form that identifies each skill a student must complete prior to the end of his clinical rotation be developed. A column for documentation of classroom completion, in-hospital completion, and field completion of each skill should be included. Students should have the "classroom" completion portion signed off prior to being able to perform such skills in the hospital or prehospital (field) environments. Appendix E provides a sample skill authorization form.

The evaluation of students in the prehospital arena is the responsibility of the field preceptor. It is important that all areas of learning be evaluated including the knowledge level (cognitive domain), level of professionalism (affective domain), and the competency of skill performance (psychomotor domain).

In order to ascertain the value of a preceptor program, students should use daily skill log forms for each day of a clinical rotation. Such a form should identify the facility at which the student completed skills, which skills were performed, the number and types of patients encountered, and any other activities the student performed during the day. A sample of a daily internship skill log is also provided in Appendix E.

SKILL GUIDELINES

Skill sheets including guidelines of how each skill is to be performed should be provided to each clinical affiliation. Depending on medical direction, training institutes may vary sequence or other procedures when performing certain skills. As such, providing detailed guidelines for each skill will ensure that students perform skills according to the standards set forth by a specific training institute, and that students are not given poor evaluations simply because they performed a skill differently than the preceptors' normal set of standards.

Obtaining Appropriate Equipment

Equipment needs often depend on class size. An instructor:student ratio of 1:6 is recommended for any practical skills training and evaluation session. Consequently, a 1:6 ratio for equipment is also recommended. Some variations may exist if all students will not practice the same skill at the same time (ie, rotating stations). Box 9.2 provides a list of EMS equipment necessary for conducting an EMT-Basic training program to the 1994 National Standard Curriculum.

Prior to the start of each class session it is important that the primary instructor determine what, and how much, equipment is needed, and make appropriate arrangements to obtain it. In addition, it is also necessary to check the equipment to make certain it is in working condition.

The primary instructor should also work with the course coordinator to acquire necessary audiovisual materials and course handouts for each session. Primary instructors should thoroughly review videos,

BOX 9.2 Equipment for Teaching the 1994 EMT-Basic National Standard Curriculum

EMS EQUIPMENT

Preparatory Module
Audiovisual materials
Anatomic manikins
Skeleton
Examination equipment:
- Exam gloves
- Stethoscope
- Blood pressure cuff
- Penlight

Lifting and moving devices:
- Stretcher
- Stair chair
- Scoop stretcher
- Flexible stretcher
- Long board
- Short board

Airway Module
Pocket face mask
Bag-valve-mask
Oxygen powered ventilation device
Oral and nasal airways
Lubricant
Suction unit (with replacement catheter)
Oxygen tank (with regulator)
Oxygen delivery devices
- Nasal cannula
- Non-rebreather mask
- Simple face mask

Intubation manikin

Patient Assessment Module
Examination equipment
EMS trip report for documentation

EMS EQUIPMENT

Medical Module
Simulated medications
- Inhaler
- Nitroglycerin bottle
- Glucose
- Epinephrine auto-injector

CPR manikins
AED unit and simulator
Defibrillation manikins
Activated charcoal
Suction equipment
Examination equipment
Obstetrics kit
Obstetrics manikin
Oxygen supplies

Trauma Module
Oxygen supplies
Trauma bag (with supplies)
- Sterile dressings
- Bandages
- Triangular bandages
- Occlusive dressing
- 4×4 gauze
- Roller bandages
- Burn kit

Splints
- Padded board splint
- Air splint
- Cardboard splint
- Traction splint
- Ladder splint
- Pillow and blanket

MAST
Examination equipment
Long spine board
Short spine board
Cervical collars
Cervical immobilization devices
Helmet (football and motorcycle)

Infants and Children Module
Examination equipment

Operations Module
Well-stocked ambulance
Triage tags

Equipment for teaching the 1994 EMT-Basic National Standard Curriculum (adapted from the 1994 National Standard Curriculum).

slides, overhead transparencies, and other visual aids at least 1 week prior to the start of class to ensure content accuracy and completeness. This allows time for the instructor to obtain an alternative form of medium if necessary.

Preparing Necessary Paperwork

Course participants should be provided with certain materials at the first class session. These include items such as a textbook, workbook, skill sheets, pocket face mask, and other equipment such as a stethoscope, blood pressure cuff, and penlight. A pocket mask prevents student contamination during CPR mannequin practice and the other equipment allows students to practice assessment techniques between class sessions.

It is recommended all such equipment be provided to each student upon entry into a program in order to increase the effectiveness of training. The cost of these items can be added to the tuition for a training program. If budget constraints prevent giving each student his own assessment equipment, it should be recommended they each purchase such equipment independently.

Additional items that should be distributed at the first class session include certain paperworksuch as a course overview, syllabus, and reading list. In keeping with ADA guidelines, it is also recommended that a job description be provided that identifies tasks that students must be able to complete in order to fulfill job requirements as a first responder, EMT, or paramedic.

Course Overview

A course overview provides general guidelines for the student on what to expect throughout the course. It should include a course description, attendance requirements, achievement requirements, course goals and objectives, a description of the grievance process, and other important information. A sample EMT-Basic course overview is provided in Appendix E.

Course Syllabus

The course syllabus should be distributed the first night of class.

The course syllabus should include an itemized list of topics for each class session and should be distributed the first night of class. A syllabus shows students what information is being presented so that they can prepare for each class session. It also allows them to know what information they've missed should they be absent from a class.

It is recommended that a disclaimer stating "Course syllabus subject to change at the sole discretion of the course coordinator or program director" be placed at the bottom of a course syllabus, just in case changes are necessary.

Reading List

Periodic "pop quizzes" help motivate students to read required information prior to class.

A reading list, like a course syllabus, should provide a list of topics for each class session. Next to each topic, a list of all required reading should be listed. This allows students to prepare adequately for each class. It should be required that students read, and be responsible for, all reading prior to each class session. By reading information prior to attending class, and re-reading information after the class, students achieve maximum benefit from courses.

Periodic "pop quizzes" help motivate students to read required information prior to class. Quizzes can range from formal exams to very informal quizlike game shows.

Sign-in Sheets

It is important that students sign in at each class session in order to document absenteeism. Sign-in sheets can be compiled into an attendance roster to see, at a glance, which and how many class sessions each student has missed. Without proper documentation, it is difficult to prove whether a student attended class sessions.

Student Class Cancellation List

Unfortunately, there are times when it becomes necessary to cancel class sessions. Most often this is due to inclement weather conditions or other instances beyond the control of administration, including snow storms, hurricanes, tornado watches, severe thunder storms, or facility problems such as no electricity, running water, or air conditioning and heater malfunctions.

Regardless of the cause of the need to cancel class, a procedure should be implemented to notify students when class is cancelled. While most institutions have a policy to notify one or two radio stations and/or make an announcement over a fire paging network, it is recommended that a phone list be developed the first night of class to notify class members individually.

> A procedure should be implemented to notify students when class is cancelled.

A phone list should include all students' names and phone numbers. For legal purposes it is necessary to obtain the permission of students prior to distributing their phone numbers. On the first night of class, ask if anyone objects to their phone number being listed; if so, delete that individual's name prior to distributing the list.

Once the list has been distributed, instruct class members on how the list works. When the administrative director or course coordinator determines it is necessary to cancel a class session, they will notify the first person on the list. That student is then responsible to phone the next person on the list, who will phone the next person, and so on. In addition to the first person on the list, the course coordinator must also notify all students who declined to have their phone number listed.

Students should also be informed that if they cannot contact the person for whom they are responsible to advise, they should phone the next person on the list, and then continue trying to reach their initial contact later.

Conducting Counseling Sessions

Occasionally during training programs, it becomes necessary to conduct counseling sessions for students with academic or behavioral deficiencies relative to a prehospital training experience. Counseling can be initiated by a student, instructor, course coordinator, administrative director, or medical director.

Students should be encouraged to contact the course coordinator for assistance with any academic difficulties, skill performance deficiencies, or personality conflicts with which they need help. In addition, the course coordinator should initiate counseling for students exhibiting problems with attendance; academic difficulties (skill performance or knowledge retention); inappropriate conduct, dress, or behavior; or any other related course matters affecting an individual's chance for successful completion of a training program.

> Students should be encouraged to contact the course coordinator for assistance with any academic difficulties, skill performance deficiencies, or personality conflicts with which they need help.

While counseling is an appropriate tool to provide students every opportunity for success within a training program, there are instances in which a counseling session may not be necessary or appropriate. Specifically, counseling sessions may not be necessary prior to the dismissal of a student as a result of:

- Failure to meet attendance policy requirements
- Academic dishonesty
- Misconduct that could endanger public safety or property

Documentation of counseling sessions should be documented immediately and accurately to include the following items:

- The reason for counseling
- Observation of the attendance, appearance and attitude of the student
- The ability of a student to meet course goals and objectives as identified by written and practical exams
- Suggestions for improvement
- A time line for the completion of corrective actions
- Consequences of noncompliance with corrective actions
- Counselor comments
- Student comments
- A date and signature of all individuals involved

Documentation should clearly support the need for counseling sessions and must be made available for review by the student. A sample student counseling form is provided in Appendix E.

> Documentation should clearly support the need for counseling sessions and must be made available for review by the student.

Maintaining Records

Maintaining student records and other course documentation is one of the most important roles of a program director. Documentation may be needed for various reasons such as discrepancies in scores, lawsuits against EMTs in the field, lawsuits against instructors or training institutes, verification of course completion, verification of instructor payments, and other purposes.

> Maintaining student records and other course documentation is one of the most important roles of a program director.

The length of time such records must be maintained can vary. It is best to obtain a legal opinion on this issue. Generally such training records must be maintained for a minimum of 7 years. Appendix E provides sample forms that can be used to maintain adequate documentation of course administrative practices and student achievement.

Course records should include the following:

- A course announcement
- A course syllabus
- Student applications
- Results of pre-entrance exams or interviews (if appropriate)
- Copies of CPR cards provided by students
- Parental consent forms (if necessary)
- Risk agreement forms
- Insurance verification documentation (if necessary)
- Instructor contracts
- Criminal history forms (if appropriate)
- Attendance rosters
- Instructor rosters
- Completed student counseling forms (if necessary)
- Incident reports (if necessary)
- Completed course evaluation forms
- Exam results (practical and written)
- Clinical rotation evaluation forms
- Skills performance verification forms
- A final course budget (income and expenses)

Instructor records should be placed in individual files and include:

- Copies of current credentials (curriculum vitae and copies of certifications)
- Instructor pay sheets
- Completed instructor evaluation forms

DECLARING CLASS DEFICIENCIES

A class deficiency is a pattern of unsatisfactory performance in a specific skill or skill area as evidenced by practical exam failures. A class deficiency could also include a knowledge deficit as evidenced by written exams in which a large number of students fail questions relative to a specific content area of instruction.

Prior to declaring a class deficiency, it is necessary to determine what percentage of a class must answer a specific question incorrectly or fail practical skills evaluations to warrant such a declaration. Generally, if 30% of a class fails to meet specific course objectives, remedial training is most likely necessary.

Once a class deficiency has been identified, the course coordinator or administrative director should analyze the course to identify the instructor(s) responsible for teaching the particular class segments in question. It is then their responsibility to notify the instructor(s) to determine whether the information was presented incorrectly or if it was misinterpreted by the students. Regardless of the cause, instructors must be informed of the incident and provided with suggestions to prevent it from occurring in the future.

Remedial training must then be provided through additional class sessions in which didactic and practical demonstrations and practice sessions are provided covering the specific course content in question. All students who did not successfully complete the written and/or practical skills portion of the exam relating to the deficiency should be required to attend remedial classes. Those students who were successful with exams should not be required to attend, but should be invited to participate.

> All students who did not successfully complete the written and/or practical skills portion of the exam relating to the deficiency should be required to attend remedial classes.

AFTER THE SESSION IS OVER

Conducting Program Evaluations

The most valuable tool instructors and administrators can use to analyze the quality and effectiveness of a training program is a course evaluation. No program is perfect; there is always room for improvement. Admitting this is the first step to improving the quality and effectiveness of training programs.

The evaluation process should include three levels: a student course evaluation, an instructor course evaluation, and an administrative review. All evaluation forms should be reviewed and compiled, with results being disseminated to all program staff involved with the course. Sample evaluation forms are provided in Appendix E.

> The most valuable tool instructors and administrators can use to analyze the quality and effectiveness of a training program is a course evaluation.

Student Course Evaluation

Student evaluation forms should ask specific questions, with an answer scale of 1 to 5, to assess the effectiveness of a training program. The following items should be included in these evaluation forms.

Stress Management For Educators

It has been well publicized that stress increases an individual's chance of a heart attack. Stress is an inherent part of life, and the field of education is no exception. Educators need to understand the effects of stress and mechanisms to decrease the negative effects of such.

While a heart attack and stroke are the most prevalent problems associated with stress, there are other effects of a stressful environment, most of which can be controlled if not prevented. These problems are indicated in Box 9.3.

The work environment often causes an individual to feel some degree of stress. In EMS training programs, instructors can become stressed for various reasons such as:

- Their full-time job causes them to be late for a class.
- They forgot their lesson plan on the kitchen table.
- The overhead projector bulb blew out and there are no replacements nearby.
- The equipment is locked in the storage room and nobody has a key.
- There are 40 people enrolled in a class and only four show up.
- Murphy is alive and well.
- Students in the back of the room are being disruptive.
- Two of four assistant instructors fail to show up to teach.
- The instructor duplicates enough handouts for 20 students, but 40 show up.
- It's the first day of class and the books still have not arrived.
- The instructor becomes ill 1 hour prior to class and cannot find a replacement.
- The instructor fails to review slides and finds during the course of instruction that they are upside down.
- No matter how hard an instructor tries, there is one student who cannot learn the information, or fails to try to the best of his ability.
- An instructor is scheduled to teach the night of his child's dance recital.
- There is a blizzard the last day of class, and no time for a makeup session because the state final exam is in 3 days.

🍎 Instructor items such as:

- Was the instructor well prepared?
- Did the instructor dress and act appropriately?
- Did the instructor maintain class interest?
- Were the audiovisual materials used by the instructor useful?

🍎 Facility items such as:

- Was the facility of adequate size?
- Was the facility conveniently located?
- Were the temperature and other environmental conditions of the facility adequate?

🍎 Coordination items such as:

- Was there sufficient training equipment and was it in working condition?

Regardless of the cause of stress, educators need to develop methods to combat its negative effects. The following remedies may be helpful:

- Set aside one evening each week as family (or significant other) night. Without fail, spend the evening in a nonstressful environment and put work out of your mind. Rent a movie, play a game, go out for dinner, take the kids roller skating. Whatever you enjoy, do it.
- Set aside 1 day per month as a "Me Day." Take the day off and do what you enjoy. Whether you plan a day trip to the casino, a walk in the park, a drive in the country, lunch with a friend, sailing, fishing, or skiing, enjoy yourself. Leave all signs of work at home; take the briefcase out of the car to remove any temptation to "review notes" while on your day off.
- Do not underestimate the power of humor. Humor is very effective in relieving stress. Watch a funny movie one night per week and feel your stress disappear.
- Exercise regularly; fitness leads to a healthier lifestyle. Exercise directs blood flow to the heart and brain, and reduces anxiety and stress.
- Do not be afraid to say no. You must make priorities in life and there has to be enough time for you. If you cannot teach a session, just say no.
- Talk with a friend or loved one. There is no shame in admitting you need help; this is the key to a successful life.
- Learn relaxation techniques. If you have a bad day, before you lose control, take a few deep breaths, go for a walk around the block, and let your mind go blank. You will be surprised at how calmly you can look at the situation after some fresh air.
- Invest in a pressure point massager; they work wonders on the muscles in the neck and low back, and make tension go away.
- At the end of a hard day, listen to relaxing music. There are relaxation tapes available, such as the soothing sound of ocean waves, or calming music such as classical music or Indian flute music.

- Were work groups of sufficient size?
- Were enough instructors scheduled to assist students with program goals and objectives?
- Did students know what was expected of them throughout the program?
- Was someone always available and willing to answer questions or offer assistance?

Curriculum items such as:

- Was enough practice time provided?
- Did the information provided make the student confident to function adequately in the field?
- Was there course content that was not covered or that should be removed? If so, what?

BOX 9.3 Negative Effects of Stress

Anxiety
Irritability
Alcoholism
Child abuse
Broken relationships
Ulcers
Stroke
Tension headaches
Diarrhea
Colitis
Hypertension
Death

Negative effects of stress.

Instructor Course Evaluation

Each instructor who participated in the program should be asked to complete an evaluation form to help determine the effectiveness of a training program. In addition, it is recommended that an informal self-evaluation session for all instructional staff involved with the training program be completed within 1 week after the conclusion of a program. Questions asked should include the following.

> It is recommended that an informal self-evaluation session for all instructional staff involved with the training program be completed within 1 week after the conclusion of a program.

- Student items such as:

    - Were students prepared for class?
    - Did students appear motivated to learn?
    - Did students participate in class activities?
    - Did students successfully meet course goals and objectives?

- Facility items as identified above.

- Coordination items as identified above.

- Organization items such as:

    - Was requested course material available?
    - Were audiovisual materials adequate?
    - Did class sessions run smoothly?
    - How can the program be improved?

Administrative Course Evaluation

The administrative course evaluation should examine multiple components of a training program to determine if the course was cost-efficient, educationally sound, and otherwise beneficial. Specific questions should include:

- How many students were enrolled in the program?
- How many students successfully completed the program?
- Were enough instructors available to teach?
- Were too many scheduled?
- Were instructors prepared for and effective with their presentations?
- Was there ample equipment in working condition?
- Is any equipment in need of repair or replacement?
- What was the total cost of the course?
- What improvements or changes are necessary for the next program?

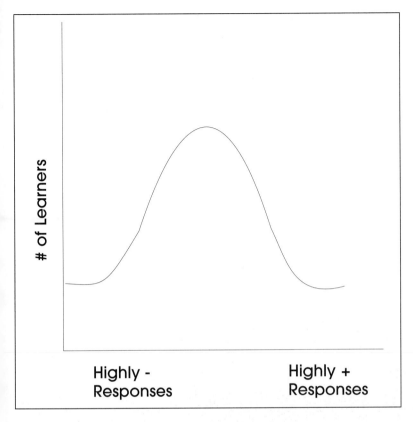

FIGURE 9.3 Normal Bell Curve for Evaluation Results

Evaluating the Evaluations

Evaluation forms should be used merely as a method for gaining understanding of how students felt about the learning experience, in order to know which areas of a training program were found to be helpful, and which should be changed for future programs. It is important to remember, however, that such evaluations are extremely subjective and require interpretation by instructors and administrators to be useful.

Reactions to training programs, as identified by course evaluations forms, usually conform to a bell curve that is slightly skewed toward the positive. A normal bell curve would indicate that given a class of 30 students, four may act very negatively about a training program, and four very positively, with the majority falling somewhere in the middle[1].

If the program was rated on a scale of 1 to 5, the average should be approximately 3.5. With such results, the chart would look similar to that in Figure 9.3. When results follow a bell curve, the program was satisfactory and administrative staff should not worry that scores were not higher; an average of 3.5 points is quite respectable.

When the scores indicate extremely favorable results, such as those shown in Figure 9.4, the instructors will most likely feel elated. Such results are sometimes caused by false feelings, such as liking the instructor or being happy the course is over, causing deceptive positive ratings. It is important that positive results be analyzed to determine which areas were effective and which were not.

When the results are negative, as identified with a bell curve similar to that in Figure 9.5, instructors and administrators should take steps to identify the cause, and take steps to ensure that problems do

Evaluations are extremely subjective and require interpretation by instructors and administrators to be useful.

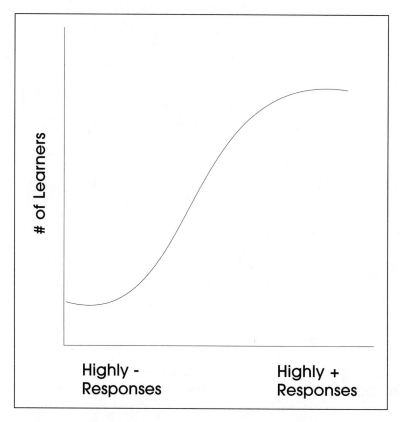

FIGURE 9.4 Positively Skewed Bell Curve for Evaluation Results

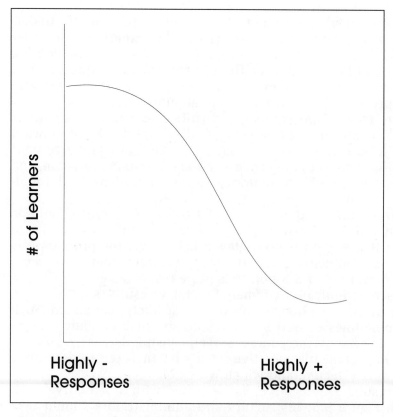

FIGURE 9.5 Negatively Skewed Bell Curve for Evaluation Results

Words To Live By

Work expands so as to fill the time available for its completion (Parkinson's Law).

The time to relax is when you don't have time for it.

Be pleasant until ten o'clock in the morning and the rest of the day will take care of itself.

People who say they sleep like a baby usually don't have any.

To err is human, but when the eraser wears out ahead of the pencil, you're overdoing it.

If you don't get what you want, want what you get.

To have a stress-free day, take a night job.

We hope vaguely, but dread precisely.

Why not put off worrying about today until tomorrow? By then it will be yesterday.

Not to decide is to decide.

Remember, no one can make you feel inferior without your consent (Eleanor Roosevelt).

Life can only be understood backwards; but it must be lived forwards (Sorenson).

(adapted from Tubesing & Tubesing, 1990[2]).

not continue in future training programs. Just as with false-positive results, false-negative scores can occur due to a student being angry he failed, or not liking a particular instructor or coordinator.

There are various reasons for negative evaluations, including the following[1]:

- *Inappropriate content* - Learners did not perceive a need for the training and, therefore, did not put much time or energy into the learning process.
- *Inappropriate design or delivery* - The choice for delivery did not promote optimal learning, such as presenting a lecture format to teach how to perform a hands-on skill.
- *Outside factors* - Outside personal factors had a negative influence on students, causing attention deficit, frequent absences from class, or a poor attitude.
- *Inappropriate selection of students* - The class may have been composed of individuals with drastically different backgrounds and experience.

Dealing With Feelings

Every instructor has had at least one bad teaching experience. It is important to understand that this is normal, and not to dwell in negative feelings. Instead, identify what elements of a particular session were inadequate and take appropriate steps to prevent them from occurring in the future.

On the other hand, if a session goes extremely well, the instructor will most likely be elated. It is important that such positive feelings do

Every instructor has had at least one bad teaching experience.

An instructor should use negative experiences to build improvements into future training programs.

not cloud the instructor's mind, making the instructor believe he is a natural presenter and does not need to prepare for future sessions. This belief could prove devastating during the next presentation.

Finally, while an instructor should use negative experiences to build improvements into future training programs, if presentations continue to result in negative feelings, feelings of anxiety, or negative evaluation results from students, the instructor should analyze whether teaching is appropriate for him. There are people who just do not make good instructors. Some instructors make excellent assistant instructors, however, but panic when placed in front of large groups. These instructors should remain assistant instructors.

ETHICAL ISSUES

A professional code of ethics for educators follows three basic principles of commitment on the part of the educator: commitment to the student, to the public, and to the profession and professional practices of the field of education.

The Student
- The instructor must not discourage students in the pursuit of learning and must not deny them access to differing points of view.
- The instructor must provide information that is not distorted by personal bias, and must present all of the information required.
- The instructor must protect students from discrimination, either against them or in their favor, on the basis of race, color, creed, national origin, sex, age, or handicap.
- The instructor must provide a safe learning environment.
- The instructor must not use a professional relationship with a student for personal gain. Dating a student may cause an ethical dilemma and may produce resentment with other students in the training program.
- The instructor must not disclose any confidential information obtained through the course of a training program.

The Public
- The instructor must not misrepresent an institution with which he is affiliated.
- The instructor must not use professional privileges for personal gain or political advancement.
- The instructor must not interfere with other instructor's rights.
- The instructor must not accept gifts or favors that may influence his judgement as an educator or offer such favors to obtain a personal gain.

The Profession
- The instructor must maintain the integrity of the profession of educators, by providing accurate and effective instruction, maintaining a positive attitude, and following the educator's code of ethics.

There are various ways to handle an instructor who fails to follow the principles identified in the educator's code of ethics. One option is to simply not contract with such instructors in the future. Another option is to give them an oral warning for the first offense, a written warning for the second offense, and suspension for subsequent infractions.

LEGAL ISSUES

Lawsuits are ever-growing in popularity in all facets of life. Commercials constantly show lawyers wishing to represent individuals in lawsuits for malpractice, negligence, and other litigation attempts. The training environment is not immune to potential litigation issues.

There are three major areas of legal liability for training departments: issues surrounding violations to individual rights, noncompliance with legally mandated training requirements, and the use of nontraditional training methods[3].

The training environment is not immune to potential litigation issues.

Student Rights

Students have certain constitutional rights that cannot be infringed upon in training programs. Instructors must be acutely aware of issues such as sexual harassment, discrimination, and harassment.

Most instructors genuinely care about their students, and tend to push students to do their best. It is essential that instructors do not push students to where an individual feels harassed or becomes emotionally unstable because of an instructor's actions. In order to decrease chances of harassment charges, instructors should treat *all* individuals equally. If an instructor makes strong expectations of some students, he must expect the same of the entire class.

Most instructors genuinely care about their students, and tend to push students to do their best.

Discrimination is the showing of partiality or prejudice in treatment (action or policy), generally directed against minority groups. For example, if three students each miss more than the maximum number of classes allowed before dismissal from a course, and the course coordinator drops only one student from the course, there may be grounds for a discrimination suit against the coordinator. Discrimination suits may be real or imagined; regardless, they can result in legal charges against an instructor.

Students have inherent rights to protect them from discriminatory practices. The Civil Rights Act protects them from discrimination based on race and sex, and the Age Discrimination in Employment Act (ADEA) protects them against discrimination based on age.

Any comments or activities by instructional staff that are considered offensive to an individual, and that allude to sex, age, race, religion, ethnic background, or handicap could result in legal claims under anti-discrimination statutes[3]. When an individual files a discrimination suit, it is not up to the individual to prove discrimination, but to the defendant to prove there was *no* discrimination.

Evaluating and Dismissing Students

No matter how hard instructional faculty may try, there are students who must be dismissed from training programs for various reasons, including academic deficiencies or behavioral problems. Regardless of the reason, appropriate documentation is necessary in order to protect instructors, administrators, and other training institute personnel adequately.

As discussed earlier in this chapter, counseling sessions should be provided when appropriate to offer students the opportunity for improvement. Certain behaviors, however, dictate immediate dismissal from a course without such counseling. With or without counseling, documentation is essential.

Whether dismissal from a training program is warranted or not, students may seek legal intervention. Possible legal infractions include libel, defamation, and harassment. To protect themselves, instructors and/or administrative personnel should adequately document steps taken to protect employee rights.

If a student is dismissed from a training program as a result of poor test or skills evaluation sessions, it is important the administrative director have validated written exams and/or have examined the evaluator to ensure accuracy with the exam process. If one evaluator finds a large number of students to be unsatisfactory when performing skills, it is necessary for the administrative staff to identify whether it is the students or evaluator whose skills are poor.

Student Confidentiality

All students have the right to privacy. Records such as test scores, notes from counseling sessions, and other private information are confidential and cannot be released without permission.

> All students have the right to privacy.

One area of concern regarding student confidentiality occurs when an individual is sent to a training session by his employer or affiliated EMS service. When someone other than the individual pays for a training program, a gray area exists regarding confidential information. For example, when a student is dropped from a course due to lack of attendance, poor test scores, or disruptive or harmful behavior, is the sponsoring agency entitled to such information? Again, a legal opinion may be needed in this matter.

Sexual Harassment

The 1964 Civil Rights Act, Title VII, Section 703, defines sexual harassment as "unwelcome sexual advances, requests for favors and other verbal and physical conduct." Furthermore, the regulations for Title IX of the 1972 Education Amendments make sexual advances and verbal and physical conduct unlawful when:

- Submission is made a term of employment or admission to a program, activity or course.
- Submission or rejection is used as a basis for decisions affecting employment or academic status.
- The harassment interferes with work or school performance or creates an intimidating, hostile, or offensive working or learning environment.

> Sexual harassment can be verbal, visual or physical in nature.

Sexual harassment can be verbal, visual or physical in nature, and occurs in a wide range of actions from inappropriate sexual comments to serious physical abuse. Any form of harassment is illegal. Instructors, students, and administrators can be victims of sexual harassment claims[4].

It has been estimated that 40% of women on a typical college campus have suffered from some form of sexual harassment. Of those who are harassed, fewer than 10% report it[4]. Most colleges and universities now have policies designed to prevent sexual harassment. The presence of such harassment is damaging to the academic integrity and professionalism of an educational institute. Those training centers not affiliated with a college or university are strongly encouraged to develop and adopt a strong policy against sexual harassment in order to maintain the integrity of training programs.

Since sexual harassment occurs at so many levels, it is sometimes difficult to identify instances of harassment. The following are some examples of sexual harassment:

- An instructor constantly tells jokes of a sexual nature and makes personal remarks about women. Several women drop the course, but it is necessary for one student to complete the course. When the student advises the instructor that she finds his jokes sexist and without humor, her grades decrease.
- An instructor constantly asks a student for a date, making the student feel uncomfortable.
- An instructor constantly makes sexist comments about women, ignoring requests to stop. The professor does not make any physical advances toward women.
- An instructor takes a special interest in a student and talks of possible jobs he could help secure following completion of the program. When they go to lunch to discuss such possibilities, the instructor propositions the student.
- A student feels threatened in class because one of her peers is involved in a physical relationship with the instructor. The student feels the relationship might affect the grades of the entire class, but especially those of the student having the relationship.

Finally, the issue of faculty and student relationships, even with adult students in which both parties agree to the relationship, must be addressed. While some institutions have policies that prohibit sexual relations between faculty and students, even with consent, others do not have such policies.

Aside from the ethical issues raised from such a relationship, it is in the best interest of all individuals involved if such relationships do not occur until the student is no longer enrolled in the training program. While the student may initially consent to a relationship, he may later claim the relationship was not one of mutual consent, thereby placing the instructor in great jeopardy.

Mandatory Training

Providing education about workplace hazards has been estimated to be the fastest growing area of liability for training personnel. These areas include haz-mat training, fire training, and communicable disease control. When someone is injured, lawyers often turn to documentation and records on how a student was trained, and by whom. Such legal claims may focus on allegations of inadequate training, use of unqualified personnel to provide such training, or a total failure to train altogether[3].

There are many regulatory agencies that impose certain statutes on training. The Occupational Safety and Health Administration (OSHA) has numerous "standards" that should be adhered to. In the event of a work-related illness or injury, OSHA will examine the records and the work environment to assess that the standards had been complied with. If not, fines and legal action may ensue. While some states are not "OSHA states" and do not follow OSHA requirements, they are still at risk for prosecution if such standards are not upheld.

In EMS training, areas such as Haz-Mat training, rescue training, CPR, AED use, and other skills that could result in harm to a patient if performed improperly are those that pose the greatest threat of liability to students and, therefore, to instructors. If a malpractice or negligence claim is prosecuted against an EMT, the defense attorney may try to prove that the EMT acted as he was taught, thereby implicating the training institute or instructors.

In order to protect training institute administrators, documentation of instructor credentials and evaluation forms must be maintained on file, as should instructor rosters that indicate who taught specific

Section 1604.11 of the EEOC's Guidelines on Discrimination Because of Sex (NEA, 1988) provides:

- A college, university, training institute, or other educational facility is ultimately responsible for the acts of its "employees" (including contracted instructors), with respect to sexual harassment. This is true regardless of whether the specific acts were authorized or forbidden by the employer, or whether or not the employer knew of such an occurrence.

- An employer is responsible for acts of sexual harassment in the workplace, with regard to conduct between fellow employees.

In EMS training, areas such as Haz-Mat training, rescue training, CPR, AED use, and other skills that could result in harm to a patient if performed improperly are those that pose the greatest threat of liability to students and, therefore, to instructors.

classes. In addition, it is essential that course content adequately cover the National Standard Curriculum and other nationally or locally accepted policies and procedures for knowledge and skill performance.

If an instructor teaches material that is inconsistent with specific scope or content requirements of the National Standard Curriculum or standards such as OSHA, there may be grounds for a lawsuit should an illness or injury result from noncompliance. In order for a lawsuit to be successful, the claimant must show that the illness or injury was the direct result of an instructor or training institute's neglectful failure to properly train the individual within the confines of the curriculum.

If an individual is hurt because a former EMT student did not know how to properly rescue him from the water, the instructor would not be liable because water rescue training is not part of the National Standard Curriculum. However, if the instructor did teach portions of water rescue within a course where it was part of the curriculum, and provided inaccurate information, he could be liable.

As with medical treatment, training is based on the "standard of care" that applies to similar training. For EMT-Basic training, the standard is the National Standard Curriculum; for CPR training, the standard is the American Medical Association guidelines; for Haz-Mat training, the standard is OSHA's Hazardous Communication Standards and for infectious disease control (communicable disease standards).

There are additional standards against which educators can be judged. While such standards generally do not mandate specific methods by which training must be accomplished, they do specify the nature and scope of training. Highly technical or high-risk skills are more susceptible to scrutiny of methods used during training. For example, if an individual inappropriately delivers a shock to himself using a defibrillator, causing injury, and it can be proven the individual received no hands-on training on how to use an AED unit, the injured person may have a legitimate claim against the instructor because such training was inadequate and ineffective[3].

Using Copyrighted Material

A copyright is a form of protection provided by the laws of the United States to authors of "original works," including literary, dramatic, musical, artistic, and certain other intellectual works. This protection is provided to both published and unpublished works. The Copyright Act gives the owner of copyright the exclusive right to do, or authorize others to do, the following[5]:

- Reproduce the copyrighted work
- Prepare derivative works based upon the copyrighted material
- Distribute copies of the work

It is illegal for anyone to violate the rights provided by the Act to the owner of a copyright. The mere ownership of a book does not give the possessor the copyright. Therefore, an instructor cannot duplicate materials contained in a book or other written materials without permission from the owner of the copyright.

The copyright for textbooks and other published written material is usually transferred to the publisher from the author of the work. In these cases, the author cannot give permission for instructors to copy material; permission must be given by the publisher.

KEY POINTS

1. An effective training program requires the skills of numerous key personnel. While instructors are the most visible, much administrative and clerical support is necessary for efficient, effective, quality programs to be conducted.

2. The training facility must be convenient, comfortable, and free of distractions. The classroom must be of sufficient size, have adequate lighting, temperature, and ventilation, and be equipped with tables, chairs, and electrical outlets.

3. One of the most important components of effective EMS training is preparation. A task analysis can help with such preparation. It involves identifying all key steps required to conduct a training program effectively and efficiently. Once key elements of a program are identified, they must be prioritized and placed into a time line in order of what tasks must be completed first. Checklists provide an effective mechanism for organizing and ensuring implementation of such tasks.

4. How and when a training program is scheduled and announced may affect the number of attendees. Sufficient time is necessary to allow for the adequate distribution of announcements.

5. All training programs have an anticipated budget including estimated income and expenses.

6. While it is optimal to use the same instructors for an entire program, it is not always possible. Methods to maintain consistency throughout a training program must be implemented when using multiple instructors.

7. The primary instructor usually has overall responsibility for individual class sessions and the presentation of information to the National Standard Curriculum. Assistant instructors help teach practical hands-on skills sessions.

8. Guest lecturers, such as emergency department physicians, CISD team members, nurses, and respiratory technicians can provide added expertise on certain topics.

9. Clinical facilities, including hospitals and field affiliation sites, provide the opportunity for students to gain experience and become proficient at performing skills.

10. Preceptors need to be knowledgeable of policies and procedures implemented by a training institute. They also need to be provided with skills sheets that identify step-by-step procedures by which students are to perform skills.

11. Students should be encouraged to contact the course coordinator for assistance with any academic difficulties, skill performance deficiencies, or personality conflicts with which they need help. In addition, the course coordinator should initiate counseling for students exhibiting problems with attendance; academic difficulties (skill performance or knowledge retention); inappropriate conduct, dress, or behavior; or any other related course matters affecting the student's chance for successful completion of a training program.

12. Maintaining student records and other course documentation is one of the most important roles of a program director. Such documentation may be needed for various reasons such as discrepancies in scores, lawsuits against EMTs in the field, lawsuits against instructors or training institutes, verification of course completion, verification of instructor payments, and other purposes. Educational facilities are usually required to maintain class records for a minimum of 7 years.

13. It is essential that instructional staff and administrators understand legal requirements that affect them. They must be sensitive to restrictions by statutes on the scope and content of training, and take measures to avoid violating student rights.

14. It is the administrator's responsibility to look at global issues surrounding a training program, to identify areas that have the potential for liability, and to develop policies and actions that minimize liabilities. Areas of concern might include instructor qualifications, adhering to state and local regulatory requirements, identifying high-risk areas for hazardous training, identifying instructors who may infringe on student rights, identifying financial hardships that may exist, or other potential problems.

15. Students have certain constitutional rights that cannot be infringed upon in training programs. Instructors must be acutely aware of issues such as sexual harassment, discrimination, and other forms of harassment.

16. The 1964 Civil Rights Act, Title VII, Section 703, defines sexual harassment as "unwelcome sexual advances, requests for favors and other verbal and physical conduct."

17. Sexual harassment can be verbal, visual, or physical in nature, and occurs in a wide range of actions from inappropriate sexual comments to serious physical abuse; any form of harassment is illegal. Instructors, students, and administrators can be the victims of sexual harassment claims.

18. Students also have inherent rights to protect them from discriminatory practices. The Civil Right Act protects them from discrimination based on sex and race, and the ADEA protects them against discrimination based on age.

KEY POINTS continued

19. A copyright is a form of protection provided by the laws of the United States to authors of "original works" including literary, dramatic, musical, artistic, and certain other intellectual works.
20. It is illegal for anyone to violate the rights provided by the Copyright Act to the owner of a copyright. The mere ownership of a book does not give the possessor the copyright. Therefore, an instructor cannot duplicate materials contained in a book or other written materials without permission from the owner of the copyright.

FOLLOW-UP ACTIVITIES

1. Identify three environments that would be acceptable for training programs, and why.
2. Identify three environments that would not be acceptable for training programs, and why not.
3. Identify five examples of sexual harassment claims that could be sought against instructors or students.

REFERENCES

1. Margolis F, Bell C. *Instructing for Results.* San Diego, CA: Pfeiffer & Company, and Minneapolis, MN: Lakewood Publications; 1986.
2. Tubesing N, Tubesing D. *Structured Exercises in Stress Management.* Deluth, MN: While Person Press; 1990.
3. Eyres P. Keeping the training department out of court. *Training.* 1990, September:59–67.
4. NEA Higher Education Advocate. *Newsletter for NEA Members in Higher Education.* Volume V, Number 11. May 9, 1988.
5. United States Copyright Office. *Copyright Basics* Document No. 1989-241-429 80.045. Washington, DC: U.S. Government Printing Office; 1989.
6. *1994 EMT-Basic National Standard Curriculum;* Lexington, KY: Department of Transportation; 1994.

10 Improving Learner Success

OBJECTIVES

Upon completion of this chapter, the reader will have sufficient information to:
1. Describe the benefit of behavior modification as it relates to the learning process.
2. Identify the process by which an instructor can identify learning deficiencies and the need for behavior modification strategies.
3. List nine types of behaviors that can cause difficulties for instructors.
4. Describe the use of positive reinforcement, negative reinforcement, and punishment as they relate to the classroom setting.
5. Provide examples of various behavior modification strategies.
6. Define extinction and overcorrection and provide examples of each.
7. Describe three benefits of the use of punishment.
8. Provide four disadvantages of the use of aversive stimuli.
9. Describe the use of response cost procedures as a behavior modification strategy and provide an example.
10. Provide examples of learning disabilities that the instructor may have to address during an EMS training program, and methods for remediating them.
11. State the difference between factual and situational multiple-choice questions, and provide an example of each.
12. Describe seven strategies that should be used by students while taking tests.
13. List 10 strategies that should be used by students in order to be better prepared for certification examinations.
14. Identify seven steps that can be taken by students to increase physical and mental preparation for certification examinations.

KEY TERMS

Aversive stimuli Negative stimuli aimed at causing a specific behavioral response

Behavior modification Interventions designed to change behavior in a measurable manner

Extinction The reduction of a behavior through the abrupt termination of the positive reinforcer maintaining the inappropriate behavior

Learning deficiency A problem that inhibits the learning process; may be behavioral, emotional, or physical

Learning disability A term describing students with physical problems that may limit their ability to perform certain tasks

Negative reinforcement The termination of an unpleasant stimulus immediately following a behavior, thereby increasing the probability of such future behavior

Overcorrection An attempt to decrease inappropriate student behaviors by requiring a student who has disturbed the environment, physically or emotionally, to restore the environment not only to its original form, but beyond

Positive reinforcement The immediate response to a behavior that increases or maintains the probability or rate of continuance of a particular behavior

Punishment The presentation of an unpleasant stimulus that decreases the future rate and/or probability of the recurrence of a particular behavior

Response cost procedures A type of behavior modification strategy that involves the presentation of a positive reinforcer for appropriate behavior and the removal of a reinforcer for inappropriate behavior

REMEDIATION OF LEARNING DEFICIENCIES

A learning deficiency is any existing problem that inhibits the learning process, and may be behavioral, emotional, or physical in nature.

No matter how effectively an instructor presents information or what instructional methods and materials are used, there are certain students who are difficult to reach. A learning deficiency is any existing problem that inhibits the learning process, and may be behavioral, emotional, or physical in nature.

In order to determine whether a learning deficiency exists, it is important to define the level of mastery that is expected from the student as well as the level of behavior the student is expected to exhibit in the classroom. Once this has been determined, the instructor must evaluate the level at which the student is performing and determine if there is a difference.

Reasons for poor performance can be varied and include both academic and/or behavioral reasons. It is important to understand, however, that these problems are solvable. All students can learn, and while some require more time than others, they can all learn. The key, however, is that they must *want* to learn.

BEHAVIOR MODIFICATION

There are many types of students who could be classified as "difficult." Some are disruptive to other students, while others are disruptive only to their own learning potential. Such students include:

- **The side-show talker** sits in the back of the room carrying on conversations, be they relevant to course topic or not.
- **The know-it-all** has been affiliated with an ambulance service for years and therefore had obtained all necessary knowledge. This student believes he knows as much as, if not more than, the instructor.
- **The whiner** has every excuse in the book as to why he does not want to do something, why he should be excused from a certain class, or why a particular test question is unfair.
- **The heckler** is the class clown. Almost all classes must deal with at least one class clown.
- **The searcher** is constantly looking for the "black and white" rules governing EMS. He may ask questions such as "why" and "what if," potentially wasting a large portion of class time.
- **The negative or hostile student** really does not want to be in class, but is required to be, either by his employment or as a means of recertification, and attempts to make the instructor miserable in the process.
- **The shy student** is usually very quiet in class and does not like to be singled out to participate in a class session. This student is generally more productive independently or in small groups.

- **The "that's not the way they do it on the streets" student** continually questions how the instructor performs emergency care techniques relative to how it is down at his ambulance station or "in the real world."
- **The cheater** is dishonest on exams or other course work. This type of student is harmful not only to him- or herself, but also to the student he is cheating from. The greatest victims, however, are the future patients the cheater will take care of in the event that he is able to complete a course by cheating through it.

Regardless of the specific type of behavior that is inhibiting a student from learning, methods for modifying behavior in order to enhance the learning process are the same. Such methods include positive reinforcement, negative reinforcement, and punishment through the use of aversive stimuli, as identified in Box 10.1.

Positive Reinforcement

Positive reinforcement is the immediate response to a behavior that increases or maintains the probability or rate of the continuance of a particular behavior. In order to be effective there must be a direct relationship between the behavior and its consequences (the reinforcer). That is, when the behavior is seen, the reinforcer must be presented.

Positive reinforcement occurs only when the reinforcer has an effect on specific behavior. The effect is dependent on several factors:

1) Student reinforcement history (what has caused motivation in the past?)
2) Student deprivation state (what is wanted but not easily or frequently obtained by the student?)
3) Perceived value of reinforcement (is it worth performing the behavior?)
4) Consistency (have reinforcements been delivered reliably and consistently in the past?)

Reinforcement is individualized in that what motivates one student to perform a certain behavior may not motivate another. If one type of reinforcer does not achieve a repeat of behavior, an alternative form of reinforcement should be attempted.

An example of the use of positive reinforcement is shown in the following scenario.

Positive reinforcement is the immediate response to a behavior that increases or maintains the probability or rate of the continuance of a particular behavior.

BOX 10.1   Types of Behavior Modification Strategies

Anticipated effect	Presentation of stimuli	Removal of stimuli
To increase the rate and/or probability of the recurrence of a behavior	Positive reinforcement	Negative reinforcement
To decrease the rate and/or probability of the recurrence of a behavior	Punishment (aversive stimuli)	Punishment (time-out)

Types of behavior modification strategies (adapted from Dembo, 1991[1]).

🍎 John lacks self-confidence and asks numerous questions rather than researching information. The instructor notices that this behavior is distracting to other students. During a break the instructor takes John aside and informs him that if he decreases the number of questions he asks to one per session, at the end of the course he will receive a blood pressure cuff.

One type of positive reinforcement involves group contingencies and peer pressure. In such situations, each member of the group must be capable of performing the target behavior. Otherwise there is a risk of subjecting students to verbal and physical abuse by classmates. For example:

🍎 An instructor offers a class party if the entire class passes the state final exam. This places pressure on slower students to succeed.

Finally, positive reinforcement only works if the reinforcer is normally deprived from the student. For example, if the reinforcer is candy, and the student usually brings large amounts of candy to class, additional candy will most likely not motivate the student. Additional examples of the use of positive reinforcement, and the effects of it, are described in Box 10.2.

Extinction

Extinction is the reduction of a behavior through the abrupt termination of the positive reinforcer that is maintaining the inappropriate behavior. For example:

🍎 Pat sits in the back of the classroom and is disruptive, often "egging on" the instructor. The instructor usually responds by focusing attention on her. Pat finds such attention positively reinforcing, and therefore continues the disruptive behavior. To cause extinction of the behavior, the instructor refrains from focusing any attention on Pat, thereby eliminating positive reinforcement of the inappropriate behavior.

> Extinction is the reduction of a behavior through the abrupt termination of the positive reinforcer that is maintaining the inappropriate behavior.

BOX 10.2 Examples of Positive Reinforcement

Behavior	Positive Reinforcer	Effect
Phil correctly answers a question in class	The instructor smiles and offers words of praise	An increased probability that Phil will answer additional questions
Carol completes assigned chapters in the workbook	The instructor reviews the workbook and offers comments for improvement	An increased probability that Carol will continue to complete homework assignments
As instructed, Jerry studied assigned materials prior to each class session	He receives 2 points extra credit on an impromptu quiz	An increased probability that Jerry will continue being prepared for class

Examples of positive reinforcement (adapted from Alberto and Troutman, 1990[2]).

Students often offer a resistance to extinction and increase the rate and/or intensity of inappropriate behavior before a significant reduction is apparent. Since the behavior will most likely get worse before getting better, it is essential the instructor not give in to the more intensive attempt to regain the positive reinforcer (most likely to be attention).

The instructor can also expect the attempted reappearance of the extinguished behavior as a means to determine if the extinction is still in effect. The re-emergence of the behavior can be terminated quickly by ignoring it. Failure to do this may result in rapid relearning by the student and may cause the negative behavior to return.

Negative Reinforcement

Negative reinforcement is the removal of an aversive stimuli immediately following a behavior, thereby increasing the probability of such future behavior. The student performs the behavior to escape or avoid an aversive stimuli. For example:

- Immediately after the instructor distributes the midterm exam Emily complains of being sick. The sickness results in Emily being sent home, thereby eliminating the aversive stimuli (the test). Such "sickness" may increase in frequency given future similar test situations.
- Chris does not like working in small groups. When divided into groups he is disruptive to the class, causing the instructor to order him to return to his desk to complete an assignment independently (thereby removing the aversive stimuli of the small group).

Instructors often inadvertently use negative reinforcement in the classroom. For example, when students whine about completing an assignment, the instructor may delete the assignment, causing students to learn that whining will result in the termination of an aversive stimuli (work). Consequently, the students whine more often.

Likewise, when reviewing exams, if students question test items they get wrong, and the instructor throws out those questions, students learn they can increase their test scores by arguing over questions, so they argue each and every incorrect answer.

For the above examples, if the instructor chooses not to eliminate an exercise or test questions when students were expecting it, they may react negatively, throwing items or whining, thereby disseminating poor attitudes throughout the class.

Punishment

Punishment involves the presentation of an unpleasant stimulus that decreases the future rate and/or probability of recurrence of a particular behavior. In order to be effective, punishment must be administered immediately following the production of an undesirable or inappropriate behavior. This can occur in two forms:

1) The removal of a desirable stimulus
2) The presentation of an undesired stimulus

Presentation of Aversive Stimuli

The presentation of aversive stimuli is a common form of punishment. It may be a natural reflex for instructors to resort to punishment when dealing with inappropriate student behavior because it has been

> Negative reinforcement is the removal of an aversive stimuli immediately following a behavior, thereby increasing the probability of such future behavior.

> Instructors often inadvertently use negative reinforcement in the classroom.

a natural form of discipline at home. This form of punishment is used often because it:

- Rapidly stops the occurrence of an inappropriate behavior and has some long-term effects. For example, students talking in the back of a room stop when the teacher yells at them.
- Facilitates learning of acceptable and unacceptable behavior or discrimination between what is safe and unsafe behavior. For example, an EMT student enters an industrial plant where a worker has collapsed, and suddenly collapses himself due to hazardous fumes. This student will learn to ensure scene safety in future situations.
- Aversive consequence of one student's inappropriate behavior becomes evident to others, thereby lessening the probability that others will engage in a similiar behavior.

Physical or other strong aversive actions are rarely, if ever, a justified form of behavior modification.

This is not to say the presentation of aversive stimuli (punishment) is recommended as a routine form of classroom management. Physical or other strong aversive actions are rarely, if ever, a justified form of behavior modification. In lesser forms, however, aversive stimuli may be indicated for long-term behavior problems with certain students who cannot be corrected by alternative means. It is essential that instructors ensure that student rights are not violated during the punishment process.

Disadvantages of Aversive Stimuli

- The student may become aggressive and strike back, causing a barrier to the learning process as well as distracting the class.
- The student may become withdrawn and completely "tune out" the instructor, thereby preventing learning.
- Since instructors are seen as a role model for students, behavior is closely observed by students. As such, the instructor's reaction may be seen as a norm, causing students to view punishment as an acceptable behavior.
- The student may only learn not to perform the inappropriate behavior in the presence of the instructor who used punishment, although he continues the behavior when the instructor is not present.

Overcorrection

Overcorrection is intended to decrease inappropriate behaviors by making a student take responsibility for his actions.

Overcorrection is intended to decrease inappropriate behaviors by making a student take responsibility for his actions. This requires a student who has disturbed the environment, either physically or emotionally, to restore the environment not only to its original form, but beyond. For example:

- John throws a piece of paper at Sue seated in front of him. Overcorrection occurs when the instructor tells John not only to pick up that paper and throw it in the trash, but also to collect all the trash in the room and dispose of it properly.
- Larry disturbs and rearranges furniture in the classroom. The instructor tells him to straighten not only those items in the immediate area that were disturbed, but all objects in the room.
- Bridget annoys or frightens another class member. The instructor tells her to apologize to all of the students, not merely those she had bothered.

Response Cost Procedures

Response-cost procedures is a type of behavior modification strategy that involve the presentation of a positive reinforcer for appropriate behavior and the removal of a reinforcer for inappropriate behavior. For example:

- Students are given 1 extra credit point for each homework assignment completed, and 1 point is taken away for each assignment not completed.

These procedures are effective without the undesirable effect associated with punishment. Rules must be explained clearly, identifying appropriate behaviors, *eg*, completing assignments and rewards for completing the behavior (1 extra credit point), as well as infractions against the behavior (loss of 1 point).

STUDENTS WITH DISABILITIES

With the adoption of the ADA in 1990, much emphasis has been placed on making modifications in both the workplace and educational facilities to accommodate individuals with disabilities. Such disabilities vary from mild to quite severe. The majority of those attending EMS training programs, however, usually require only minor modifications on the part of a training facility or instructional faculty.

The learning-disabled student is often willing to participate and usually tries extremely hard to learn. This student most often captures the hearts of instructors because he tries so hard to succeed, and yet often lacks the ability to do so on his own. The slow student does best with one-on-one learning with an instructor or tutor. With a little extra time, this type of student can succeed.

Other learning disabilities include reading problems such as illiteracy and dyslexia. Some adult learners have never learned to read or write, or can only do so at a certain level. Students diagnosed with dyslexia inadvertently mix letters in words, thereby changing their meaning. Regulations for dealing with such students vary by state; some states allow certification exams to be read to students with handicaps.

Other students are physically impaired. These students include those with visual impairments that may include sensitive eyes, difficulty seeing the board, or difficulty seeing the television when lights are on. Every possible accommodation should be provided for these students. Suggest that they sit in the front of the room; provide a handout containing the contents of the overhead transparency screens; and make appropriate accommodations for alternative lighting as necessary.

Students with hearing impairments should be provided with extra visual media during a presentation, such as instructor notes. In addition, the instructor may wish to tape a session so the student can listen to the tape at a louder volume later. Finally, there may be equipment that this type of student can use to magnify sounds such as a hearing aid or an enhanced stethoscope.

Some students may have physical problems such as arthritic hands, knees, or other joints that may make it difficult to participate actively or perform certain skills. Again, every possible accommodation should be made for physically impaired students, while following state-man-

The learning-disabled student is often willing to participate and usually tries extremely hard to learn.

Every possible accommodation should be made for physically impaired students, while following state-mandated guidelines.

dated guidelines. For example, if a student cannot kneel on the floor to perform CPR, it may be acceptable to place the mannequin on a table. During final practical exams, however, such accommodations may not be allowed since an EMT must attend to patients in the field in various positions.

PREPARING STUDENTS FOR CERTIFICATION EXAMS

How well students are prepared is sometimes as important as the knowledge they possess.

There are numerous certification exams that students must be prepared to sit for during their careers[3]. How well students are prepared is sometimes as important as the knowledge they possess. Both mental and physical preparation are extremely important in order for students to do well in certification exams.

It is necessary that instructors understand the importance of student preparation, and relay specific test-taking skills to their students during training programs in order to improve their success on exams. The following pages can be used by instructors as a means of empowering students to perform better on certification exams.

Test taking is a skill that can be learned. While some students may have a thorough knowledge of a particular content area, they might lack the ability to translate this knowledge in a testing situation. Learning test-taking skills can improve student performance on evaluations.

Exams

Since there is no penalty for guessing, students should always enter a response.

Written certification exams usually consist entirely of multiple-choice questions. Other question formats might include short-answer, true-false, or essay-type questions. Such exams are graded based on the number of correct answers, not the number of incorrect responses. Since there is no penalty for guessing, students should always enter a response. In multiple choice questions, the student has at least a 25% chance of a correct response, even if he has no idea of the correct answer.

Multiple-choice questions are comprised of two parts: the stem (question) and the responses (choices). Responses include the correct answer and three or four plausible distractors. Questions are usually factual or situational. Factual questions usually require rote learning and the ability to recall specific information while situational questions require the synthesis of information and the knowledge to determine a best response.

Here is an example of a factual multiple-choice question:

> When performing CPR, how far should the rescuer compress the victim's chest?
> a. 1/2 to 1 inch
> b. 1 to 1 1/2 inches
> c. 1 1/2 to 2 inches
> d. 2 to 2 1/2 inches

Here is an example of a situational type multiple choice question:

> You arrive on the location of a 22-year-old female patient with cold, clammy skin, slurred speech, and an intoxicated appearance. Her husband states this happened suddenly, because when he left an hour ago to get lunch, she was doing exercises. When you attempted

> to interview the patient, she was extremely combative. You should suspect the patient is most likely suffering from a(n) _____ emergency.
> a. cardiac
> b. diabetic
> c. heat-related
> d. respiratory

Regardless of the type of multiple-choice question, the first step in the selection of a correct answer is to analyze the question. To do this:

- Read the stem without reading the responses
- Understand what the question is asking
- Determine a correct response to the question
- Read all questions to select the one that is closest to the correct response.

The first step in the selection of a correct answer is to analyze the question.

When reading the question, it is important to look for key words such as:

- NOT
- RATIO
- FIRST
- NEVER
- EXCEPT
- RATE
- ALWAYS

In addition, it is essential to identify specific terms that would cause a different response. For example:

- One-rescuer versus two-rescuer CPR
- Infant versus child CPR
- Chest pain *after exertion*
- Chest pain that *radiates*
- Sudden onset
- Cool, clammy skin

Before selecting the correct answer, read all possible responses. If the correct answer is not readily apparent, exclude those choices that are obviously incorrect. Most often students can exclude two of the four possible responses, leaving a 50% chance of selecting the correct answer. If the option "all of the above" appears as a response, it is most often the correct answer.

Do not read into the question. If the question asks whether the administration of oxygen is indicated for a particular patient, do not read into the question and think "well yes, except what if the patient. . . " Your first impulse is most often the correct choice.

Studying Strategies

The most effective means for preparing academically for an exam is to study throughout a training program. Waiting until exam week and "cramming" is not productive. Specific strategies are as follows:

The most effective means for preparing academically for an exam is to study throughout a training program.

- Use course objectives when studying. State and National exams are referenced to curriculum objectives for the EMT-Basic course.
- Complete reading assignments *prior* to a particular class session.
- Attend the class session and take notes based on the instructor's presentation.
- After the training session, reread assigned chapters and notes taken in class.

- Frequently review class notes throughout the course.
- Participate in multiple short-study sessions rather than a few long sessions.
- Determine specific study preferences. Some students learn better in small groups; others do better studying solo.
- Recite information aloud to help improve retention of information.
- Prepare mental pictures of information. Visualizing key information assists with moving information into long-term memory.
- Complete practice quizzes, tests, or other aids that may be available.
- Pace study time in accordance with exam content percentages. Do not waste time studying insignificant information.

Physiologic and Mental Preparation

Taking tests is often a very stressful process.

Taking tests is often a very stressful process. Some students, especially those who have been out of school for many years, feel somewhat threatened by exams. How a student feels entering the exam process often has a great effect on a successful outcome. Anxiety is often the strongest deterrent to success.

The following physical and mental preparation strategies can help alleviate test-taking anxiety.

- Get a full night sleep prior to the exam.
- Prior to the exam, perform a few exercises. Moderate exercise increases blood supply to the brain by increasing the status of the cardiovascular system.
- Eat normal meals prior to the exam. Refrain from eating a heavy meal within 1 hour prior to a test. Immediately after eating, blood flow directed to the digestive system is increased, thereby causing drowsiness.
- Layer clothing in order to maintain a comfortable personal climate regardless of the temperature in the classroom.
- Focus on the task at hand and sit away from distractors.
- Relax and take deep breaths prior to beginning the exam.
- Be prepared and be positive.

Test-Taking Strategies

- Determine the amount of time to spend on questions. For example, if an exam consists of 100 questions and students are given 2 hours in which to complete the exam, they must complete an average of 50 questions per hour or one question every minute or so. Pacing is important.
- Determine the point value system. If each question is worth the same value (usually 1 point) as in the case of most certification exams, do not waste time on difficult questions for which the answer is uncertain.
- Use scrap paper to formulate responses and calculate answers if allowed. Make note of the questions in which the answer is uncertain and review the answer if time permits.
- When in doubt, guess, but do so logically. When the answer is not readily apparent, guess at first, write down the question number, and return to re-evaluate the answer later if time permits.
- When the exam is completed, *do not* second guess the answers or read into the questions. Remember, the first choice answer is

usually correct. Only change answers when there is a reason for a change (*ie,* the question or responses were read incorrectly the first time).

- Fill in the answer sheet correctly. Use the proper tools as directed by test moderators (*ie,* no. 2 pencils). Fill in circles completely and erase all stray marks.

- Check the test question numbers after every 10 answers to prevent a last minute panic when it is discovered that the answer to question #78 was placed in #79's space on the answer sheet.

KEY POINTS

1. No matter how effectively an instructor presents information, or what instructional methods and materials are used, there are certain students who are difficult to reach.
2. A *student deficiency* is any problem that inhibits the learning process and may consist of behavioral, emotional, or physical components.
3. There are three primary types of behavior modification strategies to handle a difficult student: positive reinforcement, negative reinforcement, and punishment.
4. *Positive reinforcement* is the immediate response to a student's behavior that increases or maintains the probability or rate of the continuance of a particular behavior.
5. The effect of a positive reinforcer is dependent on student reinforcement history, the student's deprivation state, the student's perceived value of the reinforcer, and the consistency at which reinforcements have been delivered.
6. *Extinction* is the reduction of a behavior through the abrupt termination of the positive reinforcer maintaining the appropriate behavior.
7. *Negative reinforcement* is the removal of an unpleasant aversive stimuli immediately following a behavior, thereby increasing the probability of such future behavior.
8. *Punishment* involves the presentation of an unpleasant stimulus that decreases the future rate and/or probability of the recurrence of a particular behavior. This can occur by the removal of a desirable stimulus or the presentation of an undesired stimulus.
9. The presentation of aversive stimuli (punishment) is not recommended as a routine form of classroom management. In lesser forms, aversive stimuli may be indicated for long-term behavior modification for certain disruptive students. When used, however, the instructor must ensure that student's rights are not violated.

FOLLOW-UP ACTIVITIES

1. Provide three examples each of both positive and negative reinforcements that work at 1) home, 2) work, and 3) the classroom.
2. Describe two reinforcers that may be both positive and negative.
3. Provide two examples of punishment strategies that might be used in the classroom setting.
4. Provide two examples of overcorrection techniques.
5. Provide two examples of a response-cost procedures form of behavior modification.
6. Develop a student handout consisting of helpful tips for preparing for certification exams.

REFERENCES

1. Dembo M. *Applying Educational Psychology in the Classroom,* 4th ed. White Plains, NY: Longman Publishing Group; 1991.
2. Alberto P, Troutman A. *Applied Behavior Analysis for Teachers,* 3rd ed. New York, NY: MacMillan Publishing Co; 1990.
3. *Emergency Medical Services Study Guide.* Harrisburg, PA: Pennsylvania Department of Health, Division of EMS; 1990.

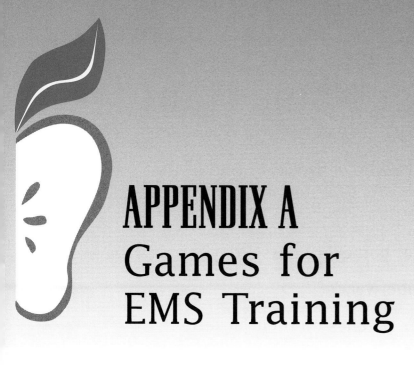

APPENDIX A
Games for
EMS Training

Scavenger Name Hunt

DIRECTIONS: Find a classmate who represents one of the following. You can use each name only once.

1. Who has their scanner on at home 24 hours a day? _____

2. Who is wearing colored underwear? _____

3. Who wears more than three patches on their jacket? _____

4. Who has broken a bone (preferably their own)? _____

5. Who has green eyes? _____

6. Who has type AB blood? _____

7. Who has been involved with EMS for more than 5 years? _____

8. Who has ever been in a hot air balloon? _____

9. Whose initials are C.P.? _____

10. Who has caused more than $1000 damage to an ambulance? _____

11. Who drives a red car? _____

12. Who is an only child? _____

13. Who has never been on an ambulance? _____

14. Who has ever performed CPR in the field? _____

15. Who is wearing mismatched socks? _____

16. Who has ever flown a plane? _____

17. Who has been hospitalized for more than 3 days? _____

18. Who does not routinely wear a seat belt? _____

19. Who never speeds? _____

20. Who is NOT certified in CPR? _____

Professionals Use the Right Words
Game Cards

Professionals Use the Right Words

Noticable distention of the abdomen caused by the accumulation of excess fluids

Game #1

Professionals Use the Right Words

Low level of sugar in the blood

Game #1

Professionals Use the Right Words

Heart attack, specifically rapid onset of anoxia and death to an area of heart muscle tissue

Game #1

Professionals Use the Right Words

Condition of elevated levels of carbon dioxide in the blood

Game #1

Professionals Use the Right Words

Condition of a patient immediately after a seizure

Game #1

Professionals Use the Right Words

Episodes of seizure activity occurring in rapid succession and considered a true emergency

Game #1

Professionals Use the Right Words
Game Cards

Professionals Use the Right Words

Condition in which the body begins using stored fat for energy; seen in out of control diabetics

Game #1

Professionals Use the Right Words

A place where infectious organisms live

Game #1

Professionals Use the Right Words

Condition of not being free of germs and foreign matter

Game #1

Professionals Use the Right Words

A medical problem with a sudden onset

Game #2

Professionals Use the Right Words

Sudden pain occurring when a portion of the myocardium is not receiving enough oxygenated blood

Game #2

Professionals Use the Right Words

Process in which plaque (fat and other foreign particles) is deposited on the inner wall of an artery

Game #2

Professionals Use the Right Words
Game Cards

Professionals Use the Right Words

Heroin, morphine, codeine, and dilantin; an overdose of which causes pinpoint pupils and respiratory depression

Game #2

Professionals Use the Right Words

Temporary condition of rapid, deep breathing that reduces the carbon dioxide level in the blood

Game #2

Professionals Use the Right Words

Blood vessel that supplies the muscles of the heart

Game #2

Professionals Use the Right Words

Profuse perspiration

Game #2

Professionals Use the Right Words

Phenobarbital, amobarbital; an overdose of which causes respiratory depression, hypotension, and dilated pupils

Game #2

Professionals Use the Right Words

Dilation of a weakened section of an arterial wall

Game #2

Professionals Use the Right Words
Game Board #1

Ascites	Hypoglycemia	Acute Myocardial Infarction
Hypercarbia	Postictal State	Status Epilepticus
Ketoacidosis	Contamination	Infection

Professionals Use the Right Words
Game Board #2

Acute	Angina Pectoris	Atherosclerosis
Narcotics	Hyper-ventilation	Coronary Artery
Diaphoresis	Barbiturates	Aneurysm

Airway Crossword Puzzle

ACROSS

1. A group of diseases and conditions in which the lungs decline in their ability to exchange gases, including emphysema, chronic bronchitis, and black lung disease.
7. A flexible breathing tube inserted through the patient's nose, into the pharynx.
10. The partial or complete collapse of the alveoli in the lungs.
13. A double-membrane sac; the outer layer lines the chest wall and the inner layer covers the outside of the lungs.
16. A container for oxygen.
19. The small branches of the airway that carry air to and from the alveoli.
22. An abnormal sound produced in the lungs as air moves through fluids in the bronchiole tree.
23. The prefix meaning below normal.
24. Any permanent, surgically made opening.
25. A drug necessary for sustaining life.
26. A whistling respiratory sound.
27. The term for breathing air in.

DOWN

3. A hand-held aid for artificial ventilation.
4. The sign for when the skin, lips, tongue, and/or nailbed colors change to blue or gray because of too little oxygen in the blood.
5. A device connected to the oxygen cylinder to provide a safe working pressure of 30 to 70 psi.
6. A device that allows control of the flow of oxygen in liters per minute.
9. A mask designed for use when low concentrations of oxygen are required.
11. Temporary suspension of breathing.
12. A device used to remove blood, secretions, or other fluids from a patient's airway.
14. Microscopic air sacs of the lungs where gas exchange takes place with the circulatory system.
15. Severe dyspnea experienced when lying down, and relieved by sitting up.
17. Movement and the lodgement of a blood clot or foreign body (fat or air bubble) inside a blood vessel.
18. Another term for the throat.
20. Coarse loud rales resting from a partial obstruction of the bronchi or bronchioles.
21. Another term for the windpipe.

Airway Crossword Puzzle

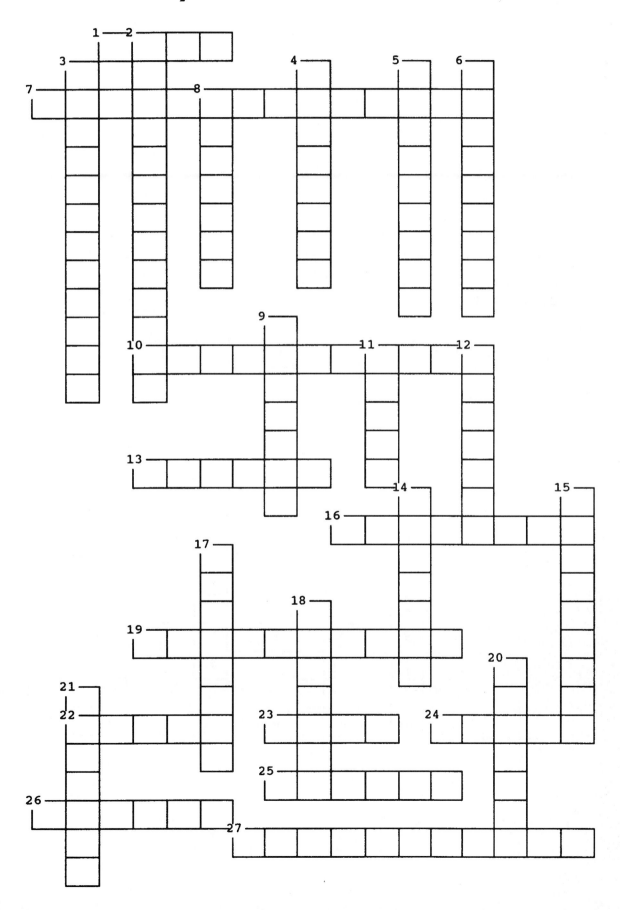

Airway Crossword Puzzle
Answer Key

Across

7. nasopharyngeal
10. atelectasis
13. pleura
16. cylinder
19. bronchiole
22. rales
23. hypo
24. stoma
25. oxygen
26. wheeze
27. inspiration

Down

1. copd
2. oropharyngeal
3. bagvalvemask
4. cyanosis
5. regulator
6. flowmeter
8. hypoxia
9. venturi
11. apnea
12. suction
14. alveoli
15. orthopnea
17. emblism
18. phari
20. rhonchi
21. trach
26. wheea

Anatomy & Physiology Crossword Puzzle

ACROSS

1. A prefix meaning fast.
2. The section of the spine that supports the small of the back.
3. A suffix meaning breathing.
4. A term meaning towards the midline of the body.
5. A prefix meaning lung.
6. The lower extension of the sternum.
7. A term referring to the front of the body.
8. The portion of the skeleton which includes the skull, spinal column, sternum, and ribs.
9. A term meaning to bend at a joint.
10. A stem word meaning stomach.
11. A term meaning away from the point of reference.
12. The major artery of the body.
13. The medical term for foot bones.

DOWN

1. A suffix meaning surgical incision.
2. A term meaning towards the side.
3. The lateral forearm bone.
4. The type of consent given when an adult is unconscious.
5. The term meaning toward the point of reference.
6. The medical term for shoulder blade.
7. The term referring to the outside.
8. The term referring to the back of the body or body part.
9. The term for lying face down.
10. The section of the spine in the lower back.
11. The dome-shaped muscle of respiration that separates the chest from the abdomen.
12. The term meaning away from the head.
13. The medical term for the chest.
14. The section of the spine in the neck.
15. A double-membrane sac lining the chest wall and lungs.

Anatomy & Physiology
Crossword Puzzle

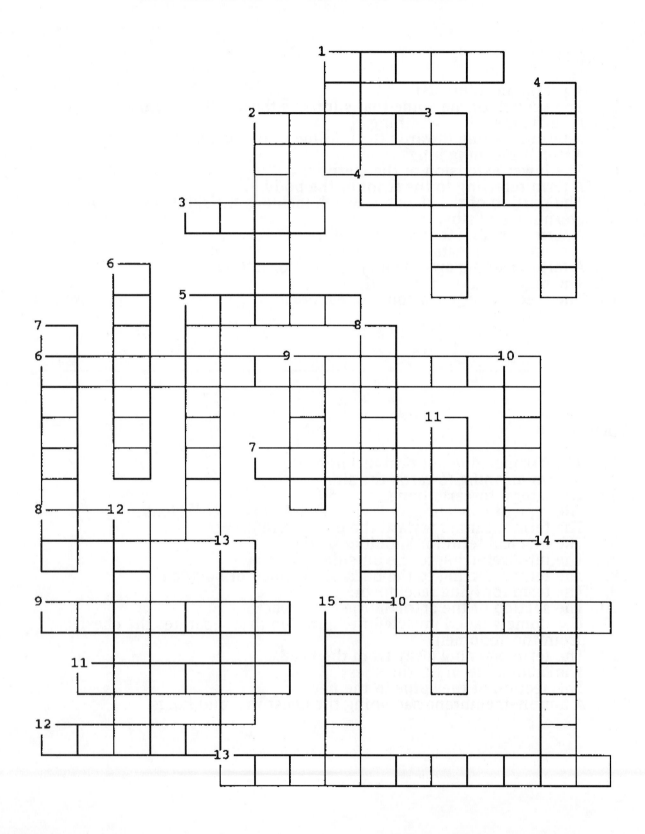

Anatomy & Physiology Crossword Puzzle Answer Key

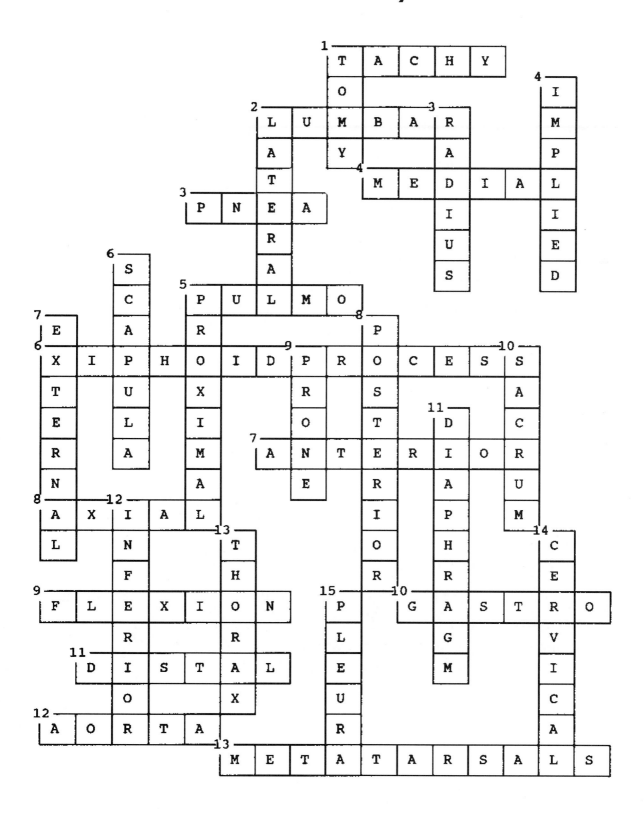

Anatomy & Patient Assessment Word-Find

DIRECTIONS: Find a word that matches each description, then find that word in the puzzle. Words can be found in any direction: left to right, right to left, top to bottom, bottom to top, diagonal forward, or diagonal backward.

Whistling respiratory sound: _ _ _ _ _ _

Difficult or labored breathing: _ _ _ _ _ _ _ _

Bluish colored skin: _ _ _ _ _ _ _ _

Rapid heartbeat: _ _ _ _ _ _ _ _ _ _ _

Movement and the lodgement of a blood clot or foreign body inside a blood vessel:
    _ _ _ _ _ _ _ _

The constant flow of blood through the capillaries: _ _ _ _ _ _ _ _ _ _

A grating noise caused by the movement of broken bone ends rubbing together:
    _ _ _ _ _ _ _ _

An atypical sound made when a patient breathes, usually indicating an airway obstruction:
    _ _ _ _ _ _ _

Lying flat in the back: _ _ _ _ _ _

Lying face down: _ _ _ _ _

Toward the midline of the body: _ _ _ _ _ _

Yellowing of the skin: _ _ _ _ _ _ _ _

The back of the body or body part: _ _ _ _ _ _ _ _ _

Abnormal sound produced in the lungs as air moves through fluids in the bronchiole tree:
    _ _ _ _ _

An instrument used to measure blood pressures:
    _ _ _ _ _ _ _ _ _ _ _ _ _ _

The process of listening to sounds that occur within the body:
_ _ _ _ _ _ _ _ _ _ _

The process of feeling any part of the body: _ _ _ _ _ _ _ _ _ _

Swelling due to the accumulation of fluids in the tissues: _ _ _ _ _ _

A sign of impaired circulation evaluated by examining the skin at the distal end of an injured limb: _ _ _ _ _ _ _ _ _   _ _ _ _ _ _

Pressure exerted on the internal walls of the arteries when the heart is relaxing:
_ _ _ _ _ _ _ _ _

Away from a point of reference: _ _ _ _ _ _

Close to a point of reference: _ _ _ _ _ _ _ _

To the side, away from the midline of the body: _ _ _ _ _ _ _

What is between the ribs, which contract during an inspiration to lift the ribs and increase the volume of the thoracic cavity: _ _ _ _ _ _ _ _ _ _   _ _ _ _ _ _

A method of opening the airway without lifting the neck or tilting the head:
_ _ _   _ _ _ _ _ _

The front surface of the body or body part: _ _ _ _ _ _ _ _ _

The anterior body cavity inferior to the diaphragm: _ _ _ _ _ _ _ _ _ _ _ _ _ _ _
_ _ _ _ _ _

The anterior body cavity located between the diaphragm and the ring of the pelvis:
_ _ _ _ _ _ _ _ _ _

The major artery of systemic circulation that carries blood from the heart out to the body:
_ _ _ _ _

The complete loss or impairment of speech usually associated with a stroke or brain lesion:
_ _ _ _ _ _ _

Temporary suspension of breathing: _ _ _ _ _

The large neck artery: _ _ _ _ _ _ _ _

The flap of cartilage and other tissues that is the superior structure of the larynx which divert fooddown the esophagus: _ _ _ _ _ _ _ _ _ _ _

The organ that attaches to the lower back of the liver that stores bile:
_ _ _ _ _ _ _ _ _ _ _

The arm bone, distal to the shoulder and proximal to the elbow: _ _ _ _ _ _ _

Anatomic term meaning away from the top of the body: _ _ _ _ _ _ _ _ _

The largest gland in the body, located in the upper right quadrant of the abdomen: _ _ _ _ _ _

The arteries that supply blood to the heart muscle: _ _ _ _ _ _ _ _ _

Anatomic term meaning toward the top of the body: _ _ _ _ _ _ _ _ _

The medial lower leg bone: _ _ _ _ _

A prefix meaning beyond normal or excessive: _ _ _ _ _

What separates the ventricle of the heart from the atrium: _ _ _ _ _ _

The portion of patient assessment that entails determining factors that may have precipitated or lead to the illness: _ _ _ _ _ _ _

What is checked to determine a head injury: _ _ _ _ _ _

The largest organ of the body: _ _ _ _

The acronym for illness that the patient has had that pertian to his current condition:
_ _ _

The acronym that indicates that the eyes are functioning normal: _ _ _ _ _ _

Anatomy & Patient Assessment Word-Find
Answer Key

DIRECTIONS: Find a word that matches each description, then find that word in the puzzle. Words can be found in any direction: left to right, right to left, top to bottom, bottom to top, diagonal forward, or diagonal backward.

Whistling respiratory sound: _ _ _ _ _ _ (Wheeze)

Difficult or labored breathing: _ _ _ _ _ _ _ (Dyspnea)

Bluish colored skin: _ _ _ _ _ _ _ _ (Cyanosis)

Rapid heartbeat: _ _ _ _ _ _ _ _ _ _ _ (Tachycardia)

Movement and the lodgement of a blood clot or foreign body inside a blood vessel: _ _ _ _ _ _ _ _ (Embolism)

The constant flow of blood through the capillaries: _ _ _ _ _ _ _ _ _ (Perfusion)

A grating noise caused by the movement of broken bone ends rubbing together: _ _ _ _ _ _ _ _ (Crepitus)

An atypical sound made when a patient breathes, usually indicating an airway obstruction: _ _ _ _ _ _ _ (Crowing)

Lying flat in the back: _ _ _ _ _ _ (Supine)

Lying face down: _ _ _ _ _ (Prone)

Toward the midline of the body: _ _ _ _ _ _ (Medial)

Yellowing of the skin: _ _ _ _ _ _ _ _ (Jaundice)

The back of the body or body part: _ _ _ _ _ _ _ _ _ (Posterior)

Abnormal sound produced in the lungs as air moves through fluids in the bronchiole tree: _ _ _ _ _ (Rales)

An instrument used to measure blood pressures: _ _ _ _ _ _ _ _ _ _ _ _ _ _ _ (Sphygmomanometer)

The process of listening to sounds that occur within the body:
_ _ _ _ _ _ _ _ _ _ _ _ (Auscultation)

The process of feeling any part of the body: _ _ _ _ _ _ _ _ _ (Palpation)

Swelling due to the accumulation of fluids in the tissues: _ _ _ _ _ (Edema)

A sign of impaired circulation evaluated by examining the skin at the distal end of an injured limb: _ _ _ _ _ _ _ _ _ _ _ _ _ _ _ (Capillary Refill)

Pressure exerted on the internal walls of the arteries when the heart is relaxing:
_ _ _ _ _ _ _ _ _ (Diastolic)

Away from a point of reference: _ _ _ _ _ _ (Distal)

Close to a point of reference: _ _ _ _ _ _ _ _ (Proximal)

To the side, away from the midline of the body: _ _ _ _ _ _ _ (Lateral)

What is between the ribs, which contract during as inspiration to lift the ribs and increase the volume of the thoracic cavity: _ _ _ _ _ _ _ _ _ _ _ _ _ _ _ _ _ (Intercostal Muscle)

A method of opening the airway without lifting the neck or tilting the head:
_ _ _ _ _ _ _ _ _ (Jaw Thrust)

The front surface of the body or body part: _ _ _ _ _ _ _ _ (Anterior)

The anferior body cavity inferior to the diaphragm:
_ _ _ _ _ _ _ _ _ _ _ _ _ _ _ _ _ _ _ _ _
    (Abdominopelvic Muscle)

The anterior body cavity located between the diaphragm and the ring of the pelvis:
_ _ _ _ _ _ _ _ _ (Abdominal)

The major artery of systemic circulation that carries blood from the heart out to the body:
_ _ _ _ _ (Aorta)

The complete loss or impairment of speech usually associated with a stroke or brain lesion:
_ _ _ _ _ _ _ (Aphasia)

Temporary suspension of breathing: _ _ _ _ _ (Apnea)

The large neck artery: _ _ _ _ _ _ _ (Carotid)

The flap of cartilage and other tissues that is the superior structure of the larynx which divert food down the esophagus: _ _ _ _ _ _ _ _ _ _ (Epiglottis)

The organ that attaches to the lower back of the liver that stores bile:
_ _ _ _ _ _ _ _ _ _ _ (Gallbladder)

The arm bone, distal to the shoulder and proximal to the elbow: _ _ _ _ _ _ _ (Humerus)

Anatomic term meaning away from the top of the body: _ _ _ _ _ _ _ _ (Inferior)

The largest gland in the body, located in the upper right quadrant of the abdomen:
_ _ _ _ _ (Liver)

The arteries that supply blood to the heart muscle: _ _ _ _ _ _ _ _ (Coronary)

Anatomic term meaning toward the top of the body: _ _ _ _ _ _ _ _ (Superior)

The medial lower leg bone: _ _ _ _ _ (Tibia)

A prefix meaning beyond normal or excessive: _ _ _ _ _ (Hyper)

What separates the ventricle of the heart from the atrium: _ _ _ _ _ (Valve)

The portion of patient assessment that entails determining factors that may have precipitated or lead to the illness: _ _ _ _ _ _ _ (History)

What is checked to determine a head injury: _ _ _ _ _ _ (Pupils)

The largest organ of the body: _ _ _ _ (Skin)

The acronym for illness that the patient has had that pertain to his current condition:
_ _ _ (PMH)

The acronym that indicates that the eyes are functioning normal: _ _ _ _ _ _ (PEARLA)

Anatomy & Patient Assessment Word-Find

```
R W Y E P U P I L S A N A L R A E P D
E A B S D E R S L A T E R A L I N T I
D U E T D E N I P U S H X D O R O H A
S S P H Y G M O M A N O M E T E R E S
S C A J S S I A L S K I E S E L P Y T
E U B I P L K A M T D E D L M H C E O
I L D M N A T S K I N I E U E U W K L
L T O R E U R E W Y N C E P D T Z U I
P A M P A T I O N F C F G N I W O R C
I T I A G A R C A Y M Y E T A P P A A
N I N L I C E R L R N B A R L M T O P
T O O P R H B O A A O A D N I R S R I
E N P A L Y N I N N I S I S O O N E L
R B E T L C O R I O S C T A A S R O L
C T L I I A R E M R U U O T P N I R A
O R V O G R O T O O F D R H N R E S R
S S I N T D T S D C R I A E E A P U Y
T H C M S I L O B M E S C T A P I T R
A Y M L U A I P A B P T N S V H G I E
L H U P R O X I M A L A I A I A L P F
M S S H H Y P E R T H L U M R S O E I
U U C G T E C I D N U A J E S I T R L
S R L S W E A T E V L A V P T A T C L
C E E U A R E S A I B I T I H T I E V
L M E W J R E D D A L B L L A G S T R
E U V R S U P E R I O R A L E S R I E
P H I S T O R Y L A M U H H M P U C S
O T C R Y S A N T E R I O R L O C K R
```

Anatomy & Patient Assessment
Word-Find
Answer Key

```
R W Y E P U P I L S A N A L R A E P D
E A B S D E R S L A T E R A L I N T I
D U E T D E N I P U S H X D O R O H A
S S P H Y G M O M A N O M E T E R E S
S C A J S S I A L S K I E S E L P Y T
E U B I P L K A M T D E D L M H C E O
I L D M N A T S K I N I E U E U W K L
L T O R E U R E W Y N C E P D T Z U I
P A M P A T I O N F C F G N I W O R C
I I A G A R C A Y M Y E T A P P A A
N O N L I C E R L R N B A R L M T O P
T O O L P R H B O A N O A D N I R S R I
E B E T A L Y N I N N I S I S O O N E L
R T L I A R E M R U O T P N I R O L A
C S V O G R O T O O F D R H N R I R A
O S I N D T S D C R I A E E A S U R Y
S H C M S I L O B M E S C T A P I T R
T Y M L U A I P A B P T N S V H G I E
A H U P R O X I M A L A I A I A L P F
L S S H H Y P E R T H L U M R S O E I
M U C G T E C I D N U A J E S I T R L
U R L S W E A T E V L A V P T A T C L
S E E U A R E S A I B I T I H T I E V
C M E W J R E D D A L B L L A G S T R
L U V R S U P E R I O R A L E S R I E
E P H I S T O R Y L A M U H H M P U C S
O T C R Y S A N T E R I O R L O C K R
```

Medical Emergencies Word-Find

Find the following words in the puzzle attached. See how many words you can find.

Edema
Dyspnea
Hyperventilation
Stroke
Congestive heart failure
Aphasia
Apnea
Asphyxia
Diaphoresis
Hypersensitivity
Pulmonary edema
Poison
Pneumothorax
Radiation
Gamma
Alpha
Beta
Hepatitis
Ipecac
Snake bites

Arteriosclerosis
Angina
Myocardial infarction
COPD
Emphysema
Cerebrovascular accident
Croup
Epiglottitis
Asthma
Anaphylaxis
Bronchitis
Heat stroke
Diabetic coma
Insulin shock
Aortic aneurysm
Third degree burn
Hazardous materials
Pancreas
Acute abdomen

Medical Emergencies
Word-Find

```
S  E  K  C  O  H  S  N  I  L  U  S  N  I  F  R  P  F  S
C  B  T  E  M  P  H  Y  S  E  M  A  T  H  A  I  U  R  T
O  E  I  R  H  E  P  A  T  I  T  I  S  E  L  L  L  X  R
N  T  N  E  M  O  D  B  A  E  T  U  C  A  P  E  M  A  E
G  A  M  B  I  P  E  C  A  C  S  R  S  T  H  P  O  R  U
E  X  O  R  L  U  S  T  R  A  C  M  R  S  A  O  N  O  F
S  P  V  O  A  I  L  C  I  U  Q  Y  E  T  R  S  A  H  L
T  A  M  V  P  S  Y  C  K  S  E  O  V  R  T  B  R  T  E
I  N  S  A  D  I  A  B  E  T  I  C  C  O  M  A  Y  O  S
V  C  Y  S  A  I  X  Y  H  P  S  A  U  K  S  E  E  M  L
E  R  R  C  O  P  D  B  A  B  E  R  C  E  L  T  D  U  A
H  E  U  U  X  A  E  N  P  S  Y  D  A  V  S  R  E  E  I
E  A  E  L  O  V  E  X  T  U  B  I  C  I  X  U  M  N  R
A  S  N  A  S  T  H  M  A  V  X  A  W  R  Q  L  A  P  E
R  N  A  R  T  E  R  I  O  S  C  L  E  R  O  S  I  S  T
T  A  C  A  R  W  E  S  T  I  S  I  L  S  A  U  A  I  A
F  K  I  C  N  A  S  T  E  T  H  N  O  S  I  O  P  T  M
A  E  T  C  P  G  E  V  R  I  C  F  S  T  S  D  N  I  S
I  B  R  I  K  L  I  U  E  T  O  A  L  R  A  I  E  H  U
L  I  O  D  E  T  A  N  G  T  E  R  U  O  H  A  A  C  O
U  T  A  E  D  E  M  A  A  O  R  C  T  K  P  P  R  N  D
R  E  B  N  C  A  B  I  W  L  A  T  S  E  A  H  T  O  R
E  S  R  T  A  D  R  A  E  G  N  I  E  V  R  O  U  R  A
A  N  A  P  H  Y  L  A  X  I  S  O  R  X  U  R  V  B  Z
I  F  A  M  M  A  R  A  M  P  E  N  S  T  I  E  S  E  A
T  H  I  R  D  D  E  G  R  E  E  B  U  R  N  S  L  L  H
V  U  H  Y  P  E  R  S  E  N  S  I  T  I  V  I  T  Y  M
L  E  S  T  E  N  N  O  I  T  A  I  D  A  R  S  L  A  G
```

Medical Emergencies
Word-Find
Answer Key

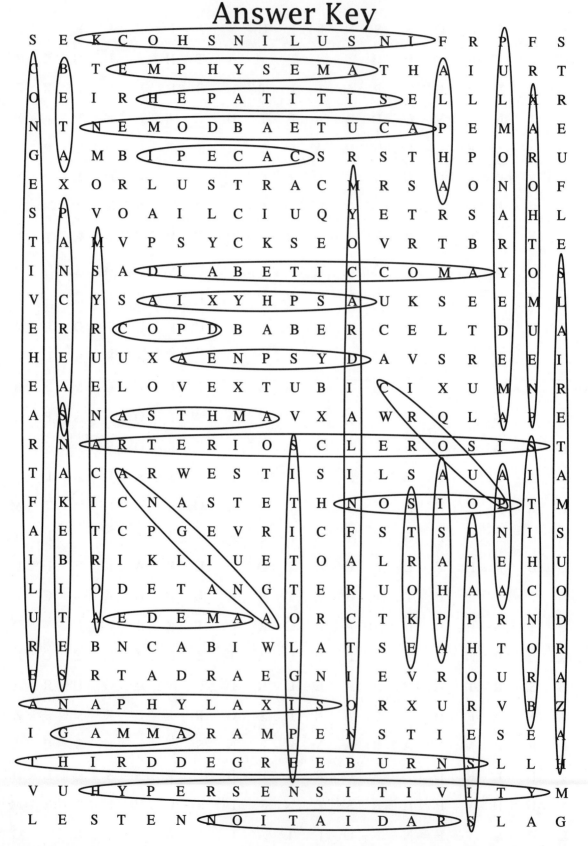

Illin' Dwarfs

Snow White arrives home one day to discover her seven dwarfs apparently suffering from various medical emergencies.

a. Sneezy suffered from a cerebrovascular accident.
b. Sleepy suffered from chronic obstructive pulmonary disease.
c. Happy suffered from angina.
d. Dopey suffered from diabetic coma.
e. Grumpy suffered from insulin shock.
f. Doc suffered from a myocardial infarction.
g. Bashful suffered from congestive heart failure.

Snow White reached this conclusion by assessing each of the dwarfs; it seems she had just finished an EMT course at the neighboring castle. See if you can be as sharp as Snow White and match the clinical findings below with the specific illnesses listed above.

1. _____ This dwarf has just come back from a jog around the forest. His pulse is rapid and he is complaining of chest pain that lasted approximately 3 minutes. His blood pressure is 160/90 and respirations are 32 and shallow.

2. _____ This dwarf is confused and stuporous. His speech is slurred and his right side paralyzed. His pulse is 132 and regular, his blood pressure is 190/120, and respirations are 14 per minute.

3. _____ This dwarf is hostile and agitated. He is wandering the room aimlessly and is acting very unlike himself. He has a history of diabetes and has just finished a new aerobics exercise. He throws rocks at Snow White when she tries to approach to take vital signs. He has a rather blank stare.

4. _____ This dwarf is having difficulty breathing, has a persistent cough, and tires easily. He is complaining of tightness in his chest, with periods of dizziness. He possesses a barrel-chest appearance and is breathing in puffs through pursed lips. His blood pressure is 130/80 and his pulse 124 and irregular. Upon auscultation of lung sounds, wheezes are heard.

5. _____ This dwarf is cyanotic, coughing up frothy pink sputum, and has swollen ankles. He is complaining of shortness of breath, anxiety, and confusion. His blood pressure is 140/90, his pulse is 110, and respirations 26 and shallow. Upon auscultation of lung sounds, rales are heard.

6. _____ This dwarf has had the flu for the past few days and has been lying around the house eating. He is complaining of dry mouth, intense thirst, and abdominal pain. His blood pressure is 100/60, his pulse 120 and weak and respirations 16 and deep. His skin is dry, red and warm.

7. _____ This dwarf is complaining of severe indigestion which started approximately 30 minutes ago. He appears anxious, irritable and unable to concentrate. His blood pressure is 100/60, his pulse is 120 and irregular, and his respirations 22 and shallow. His skin is cyanotic, cool, and clammy.

Illin' Dwarfs
Answer Key

Snow White arrives home one day to discover her seven dwarfs apparently suffering from various medical emergencies.

a. Sneezy suffered from a cerebrovascular accident.
b. Sleepy suffered from chronic obstructive pulmonary disease.
c. Happy suffered from angina.
d. Dopey suffered from diabetic coma.
e. Grumpy suffered from insulin shock.
f. Doc suffered from a myocardial infarction.
g. Bashful suffered from congestive heart failure.

Snow White reached this conclusion by assessing each of the dwarfs; it seems she had just finished an EMT course at the neighboring castle. See if you can be as sharp as Snow White and match the clinical findings below with the specific illnesses listed above.

1. __C__ This dwarf has just come back from a jog around the forest. His pulse is rapid and he is complaining of chest pain that lasted approximately 3 minutes. His blood pressure is 160/90 and respirations are 32 and shallow.

2. __A__ This dwarf is confused and stuporous. His speech is slurred and his right side paralyzed. His pulse is 132 and regular, his blood pressure is 190/120, and respirations are 14 per minute.

3. __E__ This dwarf is hostile and agitated. He is wandering the room aimlessly and is acting very unlike himself. He has a history of diabetes and has just finished a new aerobics exercise. He throws rocks at Snow White when she tries to approach to take vital signs. He has a rather blank stare.

4. __B__ This dwarf is having difficulty breathing, has a persistent cough, and tires easily. He is complaining of tightness in his chest, with periods of dizziness. He possesses a barrel-chest appearance and is breathing in puffs through pursed lips. His blood pressure is 130/80 and his pulse 124 and irregular. Upon auscultation of lung sounds, wheezes are heard.

5. __G__ This dwarf is cyanotic, coughing up frothy pink sputum and has swollen ankles. He is complaining of shortness of breath, anxiety and confusion. His blood pressure is 140/90, his pulse is 110, and respirations 26 and shallow. Upon auscultation of lung sounds, rales are heard.

6. __D__ This dwarf has had the flu for the past few days and has been lying around the house eating. He is complaining of dry mouth, intense thirst, and abdominal pain. His blood pressure is 100/60, his pulse 120 and weak and respirations 16 and deep. His skin is dry, red and warm.

7. __F__ This dwarf is complaining of severe indigestion which started approximately 30 minutes ago. He appears anxious, irritable and unable to concentrate. His blood pressure is 100/60, his pulse is 120 and irregular, and his respirations 22 and shallow. His skin is cyanotic, cool, and clammy.

The Shock of Her Life

There once was a lady washing her clothes, who saw a spider and fainted. She was in _____ shock.

When she woke up, she noticed she had been bitten by the spider; her arm and face were red and swollen and she was having a hard time breathing. She was in _____ shock.

While running to the phone to call 911, she cut her leg on a jagged piece of aluminum. She was bleeding profusely from a 2-inch laceration. She was in _____ shock.

The laceration became severely infected. She was in _____ shock.

On her way home from the hospital, she was involved in a car accident that left her paralyzed. She was suffering from _____ shock.

She later developed the flu and was vomiting and had diarrhea for days. She was suffering from _____ shock.

While getting out of the car coming home from the hospital, a tree fell on her, crushing her chest and causing her heart to fail to pump adequately. She was suffering from _____ shock.

The Shock of Her Life
Answer Key

There once was a lady washing her clothes, who saw a spider and fainted. She was in ___(Psychogenic)_____ shock.

When she woke up, she noticed she had been bitten by the spider; her arm and face were red and swollen and she was having a hard time breathing. She was in ___(Anaphylactic)___ shock.

While running to the phone to call 911, she cut her leg on a jagged piece of aluminum. She was bleeding profusely from a 2-inch laceration. She was in ___(Hemorrhagic)_____ shock.

The laceration became severely infected. She was in ____(Septic)_____ shock.

On her way home from the hospital, she was involved in a car accident that left her paralyzed. She was suffering from ____(Neurogenic)_____ shock.

She later developed the flu and was vomiting and had diarrhea for days. She was suffering from ___(Metabolic)_____ shock.

While getting out of the car coming home from the hospital, a tree fell on her, crushing her chest and causing her heart to fail to pump adequately. She was suffering from ___(Cardiogenic)_____ shock.

A Traumatic Event

Humpty Dumpty was sitting on a wall when an earthquake caused him to fall. Unfortunately, when he fell he landed on the home of the little old lady who lived in a shoe. The lady and her 12 children were home at the time and suffered a variety of injuries. See if you can match up the clinical findings with specific injuries. (Do not use any response more than once. Not all choices will be used.)

_____ Hewey complained of severe pain in his hip, with his lower leg rotated inward and his knee bent. He lacks sensation in his limb and is unable to flex his foot.

_____ Dewey is complaining of pain on the lower left side of his chest. Upon physical assessment, you find tenderness to this area and increased pain when the patient takes a deep breath. Vital signs are as follows: blood pressure = 126/70, pulse = 110, respiration = 24.

_____ Lewey is suffering from a decreased level of consciousness. His pupils are unequal, his left eye appears to be sunken, and he is suffering from projectile vomiting. His vital signs are as follows: blood pressure = 120/80, pulse = 88, respiration = 20.

_____ Larry is complaining of severe pain in his thigh area. He is in an altered state of consciousness and his one leg appears to be shorter than the other.

_____ Daryl is cyanotic with severe pain in his chest. He is extremely short of breath and his respirations are not symmetrical. His vital signs are as follows: blood pressure = 90/60, pulse = 126, respiration = 32 and shallow.

_____ His other brother Daryl is cyanotic. Upon physical examination, you notice the patient is sweating profusely and has neck vein distension. His vital signs are as follows: blood pressure = 90/80, pulse = 120 and very weak, respiration = 24.

_____ Hoky was directly under Humpty when he fell. Upon physical examination, you notice the victim is unconscious with distended neck veins, cyanosis of the head, bulging neck and shoulders, and bloodshot eyes.

_____ Poky is unconscious. Upon physical examination, you notice deformity in his forehead, unequal pupils, and fluid oozing from his ears. His vital signs are as follows: blood pressure = 88/60, pulse = 122, respiration = 28.

_____ Smokey is complaining of severe pain in the upper right quadrant of his abdomen, nausea, and extreme thirst. He is vomiting blood, is restless and lying with his legs drawn up to his chest. His vital signs are as follows: blood pressure = 100/60, pulse = 132, respiration = 26.

____ Manie is cyanotic and complaining of severe difficulty breathing. Upon physical assessment, you notice a large contusion on the right side of his chest and decreased lung sounds on that side as well.

____ Moe is lying on the floor with no sensation in his arms or legs. His vital signs are as follows: blood pressure = 116/70, pulse = 86, respiration = 18.

____ Jack is suffering from increased respiratory difficulty. Upon examination, you notice cyanosis, distended neck veins, tracheal deviation and uneven chest wall movement. Vital signs are as follows: blood pressure = 90/60, pulse = 126 and weak, respiration = 32, and lung sounds decreased on the right side.

A. Anterior hip dislocation
B. Posterior hip dislocation
C. Hip fracture
D. Fractured ankle
E. Fractured femur
F. Cervical fracture
G. Lumbar fracture
H. Neurogenic shock
I. Hemorrhagic shock
J. Open pneumothorax
K. Closed pneumothorax
L. Fractured ribs
M. Flail chest
N. Hemothorax
O. Traumatic asphyxia
P. Head injury
Q. Head injury with secondary trauma
R. Tension pneumothorax
S. Cardiac tamponade
T. Lacerated liver
U. Ruptured spleen

A Traumatic Event
Answer Key

Humpty Dumpty was sitting on a wall when an earthquake caused him to fall. Unfortunately, when he fell he landed on the home of the little old lady who lived in a shoe. The lady and her 12 children were home at the time and suffered a variety of injuries. See if you can match up the clinical findings with specific injuries. (Do not use any response more than once. Not all choices will be used.)

_B_ Hewey complained of severe pain in his hip, with his lower leg rotated inward and his knee bent. He lacks sensation in his limb and is unable to flex his foot.

_L_ Dewey is complaining of pain on the lower left side of his chest. Upon physical assessment, you find tenderness to this area and increased pain when the patient takes a deep breath. Vital signs are as follows: blood pressure = 126/70, pulse = 110, respiration = 24.

_P_ Lewey is suffering from a decreased level of consciousness. His pupils are unequal, his left eye appears to be sunken, and he is suffering from projectile vomiting. His vital signs are as follows: blood pressure = 120/80, pulse = 88, respiration = 20.

_E_ Larry is complaining of severe pain in his thigh area. He is in an altered state of consciousness and his one leg appears to be shorter than the other.

_M_ Daryl is cyanotic with severe pain in his chest. He is extremely short of breath and his respirations are not symmetrical. His vital signs are as follows: blood pressure = 90/60, pulse = 126, respiration = 32 and shallow.

_S_ His other brother Daryl is cyanotic. Upon physical examination, you notice the patient is sweating profusely and has neck vein distension. His vital signs are as follows: blood pressure = 90/80, pulse = 120 and very weak, respiration = 24.

_O_ Hoky was directly under Humpty when he fell. Upon physical examination, you notice the victim is unconscious with distended neck veins, cyanosis of the head, bulging neck and shoulders, and bloodshot eyes.

_Q_ Poky is unconscious. Upon physical examination, you notice deformity in his forehead, unequal pupils, and fluid oozing from his ears. His vital signs are as follows: blood pressure = 88/60, pulse = 122, respiration = 28.

_T_ Smokey is complaining of severe pain in the upper right quadrant of his abdomen, nausea, and extreme thirst. He is vomiting blood, is restless and lying with his legs drawn up to his chest. His vital signs are as follows: blood pressure = 100/60, pulse = 132, respiration = 26.

_K_   Manie is cyanotic and complaining of severe difficulty breathing. Upon physical assessment, you notice a large contusion on the right side of his chest and decreased lung sounds on that side as well.

_F_   Moe is lying on the floor with no sensation in his arms or legs. His vital signs are as follows: blood pressure = 116/70, pulse = 86, respiration = 18.

_R_   Jack is suffering from increased respiratory difficulty. Upon examination, you notice cyanosis, distended neck veins, tracheal deviation and uneven chest wall movement. Vital signs are as follows: blood pressure = 90/60, pulse = 126 and weak, respiration = 32, and lung sounds decreased on the right side.

A.   Anterior hip dislocation
B.   Posterior hip dislocation
C.   Hip fracture
D.   Fractured ankle
E.   Fractured femur
F.   Cervical fracture
G.   Lumbar fracture
H.   Neurogenic shock
I.   Hemorrhagic shock
J.   Open pneumothorax
K.   Closed pneumothorax
L.   Fractured ribs
M.   Flail chest
N.   Hemothorax
O.   Traumatic asphyxia
P.   Head injury
Q.   Head injury with secondary trauma
R.   Tension pneumothorax
S.   Cardiac tamponade
T.   Lacerated liver
U.   Ruptured spleen

EMS Tic-Tac-Toe Cards

EMS Tic-Tac-Toe

Which of the following is NOT a sign or symptom of breathing difficulty?

A. Shortness of breath
B. Restlessness
C. Decreased pulse rate (*)
D. Stridor

EMS Tic-Tac-Toe

Which of the following should not be done when trying to calm an emotionally unstable patient?

A. Maintain a comfortable distance.
B. Encourage the patient to talk.
C. Respond honestly to the patient's questions.
D. Hold the patient's hand to show you care. (*)

EMS Tic-Tac-Toe

What is the name for the bag of water that surrounds the fetus inside the uterus?

A. Placenta
B. Amniotic sac (*)
C. Perineum
D. Fetal sac

EMS Tic-Tac-Toe

CPR should be performed on a newborn if the heart rate is below:

A. 60 (*)
B. 40
C. 20
D. 0

EMS Tic-Tac-Toe

What is the most common cause of cardiac arrest in infants and children?

A. SIDS
B. Drowning
C. Trauma
D. Airway obstruction (*)

EMS Tic-Tac-Toe

Hardening of the arteries due to deposits on the arterial walls is called:

A. Emphysema
B. Arteriosclerosis (*)
C. Atherosclerosis
D. Pleurisy

EMS Tic-Tac-Toe

The type of injury identified by a collection of blood beneath the skin is called a(n):

A. Hematoma (*)
B. Avulsion
C. Contusion
D. Abrasion

EMS Tic-Tac-Toe

An adult patient with burns on the head, left arm, and back of left leg would have _____ % total body burns.

A. 9%
B. 18%
C. 27% (*)
D. 36%

EMS Tic-Tac-Toe Cards

EMS Tic-Tac-Toe

Which of the following is NOT a sign or symptom of shock?

A. Altered mental status
B. Increased pulse rate
C. Constricted pupils (*)
D. Nausea and vomiting

EMS Tic-Tac-Toe

Which of the following abdominal organs is solid?

A. Kidney (*)
B. Urinary bladder
C. Appendix
D. Stomach

EMS Tic-Tac-Toe

What is the medical term meaning "under the tongue?"

A. Endotracheal
B. Epidermal
C. Pericardial
D. Sublingual (*)

EMS Tic-Tac-Toe

Jaundiced skin is what color?

A. Blue
B. Ashen
C. Cherry red
D. Yellow (*)

EMS Tic-Tac-Toe

What is the normal pulse rate for an adult at rest?

A. 100-110 beats per minute
B. 80-100 beats per minute
C. 60-80 beats per minute (*)
D. 50-60 beats per minute

EMS Tic-Tac-Toe

When examining a patient with cardiac problems, how long should the EMT assess the pulse

A. 15 seconds
B. 30 seconds
C. 45 seconds
D. 60 seconds (*)

EMS Tic-Tac-Toe

The portion of the spinal column most commonly injured are the:

A. Cervical and lumbar (*)
B. Thoracic and lumbar
C. Cervical and thoracic
D. Cervical and sacral

EMS Tic-Tac-Toe

Fractures of the facial bones are dangerous because:

A. Associated bleeding is not easily controlled
B. Fractures are not easily repaired
C. Fractured bones may obstruct the airway (*)
D. Facial fractures usually cause permanent scarring

EMS Scrabble
Game #1
Trauma

CLUES:

1. The term meaning shortness of breath.

2. The bone of the upper arm.

3. The term indicating a rubbing sound from two bones.

4. A sign of a fracture (an increase in size).

5. A mnemonic for assessing pupil reaction.

6. An abnormal sound from air passing through fluid in the lungs.

1. ____ ____ ____ ____ ____ ____ ____

2. ____ ____ ____ ____ ____ ____

3. ____ ____ ____ ____ ____ ____ ____

4. ____ ____ ____ ____ ____ ____ ____

5. ____ ____ ____ ____ ____ ____

6. ____ ____ ____ ____ ____

EMS Scrabble
Game #2
Medical

CLUES:

1. The first step of the primary survey (after responsiveness).

2. A condition that constricts the bronchioles.

3. The term for a chemical that can harm the body.

4. Selling due to an accumulation of fluids in the tissue.

5. A chronic disease of the lungs.

6. The blockage or rupture of a blood vessel supplying the brain.

1. ___ ___ ___ ___ ___ ___

2. ___ ___ ___ ___ ___ ___ ___

3. ___ ___ ___ ___ ___ ___

4. ___ ___ ___ ___

5. ___ ___ ___ ___ ___ ___ ___ ___

6. ___ ___ ___ ___ ___ ___ ___

EMS Scrabble
Answer Key

Game #1

1.		D	Y	S	**P**	N	E	A
2.	H	U	M	E	R	**U**	S
3.		C	R	E	**P**	I	T	U	S
4.	S	W	E	L	L	**I**	N	G
5.		P	E	A	R	**L**	A
6.		R	A	L	E	**S**

Game #2

1.		A	I	R	W	**A**	Y
2.				A	**S**	T	H	M	A
3.			P	O	I	**S**	O	N
4.				E	D	**E**	M	A
5.	E	M	P	H	Y	**S**	E	M	A
6.						**S**	T	R	O	K	E

Beat the Reaper Cards

Beat the Reaper

Illness = Acute Abdomen

Beat the Reaper

Illness = Insulin Shock

Information required:

1. Dispatch information
2. Location
3. Signs and symptoms
4. Past medical history
5. History of present illness
6. Age and sex
7. Level or state of consciousness

Information required:

1. Dispatch information
2. Location
3. Signs and symptoms
4. Past medical history
5. History of present illness
6. Age and sex
7. Level or state of consciousness

Beat the Reaper

Illness = Angina Pectoris

Beat the Reaper

Illness = Pre-eclampsia

Information required:

1. Dispatch information
2. Location
3. Signs and symptoms
4. Past medical history
5. History of present illness
6. Age and sex
7. Level or state of consciousness

Information required:

1. Dispatch information
2. Location
3. Signs and symptoms
4. Past medical history
5. History of present illness
6. Age and sex
7. Level or state of consciousness

Beat the Reaper Cards

Beat the Reaper

Illness = Traumatic Asphyxia

Beat the Reaper

Illness = Cardiogenic Shock

Information required:

1. Dispatch information
2. Location
3. Signs and symptoms
4. Past medical history
5. History of present illness
6. Age and sex
7. Level or state of consciousness

Information required:

1. Dispatch information
2. Location
3. Signs and symptoms
4. Past medical history
5. History of present illness
6. Age and sex
7. Level or state of consciousness

Beat the Reaper

Illness = Aortic Aneurysm

Beat the Reaper

Illness = Hyperventilation Syndrome

Information required:

1. Dispatch information
2. Location
3. Signs and symptoms
4. Past medical history
5. History of present illness
6. Age and sex
7. Level or state of consciousness

Information required:

1. Dispatch information
2. Location
3. Signs and symptoms
4. Past medical history
5. History of present illness
6. Age and sex
7. Level or state of consciousness

EMS Jeopardy Cards

EMS Jeopardy
Trauma - $100

EMS Jeopardy
Patient Assessment - $200

It is the best method for controlling bleeding.

Answer: What is direct pressure?

It is a gurgling sound caused by air passing through secretions or fluids in the lower airway.

Answer: What is rales?

EMS Jeopardy
BLS - $300

EMS Jeopardy
Anatomy - $400

It is once every 5 seconds or 10 to 12 times per minute.

Answer: What is the rate of rescue breathing for an adult victim?

It is the lower (inferior) extension of the sternum.

Answer: What is the xiphoid process?

EMS Jeopardy Cards

EMS Jeopardy
Miscellaneous - $500

EMS Jeopardy
Patient Assessment - $400

It is the primary responsibility of an EMT at the scene of an emergency.

Answer: What is personal safety?

It is the normal respiratory rate of an adult at rest.

Answer: What is 12 to 20 breaths per minute?

EMS Jeopardy
Trauma - $600

EMS Jeopardy
Anatomy - $800

It is the type of open wound which is most likely to cause infection, usually from sharp, pointed objects.

Answer: What is a puncture wound?

It is the area of the lungs where gas exchange takes place.

Answer: What are the alveolar sacs?

EMS Jeopardy
Game #1

$ Amount	Fractures	Patient Assessment	Medical Emergencies	Trauma	Basic Life Support
$ 100	The type of fracture causing 3 or more fragments	A pool of blood that collects at the sight of an injury	Presents with high blood pressure, unequal pupils, and drooling	Crackling sensation of air into tissue from an open chest wound	The type of death that begins in 4 minutes without oxygen
$ 200	Partial tearing or stretching of a ligament	The normal pulse rate of an adult	The sudden blockage of coronary arteries	The only area from which an impaled object can be removed	The compression rate for 2-person CPR
$ 300	A sign indicating a basalar skull fracture, causing bruising behind the ears	The organ located in the upper right quadrant that can be lacerated by improper CPR	The type of diabetic emergency caused by not eating or excessive exercise	The best treatment for a patient who develops signs and symptoms of a tension pneumothorax	The ventilation/ compression ratio for CPR on a child
$ 400	The most effective method for immobilizing a fractured foot	The normal respiratory rate for an adult	Presents with chest pain that is relieved with nitroglycerin	Presents with severe shock, cyanosis and bloodshot, protruding eyes	The proper method for opening an airway for a patient with suspected spinal injury
$ 500	The most effective way to immobilize a fractured femur	The proper order of the primary survey	Presents with swelling of extremities and pink, frothy sputum	The best method for controlling severe bleeding	The # of ventilations per minute for rescue breathing for a child

EMS Jeopardy
Game #1
Answer Key

$ Amount	Fractures	Patient Assessment	Medical Emergencies	Trauma	Basic Life Support
$ 100	Comminuted	Hematoma	CVA	Subcutaneous emphysema	Biologic death
$ 200	Sprain	60 to 100 bpm	AMI	The chest	80 per minute
$ 300	Battle's sign	Liver	Insulin shock	"Burp" the occlusive dressing	1 : 5
$ 400	Pillow splint	12 to 20 per minute	Angina pectoris	Traumatic asphyxia	Modified jaw thrust
$ 500	Traction splint	ABCs	CHF	Direct pressure	15

EMS Jeopardy
Game #2

$ Amount	Fractures	Patient Assessment	Medical Emergencies	Trauma	Basic Life Support
$ 200	Another term for the "knee cap"	Something the patient feels and describes to the EMT	The #1 cause of death among infants	Bleeding into the sac surrounding the heart	The depth of compression for an adult victim of cardiac arrest
$ 400	The type of dislocation causing the hip to rotate away from the body	The normal pulse rate of a 1-year-old child at rest	The amount of ipecac to give a child to reduce vomiting	The type of bandage used on a patient with a pneumothorax	The most common cause of airway obstruction in a consious patient
$ 600	The connective tissue that attaches muscle to bone	Harsh, high-pitched breath sounds, indicating a partial airway obstruction	Presents with tachycardia, anxiety, pursed lips and wheezing	The most common and least serious type of brain injury	What occurs when air gets into the stomach during CPR
$ 800	Muscle spasms around a joint	The artery used to monitor blood flow to the brain	Otherwise known as a "blue bloater"	Innadequate tissue perfusion	The tequnique used to clear a foreign body obstruction
$ 1000	The preferred method for immobilizing a fractured clavicle	A tingling sensation indicating nerve or circulatory changes	A progressive disease with alveoli over-distended and trapped with air	The type of shock, usually caused by spinal injury, when blood vessel cannot constrict	Another term for the sternal notch

EMS Jeopardy
Game #2
Answer Key

$ Amount	Fractures	Patient Assessment	Medical Emergencies	Trauma	Basic Life Support
$ 200	Patella	Symptom	SIDS	Pericardial tamponade	1 to 1 1/2 inches
$ 400	Anterior dislocation	100 to 140 bpm	2 tsp	Occlusive dressing	Food
$ 600	Tendon	Stridor	Asthma attack	Concussion	Gastric distension
$ 800	Strain	Carotid	Chronic bronchitis	Shock	Heimlich maneuver
$ 1000	Sling and swath	Paresthesia	Emphysema	Neurogenic shock	Xiphoid process

EMS Family Feud Cards

Name the six different types of fractures?

1. Transverse (55)
2. Oblique (13)
3. Spiral (10)
4. Greenstick (8)
5. Impacted (8)
6. Comminuted (6)

Name the nine main duties of the EMT.

1. Emergency care (30)
2. Preparation (20)
3. Response (10)
4. Transport (10)
5. Termination of activities (10)
6. Transfer to medical facility (5)
7. Scene control (5)
8. Gaining access (5)
9. Disentanglement (5)

Name the seven differnt types of shock.

1. Hypovolemic (40)
2. Cardiogenic (20)
3. Anaphylactic (12)
4. Neurogenic (10)
5. Psychogenic (8)
6. Metabolic (6)
7. Septic (4)

Name the five solid organs in the abdominal cavity.

1. Liver (40)
2. Kidneys (20)
3. Spleen (20)
4. Diaphragm (10)
5. Pancreas (10)

Name the seven oxygen delivery devices used by EMTs.

1. Non-rebreather mask (60)
2. Nasal cannula (30)
3. Bag-valve-mask (20)
4. Demand valve (15)
5. Simple face mask (10)
6. Partial rebreather mask (10)
7. Venturi mask (5)

Name the 6 hollow organs in the abdominal cavity.

1. Stomach (30)
2. Bladder (25)
3. Large intestine (20)
4. Gallbladder (18)
5. Small intestine (10)
6. Duodenum (7)

Name 8 major methods used to control external bleeding.

1. Direct pressure (50)
2. Elevation (30)
3. Pressure points (20)
4. Splinting (15)
5. Inflatable splints (15)
6. MAST (10)
7. Tourniquet (5)
8. Pressure dressing (5)

Name 6 signs and symptoms of a myocardial infarction.

1. Radiating chest pain (45)
2. Shortness of breath (30)
3. Diaphoresis (15)
4. Pale skin (5)
5. Anxiety (3)
6. Nausea / vomiting (2)

EMS Trivia Mania
Categories

 Anatomy

 Basic Life Support

 Miscellaneous

 Medical and Environmental Emergencies

 Terminology

 Trauma

EMS Trivia Mania
Game Board

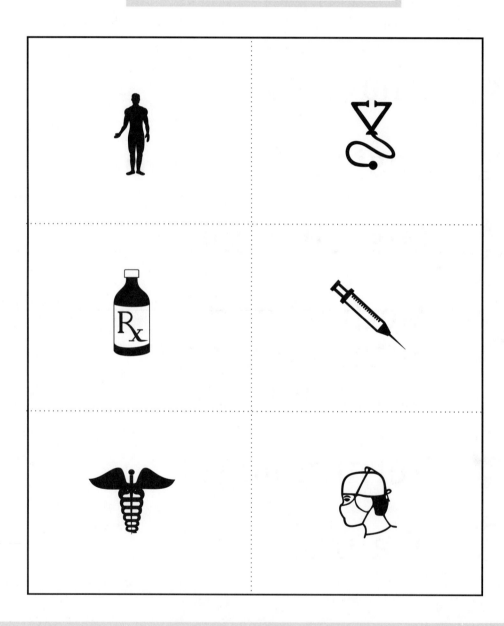

EMS Trivia Mania Cards

Card 1 (top left) — Answers

EMS Trivia Mania

- Femoral artery
- Demand-valve-mask
- Radiation
- Acute myocardial infarction
- Concussion
- Medical anti-shock trousers

Card 2 (top right) — Answers

EMS Trivia Mania

- Gallbladder
- 15:2
- Gamma
- Frostnip
- Dilate
- Golden hour

Card 1 (middle left) — Questions

- What is the main artery of the thigh?
- What type of oxygen device delivers the highest concentration of oxygen?
- What is the general term for transmission of energy?
- What is the condition that occurs when part of the myocardium dies due to deprivation of oxygenated blood?
- What is the term referring to a mild state of stupor or temporary unconsciousness, caused by a blow to the head?
- What does MAST stand for?

Card 2 (middle right) — Questions

- What is the organ that attaches to the lower back of the liver and stores bile?
- What is the ratio of compressions to ventilations for one-man CPR on an adult victim of cardiac arrest?
- Which type of radiation is extremely dangerous and is able to penetrate thick shielding?
- What is the term for the first stage of frostbite?
- What is the term meaning to enlarge or expand in diameter?
- What is the critical time period, after a traumatic injury, in which the victim's chance for survival are best if definitive treatment is provided within?

Card 3 (bottom left) — Answers

EMS Trivia Mania

- Facial artery
- 1.5 to 2 seconds
- Tonic
- Placenta
- Cyanosis
- Battle's sign

Card 4 (bottom right) — Answers

EMS Trivia Mania

- Mediastinum
- The brachial pulse
- Supplemental oxygen
- Standard of care
- Prone
- 5%

Card 3 (bottom left) — Questions

- What is the major artery supplying blood to the face?
- How long should you take to provide each breath during artificial respirations?
- What is the first phase of a convulsion?
- Exchange of blood between a mother and her fetus occurs in what organ?
- What is the term referring to when the skin, lips, and nailbeds change to blue or gray color, due to too little oxygen in the blood?
- What is the symptom of a basilar skull fracture, identified by contusions behind the victims ears?

Card 4 (bottom right) — Questions

- What is the central portion of the chest cavity containing the heart, its greater vessels, part of the esophagus, and part of the trachea?
- What is the best place to assess pulselessness on an infant?
- What is the best method for treating a victim of inhaled poisons?
- What is the term for the minimal acceptable level of emergency care to be provided, as set forth by law?
- When a patient is lying face down, he is in the _____ position.
- What percentage of a patient's available blood volume can be autotransfused by MAST?

EMS Trivia Mania Cards

EMS Trivia Mania

- Femur
- Decreases
- Hypertension
- 1/2 Pint
- Contusion
- Pulmonary edema

- What is the medical term for the thigh bone?
- As the volume of the lungs increases, the pressure inside the lungs does what?
- What condition should you suspect when you notice a prescription container of Reserpine?
- Delivery of the placenta is usually accompanied by how much blood loss?
- What is the medical term for a bruise?
- What is the absolute contraindication for the use of MAST?

EMS Trivia Mania

- Liver
- Two finger breadths above the xiphoid process
- Asthma
- Implied consent
- Hypotension
- Seal the wound

- What is the largest gland in the body?
- What is the correct hand placement for performing chest compressions on a child?
- What is the pulmonary disease in which the alveoli are obstructed by spasms?
- What type of consent allows you to treat an adult unconscious patient?
- What is the medical term for having low blood pressure?
- What is the first priority when caring for a patient with a sucking chest wound?

EMS Trivia Mania

- Upper extremities
- Reposition the head and try again
- Congestive heart failure
- Lateral recumbent
- Hyperthermia
- Anaphylactic shock

- The scapula is considered part of which body region?
- When performing CPR what should you do if you attempt to ventilate the victim but the air does not go in?
- What is the condition caused when the heart can no longer carry its normal load?
- In what position should you place a child who has had a seizure, after he stops convulsing?
- What is the medical term for an abnormally high body temperature?
- You find a victim who has just been stung by a bee and is experiencing difficulty breathing. What should you suspect?

EMS Trivia Mania

- Carotid
- Jaw thrust maneuver
- Disposable gloves
- 20
- Diastolic pressure
- Occlusive dressing

- What is the large artery in the neck?
- What is the preferred method for opening the airway of a patient with suspected spine injury?
- What is the proper control procedure for a known AIDS patient?
- A spontaneous abortion (miscarriage) occurs with the delivery of a fetus before how many weeks of pregnancy?
- What is the term referring to the pressure exerted on the internal walls of the arteries when the heart is relaxing?
- What type of dressing should you use for an open sucking chest wound?

EMS Feud Game Cards

EMS Feud

Which of the following is the most effective way to ventilate a patient with inadequate respirations due to a flail chest?

A. Assist respirations with a bag-valve-mask (*)
B. Give mouth-to-mouth ventilations
C. Immobilize the chest
D. Give oxygen by a non-rebreather mask

EMS Feud

Which injury would most likely occur to the driver of a vehicle, due to a collapsed steering column?

A. Fractured femur
B. Ruptured kidney
C. Flail chest (*)
D. Spinal fracture

EMS Feud

The deviation from accepted standard of care, resulting in further injury to a patient is called:

A. Abandonment
B. Breach of duty
C. Malpractice
D. Negligence (*)

EMS Feud

When there are hazardous materials at the scene of an emergency, where should the ambulance be parked?

A. Downhill from the scene
B. Parallel to the scene
C. Perpendicular to the scene
D. Uphill from the scene (*)

EMS Feud

The thoracic cavity contains all but which of the following?

A. Lungs
B. Heart and great vessels
C. Diaphragm (*)
D. Esophagus

EMS Feud

Which of the following is true regarding airway obstruction in burn patients?

A. Obstructions occur most commonly in the respiratory tract
B. They can be due to laryngospasm
C. They can be due to accumulation of mucus or soot
D. All of the above (*)

EMS Feud

Pain and tenderness following injury to the upper left abdominal quadrant may indicate:

A. Ruptured spleen (*)
B. Appendicitis
C. Gallbladder disease
D. Disease of the colon

EMS Feud

What is often the first sign of shock?

A. Cold, clammy skin
B. An altered mental status (*)
C. A weak, thready pulse
D. Hypertension

EMS Feud Game Cards

EMS Feud

Which of the following should be done when treating a patient with an eye injury?

- A. Apply an occlusive dressing
- B. Cover both eyes to prevent sympathetic eye movement (*)
- C. Place the patient into a head down position to facilitate drainage
- D. Avoid the use of oxygen to prevent retinal damage

EMS Feud

What should be the initial treatment for a roofer who has spilled hot tar on his leg?

- A. Attempt to remove the tar
- B. Immerse the patient's forearm in a bucket of cold water (*)
- C. Cool the burned area first and then remove the tar
- D. Rapidly transport the patient as is

EMS Feud

Often mistaken for indigestion, this heart condition is brought on by emotional stress, strenuous exercise or agitation. It is characterized by pain in the chest or arm and is known as:

- A. Angina pectoris (*)
- B. Acute myocardial infarction
- C. Stroke
- D. Chronic heart failure

EMS Feud

A substance used to absorb an ingested poison is:

- A. Syrup of ipecac
- B. Activated charcoal (*)
- C. Dilute sulfuric acid
- D. Oral glucose

EMS Feud

What care should be given to a patient covered with dry lime?

- A. Flood area with copious amounts of water
- B. Wash area with soap and water
- C. Neutralize lime with baking soda
- D. Brush lime from skin (*)

EMS Feud

What action takes highest priority in a cardiac arrest situation?

- A. Ventilation
- B. Cardiopulmonary resuscitation
- C. Defibrillation (*)
- D. Transportation

EMS Feud

Which of the following delivers the greatest CONCENTRATION of oxygen?

- A. Bag-valve-mask resuscitator
- B. Mouth-to-mouth ventilations
- C. Pocket face mask
- D. Demand valve resuscitator (*)

EMS Feud

What is the first step of the Primary Survey?

- A. Look, listen and feel for breathlessness
- B. Check for a pulse
- C. Open the victim's airway
- D. Establish unresponsiveness (*)

EMS Win, Lose, or Draw Cards

EMS Win, Lose, or Draw	Abandonment	*EMS Win, Lose, or Draw*	Abduction
EMS Win, Lose, or Draw	Cervical spine	*EMS Win, Lose, or Draw*	Diaphragm
EMS Win, Lose, or Draw	Posterior	*EMS Win, Lose, or Draw*	Kidney
EMS Win, Lose, or Draw	Puncture wound	*EMS Win, Lose, or Draw*	Skull fracture

EMS Win, Lose, or Draw Cards

EMS Win, Lose, or Draw	Primary survey	EMS Win, Lose, or Draw	Medic alert tag
EMS Win, Lose, or Draw	Biological death	EMS Win, Lose, or Draw	Abrasion
EMS Win, Lose, or Draw	Respiratory system	EMS Win, Lose, or Draw	Contusion
EMS Win, Lose, or Draw	Type III ambulance	EMS Win, Lose, or Draw	Anaphylactic shock

EMS Win, Lose, or Draw Cards

EMS Win, Lose, or Draw	Bag-valve-mask	EMS Win, Lose, or Draw	Cardiac compressions
EMS Win, Lose, or Draw	Nasopharyngeal airway	EMS Win, Lose, or Draw	Spleen
EMS Win, Lose, or Draw	Evisceration	EMS Win, Lose, or Draw	Hemothorax
EMS Win, Lose, or Draw	Pulmonary edema	EMS Win, Lose, or Draw	Triage tags

EMS Win, Lose, or Draw Cards

EMS Win, Lose, or Draw

Cardiac tamponade

EMS Win, Lose, or Draw

Insulin shock

EMS Win, Lose, or Draw

Seizures

EMS Win, Lose, or Draw

Second degree burns

EMS Win, Lose, or Draw

Hypothermia

EMS Win, Lose, or Draw

Septic shock

EMS Win, Lose, or Draw

Flail chest

EMS Win, Lose, or Draw

Traumatic asphyxia

EMS Anybody's Guess Cards

Diagnosis

Increasing difficulty breathing

Bulging neck veins

Uneven chest movement

Tracheal deviation

Tension Pneumothorax

Diagnosis

Impaired pupil reaction

Severe abdominal cramps

Burns around mouth

Altered level of consciousness

Poisoning

Diagnosis

Marked anxiety

Dizzy and lightheaded

Rapid respirations

Numbness and tingling

Hyperventilation

Diagnosis

Cyanosis around lips

Rapid pulse, low blood pressure

Squeezing sensation in chest

Itching and burning skin

Anaphylactic Shock

EMS Anybody's Guess Cards

Diagnosis

Distended neck veins

Hemoptysis

Swollen, cyanotic face

Bloodshot, protruding eyes

Traumatic Asphyxia

Diagnosis

Intense thirst

Labored respirations

Severe abdominal pain

Acetonic odor to breath

Diabetic Coma

Diagnosis

Headache

Irritability and confusion

Difficulty breathing

Cherry red skin color

CO Poisoning

Diagnosis

Altered LOC

Slow, bounding pulse

Unequal pupils

One-sided weakness

CVA

APPENDIX B
Components of
an EMS System

An EMS system is composed of individuals with various levels of training. The specific makeup of levels of services varies from state to state. While some states use a "tiered" approach, with BLS providers responding to noncritical emergencies and ALS providers responding to life–threatening emergencies, other states use a system whereby ALS providers respond to all requests for emergency care.

With the implementation of National Standard Curriculum for first responders, EMTs, and paramedics, the level of training emergency responders receive will be consistent from state to state. As shown in Figure B.1, the medical command physician maintains overall responsibility for individual EMS providers. These individuals may be a sole county medical command physician or hospital medical directors from whom responders receive medical command.

ALS providers include EMT–Paramedics and, in some states, prehospital registered nurses. These individuals provide life–saving techniques both on the ground, and in the air in both fixed wing and helicopter transport to hospitals and trauma centers.

At the basic life support level, the common form of certification is as an EMT. Various states provide intermediate levels between an EMT and EMT-Paramedic by providing additional training in specific life–saving techniques to meet regional needs. For example, wilderness training may be provided to individuals in areas of the country with high levels of wilderness related emergencies.

Some states certify EMTs at the Basic level in accordance with the Department of Transportation EMT–Basic training program. Others augment that training for certification as an EMT–Cardiac, by including training in the recognition of abnormal cardiac rhythm and subsequent defibrillation or cardioversion. Still other states provide certification as an EMT–Trauma by including additional training in advanced skills for handling victims of traumatic injuries.

A more common advanced level training is in the form of certification as an EMT–Intermediate. These emergency responders receive training in advanced skills such as intubation, intravenous fluid replacement and the administration of certain medications.

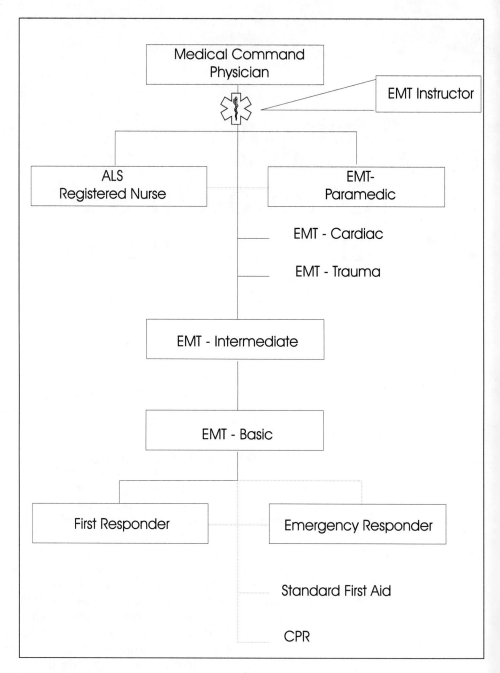

FIGURE B.1 Components of an EMS System

The EMT–Basic training program is comprised of those basic skills necessary for an emergency responder to handle nonserious and certain life threatening emergencies and assist to ALS providers with the treatment of critically ill or injured patients. The 1994 EMT–Basic National Standard Curriculum has incorporated certain advanced skills into basic training; skills such as AED and patient–assisted medication administration for certain drugs.

Another key element of the BLS system are those individuals most likely to be the first to appear at the scene of an emergency situation. There are two training programs for these individuals: the Department of Transportation National Standard Curriculum's First Responder and the American Red Cross' Emergency Responder. Both training programs provide approximately 40 hours worth of training in techniques such as CPR, bleeding control, and immobilization techniques, which responders should be able to perform, with minimal equipment, prior to the arrival of an ambulance.

The lay public can also serve a vital role in the EMS System. Training in CPR and standard first aid for the general public aids in decreasing mortality and morbidity as well as reducing necessary rehabilitation time due to the rapid treatment of life–threatening problems and prevention of more severe injuries.

At the forefront of the EMS system of emergency providers are those EMT instructors committed to providing essential training. While medical direction is important in EMS education, it is the instructional staff that imparts knowledge on emergency service responders.

APPENDIX C
Creating Scenarios

One of the most important elements an instructor can provide students with is a realistic environment in which to perform emergency care techniques. While students progress through learning, demonstration, and practice of skills, it is essential that students "get a feel" for the emergency environment prior to being placed in a true emergency situation. Providing realism in an EMS training program can provide a simulation of an emergency environment without putting a victim or the student in jeopardy.

One of the best methods to provide such realism is through the use of moulage (the use of makeup and props to simulate an illness or injury). A victim with a piece of tape marked "deformity" placed on the thigh will not provide the same realistic effect as a simulated bruised and swollen thigh. The techniques for applying moulage are easy to learn and ultimately increase the effectiveness of practical skills training.

Writing a Scenario

The first step in creating a successful scenario is to determine the skill to be evaluated, the illness or injury that would require the use of such a skill, and the mechanism of injury from which it would result. For example, if the skill to be used is C–spine immobilization, a common injury requiring such immobilization is neck pain and a common mechanism of injury is an automobile accident.

The next step in creating the scenario is to determine the victim's past medical history, present or past medications, allergies, or other information that could be relevant to the emergency situation. History, medications, or other information need not necessarily be related to the illness or injury at hand.

Once the illness or injury has been determined, it is necessary to identify vital signs that would be appropriate. Vital signs should also include a set that would result from inappropriate treatment so that the evaluator can use them should students mistreat the victim.

Programming the Victim

The next step in creating an effective scenario is to program the victim. The victim needs to become actively involved in the illusion process in order to create a realistic environment. The victim must act and react appropriately according to the treatment students provide, whether accurate or not.

The victim should be programmed with information such as:

- What is the injury?
- What is the history of the present illness or injury?
- Where was the individual when the illness or injury occurred?
- How long ago did the illness or injury occur?
- How might the illness or injury affect the individual's life?
- Where does it hurt?
- Does anything make it feel better or worse?
- What might happen if the situation is not handled appropriately?

A victim information sheet such as that provided in Box C.1 can assist in preparing the victim for a scenario. The sheet should include a description of the scenario, moulage and props needed, and acting directions for the victim.

It is essential that the victim act and react appropriately when treatment is provided. For example, if the victim has a deformed thigh, and the student applies a traction splint appropriately the victim should sigh with relief when adequate traction is provided. Likewise, if the patient is complaining of difficulty breathing and the student does not apply high flow oxygen, the victim should become increasingly short of breath and increase the rate of respirations.

Creating the Environment

Setting the stage for an emergency situation simulation is extremely important to increase realism. Environmental considerations include the location of a scenario, required props, appearance of clothing, and layout of the room. If the scenario implies the victim has been drinking, empty beer cans or alcohol bottles should be spread around the room, and alcohol should be sprayed on the victim to make it smell as though he had been drinking.

If the scenario implies a fight, the use of a weapon such as a bloody knife or a gun, bat, or other weapon can also add to realism of the situation. These props should help the student identify the mechanism

BOX C.1 Sample Victim Information Sheet

SCENARIO	MOULAGE	PATIENT PROGRAMMING	VICTIM
#1 – Bar fight	Laceration above the right eye Impaled knife in the upper right quadrant Pale and diaphoretic skin Alcohol on breath	Agitated Loses consciousness after the completion of the complete survey, or 4 to 5 minutes into the scenario if a complete survey is not done.	John Doe

Sample victim information sheet

of injury or provide additional clues regarding the emergency situation, history of the illness, or other important information. If the scenario involves drugs, paraphernalia such as a syringe, tourniquet, or confectioner's sugar can be used as effective props.

The presence of a bystander such as an obnoxious boyfriend or concerned parent can also add realism in the scenario by increasing the tension and stress associated with the emergency situation.

APPENDIX D
Organizations Associated With EMS

American Academy of Ophthalmology
P.O. Box 7424
San Francisco, CA 94120–7424
(415) 561–8500

American Academy of Orthopaedic Surgeons (AAOS)
6300 N. River Road
Rosemont, IL 60018
(800) 626–6726
   Concerned with continuing education for Orthopaedic Surgeons, Allied Health Professionals and the general public. Publishes Emergency Care and Transportation of the Sick and Injured.

American Ambulance Association
3814 Auburn Blvd., Suite 70
Sacramento, CA 95821
(916) 483–3827
   A national organization for operators of private ambulance services which provides members with educational opportunities and legislative representation.

American Burn Association (ABA)
Medical Center
Valhalla, NY 10595
(914) 285–8660
   Works to stimulate and sponsor research in the treatment and prevention of burns.

American College of Emergency Physicians (ACEP)
P.O. Box 619911
Dallas, TX 75261–9911
(972) 550–0911
   Organization dedicated to improve the quality of medical care provided in emergency departments.

American College of Healthcare Executives
1 North Franklin Street, #1700
Chicago, IL 60606
(312) 424–2800

American College of Surgeons. Committee on Trauma (ACS)
633 North St. Clair Street
Chicago, IL 60611
(312) 202–5000
Committee concerned with all phases of emergency care provided by rescue and ambulance service personnel as well as in hospital emergency departments.

American Heart Association
Committee on Emergency Cardiac Care
7320 Greenville Ave.
Dallas, TX 75231
(214) 373–6300
Helps promulgate national criteria regarding basic life support and advanced cardiac life support practices. Develops CPR standards and training materials.

American Hospital Association
P.O. Box 92683
Chicago, IL 60675–2683
(800) AHA–2626

American Medical Association (AMA)
Commission on Emergency Medical Services
515 North State Street
Chicago, IL 60610
(312) 464–5000
Responsible for the identification and implementation of educational programs for physicians and allied health professionals in emergency medical services.

American Public Health Association (APHA)
Injury Control and Emergency Services Forum
1015 Fifteenth Street, NW, Suite 300
Washington, DC 20005
(202) 789–5600
Provides a forum for the discussion of issues, needs and priorities for EMS organizations in order to increase the effectiveness of injury reduction practices. Publishes the American Journal of Public Health.

American Red Cross
Audiovisual Loan Library
5816 Seminary Rd.
Falls Church, VA 22041
(703) 379-8160

Health and Safety Division
8111 Gate House Road
Falls Church, VA 22042
(703) 206–6000

Provides certified basic training in personal safety, first aid, and emergency care including CPR.

American Society for Training and Development (ASTD)
1640 King Street
Box 1443
Alexandria, VA 22313-2043
Publishes Training and Development Journal.

American Society for Testing of Materials (ASTM)
100 Barr Harbor Drive
West Conshohocken, PA 19428
An organization established for the development of standards, test methods, definitions, practices, classifications and specifications. Committee F–30 on Emergency Medical Services serves to develop standards through the voluntary cooperation of organizations, agencies and individuals committed to ensuring the highest quality of the Emergency Medical Services System.

American Trauma Society (ATS)
8903 Presidential Parkway, #512
Upper Marlboro, MD 20772
(800) 556–7890
Dedicated to assisting with the reduction of suffering, death and disability associated with injuries by promoting the prevention of injury and improvement of trauma care through educational services.

Audio Digest Foundation
1577 E. Chevy Chase Dr.
Glendale, CA 91206
(818) 240–7500

Center for Disease Control
1600 Clifton Road, NE
Atlanta, GA 30333
(404) 488–4656
A Federal Agency charged with protecting the health of the citizens in the United States by providing leadership and direction in the prevention and control of diseases and other preventable conditions.

Disaster Research Center
University of Delaware
Newark, DE 19716
(302) 831–6618
An organization established to study the reactions of groups and organizations in community–wide emergencies, focusing on planning for and response to large–scale community crisis.

Dive Rescue, Inc.
201 North Link Lane
Fort Collins, CO 80524-2712
(970) 482–0887

Emergency Nurses Association
216 Higgins Road
Park Ridge, IL 60068-5736
(847) 698–9400
A professional organization for nurses providing emergency care, promoting the improvement of emergency care through professional development.

Federal Communications Commission

1919 M Street, NW
Washington, DC 20554
(202) 418-0200

An agency responsible for policy development, licensing and the regulation of the radio communication component of the Emergency Medical Services System.

Federal Emergency Management Agency (FEMA)

Federal Center Plaza
500 C Street, SW
Washington, DC 20472
(202) 646-2500

An agency responsible for the coordination of response activities for natural and manmade disasters. FEMA serves as the President's policy development and advisory arm on civil preparedness matters and is concerned with all aspects of emergency health, medical, and human-service preparedness.

International Association of Fire Chiefs

4025 Fair Ridge Drive
Fairfax, VA 22033
(703) 273-0911

Dedicated to ensuring adequate knowledge, skills, and professional attitudes for fire fighters in an effort to maximize the effectiveness of response to emergency situations.

International Fire Service Training Association

Oklahoma State University
930 N. Willis Street
Stillwater, OK 74078
(405) 744-5723

International Rescue and Emergency Care Association

8630M Guilford, Suite 319
Columbia, MD 21046
(800) 221-3435

Promotes the recognition and establishment of organized rescue and emergency care techniques through training. Publishes the Rescuer magazine.

Joint Commission on Accreditation of Healthcare Organizations

1 Renaissance Blvd.
Oakbrook Terrace, IL 60184
(708) 916-5600

Lakewood Publications, Inc.

50 S. Ninth St.
Minneapolis, MN 55402

Publishes Training, The Magazine of Human Resources Development

National Association of Emergency Medical Technicians (NAEMT)

102 W. Leake St.
Clinton, MD 39056
(601) 924-7744

A professional association of EMTs and EMT-Paramedics, promoting continuing education and professionalism for EMS providers and working toward the recognition of uniform certification standards.

National Association of State Emergency Medical Services Directors (NASEMSD)
1947 Camino Vida Rosa, Suite 200
Carlsbad, CA 92008
(619) 431-7054
An association dedicated to the improvement of the quality of emergency medical care through the coordination of the development of EMS systems throughout the country.

National Council of State Emergency Medical Services Training Coordinators (NCSEMSTC)
Iron Works Pike
Lexington, KY 40578-1910
(606) 231-1960
Dedicated to the improvement and standardization of EMS training, certification, recertification, revocation, and reciprocity through uniform nationwide standards.

National Disaster Medical System
5600 Fishers Lane
Rockville, MD 20857
(301) 443-4893

National Flight Nurses Association
6900 Grove Road
Thorofare, NJ 08086
(609) 384-6725
An association dedicated to the improvement of the quality of aeromedical health care through the establishment of high standards for training and continuing education of health-care professionals involved with aeromedical transport. Publishes The Journal of Aeromedical Health Care.

U.S. Department of Transportation (DOT)
National Highway Traffic Safety Administration
EMS Division
400 7th Street, SW
Washington, DC 20590
(202) 366-5440
An agency that promotes the development of guidelines and standards for all components of comprehensive emergency medical services which impact on the effectiveness of care for persons injured on the highways. This organization assists with the development and implementation of various training programs including First Responder, EMT, EMT- Paramedic, EMT-Refresher, FR-Refresher, and EVO courses.

APPENDIX E
Sample Forms

AMERICANS WITH DISABILITIES ACT

ACCOMMODATION POLICY

Purpose: To provide a description of policies, procedures and responsibilities for implementing provisions of the Americans with Disabilities Act of 1990 (ADA) P.L.101–336.

Scope: The information provided herein applies to all prehospital EMS personnel.

Objectives:

1. Identify a uniform method for identifying persons who qualify for an accommodation under this Act.

2. Identify a uniform method for making accommodations under this Act.

3. Ensure that all prehospital EMS personnel are aware of certification requirements of which the program entails, to include:

    a. Necessary Qualifications
    b. Competency Areas
    c. Description of Tasks

Policy:

A. Admissions/Registration

    1. No discussion of, screening for, or other form of inquiry concerning potential disabilities shall be performed prior to a student's admission to a training program. No inquiry may be made of a prospective student about any disability. Aptitude or diagnostic testing may only be performed and utilized when it is required of ALL students.

    2. The registration process will include distribution of a Student Overview that includes course specific performance and certification requirements. Students will be given an opportunity to ask questions about the material contained in the overview. Each student will be required to sign a statement indicating he has read and understands the content of the Student Overview and Functional Position Description.

    3. The Functional Position Description and Course Overview will be provided to all students at the time of class registration.

    4. No individual shall be excluded from participation in a training program or from becoming eligible for state certification on the basis of a disability. Individuals unable to perform all required skills may audit programs and receive certificates of attendance.

B. Practical skills evaluations as required for successful course completion and/or certification:

1. No accommodation will be made in a training program that is not reasonably available in a pre-hospital environment.

2. Students may use performance aids that could be readily available and easily accessible to them in the prehospital setting. It is the responsibility of the student to provide any personal aids deemed necessary and appropriate. Examples of such devices include amplified stethoscopes, glasses, artificial limbs, and hearing aids.

C. Written examinations as required for successful course completion and/or certification.

Reasonable and appropriate accommodations for the written component of the certification process for individuals with disabilities:

1. Individuals who request special accommodations on the written examination due to a disability will be permitted to take the standard format of the examination but receive an extended amount of time in which to complete the examination.

2. Students must identify their request for modification of the standard course written exam format to the Course Coordinator 2 weeks prior to scheduled exams. The Course Coordinator shall make course exam accommodations consistent with certification exam accommodations (additional time).

ATTENDANCE ROSTER

Class Number: _____
Course Title: _____
Registration Date: _____

Course Coordinator: _____
Location: _____
Number Registered: _____

DATE (Month/Day)

NAME																			
1.																			
2.																			
3.																			
4.																			
5.																			
6.																			
7.																			
8.																			
9.																			
10.																			
11.																			
12.																			
13.																			
14.																			
15.																			
16.																			
17.																			
18.																			
19.																			
20.																			

APPLICATION FOR ENROLLMENT

Personal Information

Full Name: _____

Street, Apt.#: _____

City, State, Zip: _____

Home Phone: _____

Work Phone: _____

Date of Birth: _____/_____/_____

Social Security Number: _____–_____–_____

Affiliation/Company: _____

Station #: _____

County of Residence: _____

Education Level: (Circle highest level of years completed)

1 2 3 4 5 6 7 8 9 10 11 12 13 14 15 16 17 18

OFFICE USE ONLY

Received on:

Prerequisite check:

Payment:
_____ Company Check   _____ Cash
_____ Personal Check   _____ LOI
_____ Money Order   _____ Purchase Order
_____ Amount Received   _____ Date Forewarded

Student Rejected:
_____ Under age requirement
_____ Lacks authorized signature
_____ Lacks prerequisites
_____ Form not complete
_____ Lacks sufficient funds
_____ Class full
_____ Class canceled

Course/Program Information

Course Title: _____   Course #: _____

Location: _____   Start Date: _____/_____/_____

Company Officer Authorization

I certify that the above student meets the prerequisites and age requirements to participate in this course. I further verify that the above listed individual is an active member of this company and is covered by workman's compensation while participating in this course.

Does your organization agree to provide payment for this student? _____ Yes _____ No

_____   _____

Signature of Officer (Name and Title)   Date

Criminal History

Have you ever been arrested and/or convicted of a misdemeanor or felony? _____ Yes _____ No

A conviction offense is not a bar from certification examinations in all cases; each case is considered on its own merits. If "yes," the applicant may be required to provide an original State Police "Criminal Record Check." In some cases, the applicant will be required to provide additional documentation. A positive criminal history does not prevent anyone from enrolling in a training session, but may prevent ability for state certification.

Student Signature

I verify, to the best of my knowledge, the above information is accurate and correct. I further agree that if I am not affiliated with an organization, I agree to provide my own insurance. I also certify that I meet the age requirements and prerequisites of the above registered course and understand that any falsification of information may lead to my rejection for class participation.

I further agree that upon my acceptance, I will report for the identified course of instruction at the appropriate time and starting date posted for the course; and if circumstances beyond my control prevent me from attending the course, I will notify the Chester County DES Training Division as soon as this becomes known to me.

_____   _____

Signature of Student   Date

Payment (check appropriate method)   Amount of payment _____

_____ Company Check   Check #: _____
_____ Personal Check   Check #: _____
_____ Money Order   M.O. #: _____
_____ Cash
_____ Letter of Intent (LOI)
_____ Purchase order

EMT–BASIC COURSE SYLLABUS

Lesson #	Date/Time	Lesson	Primary Instructor
1.1		Introduction to emergency medical care	
1.2		Well–being of the EMT–Basic	
1.3		Medical/legal and ethical issues	
1.4		The human body	
1.5		Baseline vital signs and sample history	
1.6		Lifting and moving patients	
1.7		Evaluation: preparatory module	
2.1		Airway	
2.2		Practical skills lab: airway	
2.3		Evaluation: airway module	
3.1		Scene size–up	
3.2		Initial assessment	
3.3		Focused history and physical exam (trauma)	
3.4		Focused history and physical exam (medical)	
3.5		Detailed physical exam	
3.6		Ongoing assessment	
3.7		Communications	
3.8		Documentation	
3.9		Practical skills lab: patient assessment	
3.10		Evaluation: patient assessment module	
4.1		General pharmacology	
4.2		Respiratory emergencies	
4.3		Cardiovascular emergencies	
4.4		Diabetes/altered mental status	
4.5		Allergies	
4.6		Poisoning/overdose	

Lesson #	Date/Time	Lesson	Primary Instructor
4.7		Environmental emergencies	
4.8		Behavioral emergencies	
4.9		Obstetrics/gynecology	
4.10		Practical skills lab: medical/behavioral and OB/GYN	
4.11		Evaluation: medical/behavioral and OB/GYN	
5.1		Bleeding and shock	
5.2		Soft tissue injuries	
5.3		Musculoskeletal care	
5.4		Injuries to the head and spine	
5.5		Practical skills lab: trauma	
5.6		Evaluation: trauma module	
6.1		Infants and children	
6.2		Practical skills lab: infants and children	
6.3		Evaluation: infants and children	
7.1		Ambulance operations	
7.2		Gaining access	
7.3		Overviews	
7.4		Evaluation: operations	
8.1		Advanced airway	
8.2		Practical skills lab: advanced airway	
8.3		Evaluation: advanced airway	

EMERGENCY MEDICAL TECHNICIAN OVERVIEW

ROLES AND RESPONSIBILITIES

A certified EMT is authorized to provide (BLS) services including but not limited to rescue, triage, and the transfer and transport of both emergency and nonemergency patients in accordance with the current Department of Transportation EMT National Standard Curriculum.

An EMT's scope of practice shall be limited to the above listed activities except where the Secretary of Health (Secretary) authorizes an EMT to perform additional activities.

RULES OF CONDUCT

1. Appearance

   Students must exhibit good personal hygiene. Each student must be neat, clean, and wear clothing appropriate for the material being covered. All students will be required to wear appropriate protective gear during the vehicle rescue portion of instruction; this includes a turnout coat, helmet, gloves, bunker pants with boots or 3/4 boots (where applicable).

2. Behavior

   Students must maintain a positive attitude, professional manner, and behavior appropriate to a classroom setting. In addition, students will obey all rules and regulations of the training facility.

3. Drugs/Alcohol

   Students displaying abusive behavior or other behavior normally associated with drug or alcohol usage shall be dismissed from the class which will count as an absence. The student must be counseled before returning to the class.

4. Academic Dishonesty

   Academic dishonesty includes, but is not limited to, cheating, plagiarizing, bribery, fabrication of information or citations, facilitating acts of academic dishonesty by others, having unauthorized possession of examinations, submitting the work of another person or work previously used without informing the instructor, or tampering with the academic work of other students.

STUDENTS' RIGHTS AND RESPONSIBILITIES

1. Student Rights

   a. The student has a right to competent instruction, course counseling, and adequate facilities, and in all areas he has the right to expect the highest degree of excellence possible within the resources of the Training Institute.

b. The student has a right to protection from unreasonable and capricious actions by faculty and administration.

c. Each student has the right to be considered for admission without regard to age, sex, ancestry, religious or political belief, or country of origin.

d. Each student has the right to know the rules by which s/he is governed through the medium of a clear and precise written explanation of the rules.

2. Student Responsibilities

a. The student has the responsibility to devote himself to the serious pursuit of learning and to respect the rights and opinions of others, including faculty, administration, and fellow students.

b. The student has the responsibility to comply with any and all the rules governing participants of training programs.

c. The student has the responsibility to support academic integrity.

d. The student has the responsibility to conduct himself in accordance with generally accepted standards of conduct as embodied in society's laws and regulations.

e. Each student has the responsibility to respect innovation and individual differences and to conduct himself so as not to violate the rights of other students and members of the administration and faculty.

COURSE REQUIREMENTS

1. Aptitudes

a. Vision

Students must have visual acuity sufficient to (1) distinguish visual color discrimination when examining patients and (2) determining by appearance diagnostic signs that require immediate detection and proper action.

b. Hearing

Students must have hearing acuity sufficient to receive verbal directions and instructions and to distinguish diagnostic signs.

c. Reading/Writing

Students must have the ability to read and write English sufficiently to read items such as prescription bottles, and to write English sufficiently to complete patient record forms and examination reports.

d. Physical

Students must have the ability to perform the skill objectives as outlined in the National Standard Curriculum.

All students must have the aptitudes as listed above when taking the practical skills examination for state certification. Medical problems must be resolved prior to taking practical examinations.

NOTE: In accordance with the American Disabilities Act (ADA), any requests for accommodations must be submitted in writing, within two weeks after the course begins.

2. Attendance

a. Each student shall be permitted to miss a total of twelve (12) hours. Any hour, or portion thereof, missed, which exceed twelve (12) hours will result in the student being dismissed from the course.

3. Clinical Time

All EMT students, with the exception of critical care(*) hospital personnel, are required to spend 10 hours training in a local hospital. Such experience shall be spent in the hospital's emergency department. Additionally, the student should be exposed (via a brief tour) to such areas as CCU, ICU, OR, and OB. Clinical experience must be completed prior to the written examination for state certification.

(*) Critical care hospital personnel enrolled in EMT training programs are to spend ten hours with an active ambulance service in lieu of the in-hospital experience.

4. Interim testing

a. Students must pass the midterm and final course exam with not less than 70% on the written interim exam. One retest is permissible for each exam and must be passed with a 70% or greater.

b. Students must pass the midterm and final course practical skill examinations (scenario based). One retest is permissible for each practical skill test.

CAUSES FOR DISMISSAL

1. A student may be immediately dismissed from a course for:

a. Failure to maintain a 70% on the written midterm or final course exam.

b. Failure of midterm or final course skill tests, subject to retest policy.

2. A student will be immediately dismissed from a course for:

   a. Failure to meet attendance requirements.

   b. Academic dishonesty.

   c. Misconduct which could endanger public safety/property.

3. The following are subject to one counseling session prior to dismissal. Any additional infraction will result in automatic dismissal from the course:

   a. Behavioral misconduct.

   b. Inappropriate hygiene.

4. Any of the above reasons must be documented in writing by the course coordinator and sent to the administrative director within 7 days of the student being dismissed.

CRIMINAL HISTORY

All students are required to complete a criminal history form. Any applicant who has been arrested and/or convicted of a felony or misdemeanor is required to obtain a criminal history report from the State Police Department, and submit it for processing.

The State Department of Health has the right to refuse certification for conviction of certain offenses. A positive criminal history does not prevent any student from attending training, however, may prevent the ability to take the state certification examination process. All criminal history forms must be approved prior to processing state certification examinations.

CERTIFICATION REQUIREMENTS

To be eligible for the written and practical skill examinations developed by the Department for Emergency Medical Technician, persons must have:

1. Successfully completed an approved basic EMT training course

2. Current CPR certification

GRIEVANCE

Complaints regarding instructors, course administration, and course content shall be submitted in the following manner:

1. An individual must present the complaint to the course coordinator. The course coordinator will discuss the complaint and review policies with the individual to determine if a particular problem is defined and explained.

2. If still unsatisfied, the individual may present the complaint to the training institute in writing. The training institute will review the complaint and discuss the complaint with the course coordinator. The training institute will notify the individual of the outcome of the investigation.

3. If the proposed resolution by the training institute is unsatisfactory, the individual may submit the complaint in writing to the Department. The Department will review the complaint, make a determination and notify, in writing, the individual, the training institute, and course coordinator of the decision reached.

4. Without satisfactory results by the regional council, the individual may submit the complaint in writing to the Division.

   The Division will review the complaint and make a determination. The Division will notify, in writing, the individual and the administrative director of the decision reached.

PRACTICAL EXAMINATIONS

1. <u>Candidate Prerequisites</u>

   a. Be at least 16 years of age

   b. Successfully complete a training program approved by the Department, or previously certified to the level of the certification exam

   c. Possess current CPR card

   d. Complete and submit skill verification forms

   e. Complete field and/or clinical time

2. <u>Major Examination Areas</u>

   a. Patient assessment

   b. Basic life support

   c. Extremity fractures

   d. Soft tissue

   e. Central nervous system

    f.   Patient lifting and moving

    g.   Childbirth

    h.   Thoracic injuries

    i.   Medical antishock trousers

    j.   Medical emergencies

    k.   Oxygen therapy

    l.   Adjunctive equipment

3. Absence

Persons who do not attend scheduled practical examinations must make arrangements to complete the practical examination at another regularly scheduled exam.

4. Leaving Test Site

After the testing begins, any student leaving a test site prior to completion of all stations without prior permission of the coordinator (or designee) will be considered having FAILED the test. Acceptable reasons for leaving the test site shall include, but are not limited to personal illness, injury, or family emergencies, which must then be documented in writing within 3 working days.

5. Time Constraints

Students shall inform the regional coordinator or designee of any time constraints.

    a.   Time constraints must be identified by the student prior to starting the examination.

    b.   Under normal circumstances, students will be scheduled so that they are oriented and tested within three (3) hours.

6. Scoring

    a.   Satisfactory Grade

        The candidate is able to identify the problem or task presented. The candidate is able to select and prioritize appropriate treatment. The candidate is able to demonstrate appropriate treatment or skills within the established objectives.

b. Unsatisfactory Grade

The candidate is unable to identify the problem or task presented. The candidate is unable to demonstrate appropriate treatment or skills within the established objectives. The student performed task(s), treatment, or skill(s) that adversely affect patient outcome.

Please complete the following information and return it to the instructor at the first class.

Name _____

Address _____

Phone (Home) _____ (Work) _____

Affiliate _____

I verify that I have read the EMT syllabus and overview and comprehend what is expected of me.

Name _____ Date _____

Signature _____

(Adapted from the Pennsylvania Department of Health Course Overview. Some material may not be applicable in certain states.)

FINAL INSTRUCTOR ROSTER

Course Number: _____

Coordinator: _____

County: _____

Registration Date: _____

LESSON	DATE	PRIMARY	SECONDARY	SECONDARY	SECONDARY	SECONDARY	SECONDARY

FUNCTIONAL POSITION DESCRIPTION FOR THE EMERGENCY MEDICAL TECHNICIAN

INTRODUCTION

The following is a position description for the Emergency Medical Technician (EMT). This document identifies the qualifications, competencies and tasks expected of the EMT.

QUALIFICATIONS FOR CERTIFICATION

- Apply and successfully complete a state approved EMT training program,

- Be a minimum of 16 years of age upon enrollment, and

- Successfully complete certification examinations.

- Have the ability to hear, read, write, communicate, and interpret instructions in the English language.

- Demonstrate competency in handling emergencies using basic life support equipment in accordance with the objectives in the U.S. Department of Transportation National Standard Curriculum for EMT and other objectives identified include having the ability to:

  ▶ Verbally communicate in person and via telephone and telecommunications; communicate the status of a patient to other EMS providers and hospital staff; and hear via telecommunications, telephone and patient/bystanders voice.

  ▶ Lift to a height of 33 inches, and carry and balance a minimum of 125 pounds.

  ▶ Use good judgement and remain calm in high–stress situations.

  ▶ Read training manuals, books and road maps.

  ▶ Accurately discern street signs and address numbers.

  ▶ Verbally interview patients, family members, and bystanders and hear their responses.

  ▶ Document, in writing, all relevant information in prescribed format.

  ▶ Verbally communicate status of patients to co–workers and hospital staff, and answer oral questions.

  ▶ Demonstrate manual dexterity, with the ability to perform all tasks related to quality patient care.

▶ Bend, stoop, crawl, and walk on uneven surfaces.

▶ Function in varied environmental conditions such as lighted or darkened work areas, and extreme heat, cold, and moisture.

DESCRIPTION OF TASKS

The EMT may function alone or as a member of a multimember team. Tasks which the EMT may perform include the following:

- Receive calls from a dispatcher, verbally acknowledge the call, read road maps, assist in the identification of the most expeditious route to the scene, and observe traffic ordinances and regulations enroute to and from the emergency scene.

- Upon arrival at the scene, insure the vehicle is parked in a safe location; perform a size–up to determine scene safety, mechanism of injury or illness, determine the total number of patients, and request additional help if necessary.

- In the absence of law enforcement, create a safe environment for the protection of the injured and those assisting in the care of patient(s).

- Determine the nature and extent of illness or injury, take pulses, blood pressure by auscultation and palpation, visually observe changes in skin color, and establish a priority for emergency care. Based on assessment findings, render emergency care to adults, infants, and children.

- Establish and maintain an airway, ventilate patients, perform cardiac resuscitation, use automated external defibrillators, provide prehospital emergency care of single and multiple system trauma such as controlling hemorrhage, treatment of shock (hypoperfusion), bandaging wounds, and immobilization of painful swollen and deformed extremities.

- Manage medical patients to include assisting in childbirth, management of respiratory, cardiac, diabetic, allergic, behavioral and environmental emergencies, and suspected poisonings.

- Search for medical identification emblems, bracelets, or cards that provide emergency care information. Additional care is provided based on assessment of the patient and obtaining past medical information.

- Assist patients with prescribed medications including sublingual nitroglycerine, epinephrine auto injectors, and hand-held aerosol inhalers.

- Administer oxygen, oral glucose, and activated charcoal.

- Reassure patients and bystanders by working in a confident, efficient manner and avoid mishandling patients and undue haste while working expeditiously.

- Where extrication is required, assess the extent of injury and give all possible emergency care and protection to the patient. Use recognized techniques and equipment to remove patients safely.

Radio dispatchers for additional help as necessary. Following extrication, provide additional medical care and triage injured victims in accordance with standard emergency procedures.

- Comply with regulations on the handling of crime scenes and prehospital death by notifying appropriate authorities and arrange for protection of property and evidence.

- Carry and lift the stretcher, placing it in the ambulance and see that the patient and stretcher are secured. Continue care enroute to the appropriate facility.

- Determine the most appropriate facility for patient transport unless otherwise directed by medical control. Report the nature and extent of injuries, the number of patients being transported, and the destination of patients to ensure prompt medical care in accordance with local protocols.

- Observe and reassess the patient enroute, and administer care as directed by medical control. Assist with lifting and moving the patient and appropriate equipment from the ambulance into the emergency facility.

- Report verbally and in writing, observations and emergency treatment given to the patient, at the scene and in transit, to the receiving staff for record keeping and diagnostic purposes. Upon request, provide assistance to the receiving facility staff.

- After completion of the call, restock and replace patient care supplies, clean all equipment following appropriate decontamination and cleaning procedures, make careful examination of all equipment to ensure availability of the ambulance for the next call. Maintain the ambulance in an efficient operating condition.

- Attend continuing education and refresher training programs as required by employers' medical direction and/or the certifying agency.

- Meet qualifications within the functional position description of the EMT.

Student's Name: _____

(Please Print)

At the second session of any Emergency Medical Technician (EMT) course, each student must sign one of the following statements:

I have read and understand the functional job description of an EMT and have no conditions which would preclude me from safely and effectively performing all the functions of the level of EMT for which I am seeking certification.

_____   _____

Signature   *Date*

I have read and understand the functional job description of an EMT and will be submitting a request for an accommodation for the written certification examination. I understand I must submit appropriate documentation no later than two weeks prior to the EMT certification exam.

_____   _____

Signature   *Date*

INCIDENT REPORT

Date/Time of Incident: _____

Name of Person Completing this Form: _____

Briefly describe the incident:

_____

_____

_____

_____

_____

_____

Describe any action taken:

_____

_____

_____

_____

_____

_____

Describe any notifications made:

_____

_____

_____

_____   _____

         (Signature)   (Date)

PARAMEDIC SKILLS AUTHORIZATION FORM

Student: _____

SKILLS	DATE SUCCESSFULLY COMPLETED		
	Classroom	Hospital	Field
Vital signs			
Patient assessment (trauma)			
Patient assessment (medical)			
Documentation			
Application of airway adjuncts			
EOA/EGTA insertion			
Endotracheal intubation (adult)			
Endotracheal intubation (infant)			
Nasotracheal intubation			
Intraosseous insertion			
NG tube insertion			
Phlebotomy			
Peripheral IV			
MAST application and inflation			
MAST deflation			
External jugular insertion			
Discontinuation of IV			
Medication administration SQ route			
Medication administration IM route			
Medication administration IV route			
Medication administration ET route			
Medication admin. IV piggyback			

SKILLS	DATE SUCCESSFULLY COMPLETED		
	Classroom	Hospital	Field
Patient assessment (OB)			
Patient assessment (GYN)			
Patient assessment (pediatric)			
Draw medication from vial			
Draw medication from ampule			
Draw medication from tubex			
Draw medication from pre-filled			
Relieve FAOB (adult conscious)			
Relieve FAOB (adult unconscious)			
Relieve FAOB (child conscious)			
Relieve FAOB (child unconscious)			
Relieve FAOB (infant conscious)			
Relieve FAOB (infant unconscious)			
Perform adult CPR			
Perform child CPR			
Perform infant CPR			
Perform cricothyrotomy			
Insert transtracheal jet			
Perform ET suctioning extubation			
Suction			
Perform chest decompression			
Recognize & treat dysrhythmia			
Perform cardiac monitoring			
Perform defibrillation			
Perform cardioversion			
Apply external pacing			
Perform carotid sinus massage			
Serve as mega code team leader			

SKILLS	DATE SUCCESSFULLY COMPLETED		
	Classroom	**Hospital**	**Field**
Apply short backboard			
Apply long backboard			
Perform rapid extrication			
Treat soft tissue injuries			
Apply splinting devices			
Apply sling/swathe			
Apply traction splint			
Insert urinary bladder catheter			
Apply rotating tourniquets			
Perform cephalic breech delivery			
Perform scalp IV insertion			
Perform psychiatric intervention			
Perform EOA/EGTA extubation			
Use magill forceps			
Remove helmet			

PARAMEDIC STUDENT DAILY LOG FORM

Student: _____   EMT #: _____

Preceptor: _____   EMT #: _____

Date/Time On Duty: _____   Date/Time Off Duty: _____

Type of Calls: (Identify the # of patients treated in each category, by chief complaint)

_____ Adult   _____ Pediatric   _____ Neonatal

_____ Cardiac   _____ Cardiac arrest   _____ Respiratory distress

_____ Diabetic   _____ Seizure   _____ Other medical complaint

_____ Overdose   _____ Anaphylaxis   _____ Maternity

_____ Psychological   _____ Traumatic injury   _____ Other (explain) _____

Skills Performed by Student: (Identify the # of attempts and successful completion of each skill)

SKILL	U	S
Patient assessment		
IV insertion		
Intraosseous insertion		
Calculate IV drip rate		
Draw blood		
Medication administration		
Calculate dose		
Administer IV route		
Administer IM route		
Administer SQ route		
Administer SL route		

SKILL	U	S
Intubation		
EOA/EGTA intubation		
External pace		
Defibrillation		
MAST application		
Communication		
Chest decompression		
Needle cricothyrotomy		
EKG interpretation		
Lead placement		
Other		

Other Activities Performed: _____

_____

Student Signature: _____   Preceptor Signature: _____

PARENTAL CONSENT FORM

Course Number: _____   Date: _____

Coordinator: _____

Student's Name: _____   Date of Birth: _____

Address: _____

City: _____   State: _____   Phone No: _____

Course Location: _____

I, _____ a parent or guardian of _____, understand that my son/daughter is interested in enrolling in an Emergency Medical Training course offered by _____. I realize this is a course dealing with Human Anatomy and Physiology, and will require working closely with and physically examining other students. My son/daughter will be taught how to handle emergencies such as: Respiratory and Cardiac Arrest, Choking, Severe Bleeding, Emergency Childbirth, and Vehicle Rescue.

The intent of this course is to train and certify personnel in emergency procedures. Therefore, I understand he/she will be taught all the skills required in an Emergency Medical Services Course to function independently, possibly on a Basic Life Support Ambulance. To accomplish this, he/she will have to meet or exceed the requirements for course completion and certification to be certified as a First Responder or Emergency Medical Technician in the State of _____.

Thus, I do therefore permit _____ to enroll in this course of instruction beginning on: _____ .

Parent or Guardians Signature: _____   Date: _____

STUDENT COUNSELING FORM

Student: _____   Date: _____

Reason for Counseling:

_____ Routine   _____ Student Initiated   _____ Institute Initiated

General Observations:

1. Attendance:

    _____ Punctual   _____ Habitually Late

    _____ Occasionally Tardy _____ Other

    _____

    _____

2. Appearance:

    _____ Neat and Clean   _____ Unkept   _____ Other

    _____

    _____

3. Attitude:

    _____ Willing, Eager, and Pleasant   _____ Other

    _____

    _____

4. Is student experiencing difficulty meeting course demands?

    _____ Yes   _____ No

    _____

    _____

Corrective Action Needed:

1. Describe action necessary:

    _____

    _____

2. Timetable for completion/review of corrective measures:

    _____

3. Date for next counseling session:

    _____

Counselor's Comments:

_____

_____

Student's Comments:

_____

_____

_____

I have read and understand the above information as it has been presented to me. My signature does not necessarily mean I agree with all the materials listed, but it acknowledges that I have read the material.

Student: _____   _____
                         (Print Name)   (Signature)

Counselor: _____   _____
                         (Print Name)   (Signature)

GLOSSARY

Active listening   A type of communication in which instructors summarize and paraphrase what students say so the students feel they have been understood

Acronym   Mnemonics that use the first letter of each word of a list to form a word

Administrative director   The individual responsible for the overall administration of a training program; sometimes referred to as the program director

Affective domain   One of the categories of educational objectives for student attitudes, values, and emotional growth; this domain includes the following five basic categories: receiving, responding, valuing, organizing, and characterization of a value

Affective strategies   Learning strategies directed toward improving the successful attainment of objectives targeted toward the affective domain; such strategies include focusing student attention, maintaining motivation, and managing time in an attempt to improve student involvement

Andragogy   The methodology of lifelong education for adults

Anxiety   The emotional state associated with apprehension and fear

Aptitude test   A test used to predict how well a student will learn unfamiliar material

Assistant instructor   An individual who assists a primary instructor with skills instruction; also referred to as practical skills instructor or lab instructor

Automaticity   The result of overlearning behaviors to the point that they can be carried out without conscious thought

Aversive stimuli   A negative stimulus aimed at causing a specific behavioral response from an individual

Baseline   The natural occurrence of behavior before intervention

Behavioral objective   A statement regarding specific changes educators intend to produce in student behavior

Behavior disorder   A category in special education for students exhibiting one or more of the following behaviors over a substantial period: inability to learn not related to intellectual, sensory, or health factors; difficulty with interpersonal relationships; inappropriate behavior or moodiness

Behavior modification   Interventions designed to change behavior in a precisely measurable manner

Beta   A 1/2 inch videocassette format not compatible with the VHS format

Bullet   In text, a circle, star, or other symbol used to emphasize a line or word

CD-I (compact disc interactive)   An interactive product that delivers still images, audio, graphics, and data; it is a closed-system box designed to connect to a home television or some other monitor, similar to that of a VCR

CD-ROM (compact disc read only memory)   A format of standard laser disc that stores a large amount of information and requires a CD drive in a computer system; each 4.72 inch disc stores approximately 650 megabytes of digital data; information cannot be written to or stored on the disc

Chunking   Organizing information into small sections of material in order to make the delivery more easily understood and remembered

Classroom management   Instructor behaviors and activities that encourage learning in the classroom

Clinical facility   An institution or agency that, in coordination with an accredited training institute, provides medical direction and continual assessment of student performance for in-hospital observation and skill performance

Coaching   A program of test preparation to increase exam results

Cognitive domain   One of six categories of educational objectives: knowledge, comprehension, application, analysis, synthesis, and evaluation

Cognitive style   The way in which students respond to perceptual tasks

Communication   The process by which information is exchanged between two or more individuals

Computer-aided instruction   Instruction that uses the computer as an instructional media

Computer-based instruction (CBI)   The use of a computer as a tutor to present information, provide students the opportunity to practice what they learn, evaluate student achievement, and provide additional instruction

Conceptual tempo   A cognitive style referring to the speed at which students respond to a task and the number of errors they make in their responses; usually referred to as impulsive or reflective

Condition   Part of an instructional objective that describes any materials, restrictions, or requirements, placed on a student when attempting to meet such objectives

Consultation triad   An instructional strategy in which teams of three students participate in practice exercises

Content validity   The extent to which a test is representative of a defined body of knowledge

Correlation   A measure of the degree of relationship between two variables

Creativity   The capacity of student to produce a novel or original answer, product, or method of doing something

Criteria   The element against which a student is judged to determine if he or she has successfully met the terms of an instructional objective

Criterion-referenced assessment   Measurement in which a student's score is interpreted against a defined body of student behavior or to some specified level of performance

Criterion-referenced testing   A testing procedure in which a student's performance is based on whether specific objectives have been achieved

Culture   The way in which a group of people think, feel, and react in order to solve problems of living in their environment

Decoding   The process of translating a symbol back into its original form, such as translating a letter into its sound or a word into its meaning

Defamation   The act of attacking or injuring the reputation or honor of an individual by false and malicious statements

Demonstration   An instructional strategy in which instructors show to students the steps involved with a particular skill for training purposes

Diagnostic test   A test used to measure student strengths and weaknesses in a given area

Disability   A term describing a physical problem or problems that limit a student's ability to perform certain tasks

Discipline   The degree to which students behave appropriately, are involved in classroom activities, and are task-oriented

Discovery learning   The learning of new information largely as a result of the student's own efforts

Discrimination   The showing of partiality or prejudice in treatment generally directed against a minority group

Distractor   An incorrect option or possible response on a multiple-choice item

Education   The general acquisition of information in order to better oneself; the process by which one learns study habits, problem solving, and general principles that govern the learning process throughout one's life; education alone, however, will not prepare someone for a specific vocation

Empathetic understanding   Sensitivity to and awareness of the feelings, motives, attitudes, and values of others

Encoding   The short-term memory process of transforming incoming information into episodic form and associating it with old knowledge for storage in long-term memory

Entry behavior   The knowledge, skills, or attitudes that a student brings into a new learning situation

Essay item   A test format that requires students to structure long written responses

Evaluation   The process of obtaining information to form judgements so that educational decisions can be made

Excess baggage   Outside problems that when brought into the classroom may distract the student from effective reception and processing of information, thereby minimizing learning

External locus of control   A feeling that one has little control over one's fate and the failure to perceive a cause-and-effect relationship between actions and consequences

Extinction   The reduction of a behavior through the abrupt termination of the positive reinforcer maintaining the inappropriate behavior

Extrinsic motivation   Motivation influenced by external events such as grades, points, or money

Field affiliation   A licensed ambulance service that, in coordination with an accredited training institute, provides continual assessment of student performance of prehospital observation and skill performance

Field-dependent   A cognitive style in which a student is distracted by or sensitive to background elements

Field-independent   A cognitive style in which a student is capable of overcoming the effects of distracting elements when attempting to differentiate relevant aspects of a particular situation

Field internship   The portion of required training during which a student obtains a supervised learning experience on a licensed prehospital emergency care unit

Formative evaluation   The measurement of student achievement before, during, and after instruction for the purpose of planning instruction or assessing student progress

Frequency distribution   A table that summarizes how often each score on a test occurs

Fun   An enjoyable or pleasurable experience; a source of amusement or merriment

Game   Any form of play, amusement, or recreation involving physical or mental competition under a specific set of rules

Goal structure   The way in which students relate to one another and to the instructor while working toward the attainment of instructional goals; includes cooperative, competitive, and individualistic goal structures

Grammatical clue   A flaw in wording or punctuation that directs the examinee to the correct answer

Group discussion   An "open forum" of group interaction to talk about problem solving issues

Guessing   A conjecture, often at random, made when the correct answer to a question is not known

Halo effect   An effect that can enter into the scoring of essay items, whereby there is a tendency to give higher scores to those known to be good students and lower scores to those known to be poor students, independent of the quality of responses

Handicapped   A term describing individuals who have a physical disability or behavioral characteristic so severe that they are hindered in educational situations and require special assistance to profit from instruction

Harassment   The act of troubling, worrying, or tormenting by repeated attacks or actions

Hearing-impaired   An individual with a hearing loss significant enough to require special education or training; the term includes both deaf and hard-of-hearing individuals

Hemisphericity   The identification of two halves of the human brain, each controlling different functions; the right hemisphere appears to be primarily responsible for spatial relationships and imagination, while the left is primarily responsible for verbal abilities and sequencing

Hierarchy of needs   Maslow's classification of human needs

Impulsive   A dimension of conceptual tempo, describing rapid responders who make a moderate number of errors

Instructional goals   Statements describing the major purpose of a training program

Intelligence   The capacity that allows a student to learn, solve problems, and/or interact successfully with his or her environment

Intelligence quotient (IQ)   The ratio of mental age to chronological age, multiplied by 100 (100 x [MA/CA])

Interactive video   The use of a videotape player and a computer interface to function in coordination in order to provide interactive training

Interactivity   A balance of control of learning between instructors and students, resulting in some type of interaction from both

Interface   A card that, when installed into a computer, allows for information contained on a videodisc or videotape to be viewed on a computer screen

Internal locus of control   A feeling of control over one's fate and the belief that effort and reward are connected

Intrinsic motivation   Motivation influenced by personal factors such as satisfaction or enjoyment

Item analysis   The process of analyzing single test questions

LCD panel   A device that allows text and graphic information to be displayed from a personal computer onto a large screen or wall, using a standard overhead projector as the light source; allows large groups of people to view the computer display and images at one time

Learning style   Similar to cognitive styles, these are individual differences that influence the way in which a student learns and processes information

Learning   An active process of communication between students and instructors, resulting in the gaining of knowledge and mastering of information; results in a relatively permanent change or modification in behavior as a result of experience or training

Learning Deficiency   A problem that inhibits the learning process; may be behavioral, emotional, or physical

Learning disabilities   A wide variety of disorders in which a student has learning problems that cannot be attributed to emotional difficulties, retardation, or sensory impairment

Learning style   Individual differences that influence learning in classroom situations

Lesson plan   A detailed outline of the objectives, content, procedures, techniques, and evaluation of a single instructional session

Libel   A false and malicious written or printed statement, or any sign or picture that accuses another of immoral or unlawful conduct, thereby exposing an individual to public ridicule, or injures an individual's reputation in any way

Locus of control   An individual's perception of whom is responsible for the outcome of events and behavior in their lives

Longevity   A learning principle stating that reinforcement and practice leads to retention of information and skills

Long-term memory   The part of information processing system that retains encoded information for long periods

Malpractice   Unprofessional treatment or neglect, misconduct, or improper practice in any professional or official position

Mastery learning   An instructional strategy that allows students to study material until they master it

Matching format   A test item consisting of a two-column format—item and response—that requires students to make a correspondence between the two

Mean   An arithmetic average of a group of scores

Median   The midpoint in a distribution; the 50th percentile

Megabyte   One million bytes of information

Megahertz (MHz)   Millions of cycles per second, referring to the speed of a microprocessor unit of a computer

Metacognition   Knowledge of one's own cognitive processes and the ability to regulate those processes

Mnemonic   Technique that links new data and visual images or semantic knowledge in order to improve recall of information

Mode   A measure of the most frequently occurring score on an examination

Multimedia   The integration of more than one form of medium, often referring to the use of multiple forms of media centrally controlled and coordinated, usually by a computer

Multiple-choice format   A test format in which the examinee selects the correct answer from a list of possible options

Multi-screen   The projection of images onto several image areas

National standard curriculum   The current edition of a specific national training program adopted by the Department of Transportation, and amendments or revision thereto

Negative reinforcement   The termination of an unpleasant stimulus immediately following a behavior, thereby increasing the probability of such future behavior

Negative skewness   Asymmetry of test scores in which most scores in a distribution are high

Negligence   Failure to use a reasonable amount of care resulting in injury or damage to another

Noise   Anything that interferes with the accurate transmission of a message

Normal distribution   A bell-shaped, symmetric distribution of scores, normally found in test results

Normal distribution curve   A symmetric distribution of test scores in which most scores lie in the center and scores decline in frequency as they move away from the center

Norm-referenced evaluation   A rating based on a student's performance when compared with the performance of others on the same exam

Objective   A statement regarding the specific changes educators intend to produce in student behavior as a result of instruction

Oral tests   Exams in which both questions an answers are given out loud

Overcorrection   An attempt to decrease inappropriate student behaviors by requiring a student who has disturbed the environment, physically or emotionally, to restore it not only to its original form, but beyond

Overlearning   Continuing practice or drill to the point at which a skill becomes an automatic

Paradigm   A pattern, example or model that describes the boundaries by which one lives; it is within such boundaries that a student looks at situations or ideas that are most comfortable; similar to "tunnel vision," it is often beneficial to look at issues from a different perspective

Pedagogy   The methodology of formalized education of children

Perceptual modalities   Any one of the sensory channels through which a student receives information

Performance   The behavior a student should be able to perform as a result of training, relative to instructional objectives

Performance test   A non-paper and non-pencil test that requires students to engage in some type of process or skill performance

Positive skewness   Asymmetry of test scores in which most scores in a distribution are low

Positive reinforcement   The immediate response to a behavior that increases or maintains the probability or rate of the continuance of a particular behavior

Preceptor   An individual who evaluates a student's performance in a prehospital or in-hospital clinical facility

Primacy   The way you learn something the first time is the way you learn it best

Probing   A strategy of trying to get a student to reach a correct answer; may involve restating the question or asking related questions to help the student

Programmed learning   An instructional procedure in which material is arranged in a particular sequence and in small steps; programs require students to respond and provides immediate evaluation and feedback

Prompting   The presentation of additional stimuli to increase the probability an appropriate response will occur

Psychomotor domain   Another of three domains of learning, primarily affecting the physical ability to perform skills or other type movement

Punishment   The presentation of an unpleasant stimulus that decreases the future rate and/or probability of the recurrence of a particular behavior

Puzzle   A question or problem that exercises one's mind to test cleverness, skill, or knowledge

Range   The difference between the highest and lowest scores in a distribution

Reading difficulty   The level of reading ability required to understand test questions

Recency   A learning principle stating that what a student learns last is what he or she will most likely remember

Recitation   The term referring to a series of questions teachers ask to elicit student responses

Reflective   A dimension of conceptual tempo describing students who are slower to respond, thereby tending to make fewer errors

Relevance   The correlation between test items and the content area to be assessed

Reliability   The extent to which a test is consistent in measuring what it is intended to measure

Resolution   The clarity or graininess of a video or computer image as measured by lines or pixels; the smallest resolvable detail in the image

Response-cost procedures   A type of behavior modification strategy that involves the presentation of a positive reinforcer for appropriate behavior and the removal of a reinforcer for inappropriate behavior

Reward   An object, stimulus, or outcome that is perceived as being pleasant

Rote learning   The learning of disconnected or arbitrary verbal material (eg, a list of chronological information)

Self-actualization   Maslow's term for the psychological need to develop one's capabilities and potential in order to enhance personal growth

Self-concept   The total organization of perception that an individual has of himself; often used interchangeably with self-esteem

Self-efficacy   The belief that one can successfully execute the behavior required to produce a particular outcome

Self-esteem   The value or judgement an individual places on his or her behavior; often used interchangeably with self-concept

Self-fulfilling prophecy   A phenomenon in which an instructor's expectations lead to differential behavior by the instructor toward certain students; the teacher's attitude may help produce the "expected" behavior in the students

Shaping   A technique whereby students are taught to perform complex behaviors by analyzing the desired behavior and dividing it into small, easily identifiable behaviors that can be readily reinforced

Short-answer format   A test item for which the student must provide a brief response to the stem questions, usually consisting of a word or phrase

Short-term memory   The part of information processing in which conscious mental activity is carried out; in-

formation is held in short-term memory for only a few seconds

Simulation   A well-defined exercise designed to make a practice session as realistic as possible

Slides   A piece of film, usually containing an image, which when projected through a light source is enlarged and viewed from the screen; refers to the traditional 2 x 2 inch 35-mm film or overhead transparency film

Slide show presentation   A feature offered by some presentation software packages that allows for slides to be shown automatically on the computer screen, in either a predetermined sequence or at random

Socioeconomic status (SES)   A ranking to determine social position in a society; in the United States, SES is determined by objective indices such as occupation, educational background, and material resources

SQ3R system   A system for improving comprehension and retention of text material; students are encouraged to Survey material, develop Questions about it, Read and Review the test and, finally, practice Recalling the important points of the text

Standard deviation   A measure of the spread of scores around the mean of the distribution

Standard of care   The level of conduct expected of similarly trained professionals in a given field

Standardized test   A test commercially prepared by measurement experts who have carefully studied all test items used in a large number of training programs

Stem   The portion of a multiple-choice test item that consists of an incomplete statement or question and is followed by a list of options

Storyboard   A visual outline of media design

Stress   An unpleasant personal condition produced by a stimulus

S-VHS (Super-VHS)   A videotape format that provides for better resolution and less noise than standard VHS tapes

Task analysis   The identification of subordinate skills and knowledge that students must acquire in order to achieve educational objectives

Taxonomy of educational objectives   A classification system that divides objectives into three domains: the affective, cognitive, and psychomotor

Teaching   A system of actions intended to induce learning

Test   A measurement containing a series of questions, each of which has a correct answer

Test anxiety   A psychological state of stress caused by a testing situation

Test bank   A set of test questions from which exams can be created to match course objectives

Training   The process of acquiring specific knowledge and skills necessary to perform a skill or task; common in the industry in order to prepare workers for specific tasks; designed to affect performance by teaching skills

Training institute   An educational institution approved by state or other regulatory authorities to provide emergency medical services training

True-false format   A test format in which examinees indicate whether a statement is correct (true) or incorrect (false)

Validity   The extent to which a test measures what it is intended to measure

VHS (Video home system)   The most popular 1/2-inch consumer videotape format

Videoconferencing   The use of a specialized audio-visual system and satellite telecommunications, which allows for groups at remote locations to participate in the same meeting or seminar at the same time

Virtual reality   An extensive gamut of technologies used in an attempt to merge physical senses and actions with computer-generated images in order to create a perception of realism

Visual impairment   A difficulty in clearly distinguishing forms or discriminating details by sight at a specific distance, resulting in the need for special methods and materials

Vivacy   A learning principle stating the more vivid the experience, the more likely the student is to learn and remember it

BIBLIOGRAPHY

Alberto P, Troutman A. *Applied Behavior Analysis for Teachers,* 3rd ed. New York; Macmillan Publishing Co.; 1990.

Barbe W, Swassing H, Milone M. *Teaching Through Modality Strengths.* Columbus, OH: Zaner-Bloser, Inc.; 1979.

Bard R. *Trainer's Professional Development Book.* San Francisco: Jossey-Bass; 1987.

Bergeron R. The uses of colors to enhance training communications. *Performance and Instruction.* 1990; August:34–37.

Birnbauer H. *Training for Trainers: Increasing the Effectiveness of On-the-Job Training Instructors.* Bensalem, PA: Institute for Business and Industry; 1981.

Bjorklund D. *Children's Thinking: Developmental Function and Individual Differences.* Pacific Grove, CA: Brooks/Cole; 1990.

Bloom B, Englehart N, Furst E, Hill W, Krathwohl D. *Taxonomy of Educational Objectives: Handbook I, Cognitive Domain.* New York: McKay; 1956.

Borsook T, Higginbotham-Wheat N. *Interactivity: what is it and what can it do for computer-based instruction?* Educational Technology. 1991; October:11–17.

Bourn S. *Building Blocks for the Adult Learner.* Paper presented at the EMS Today Conference; Albuquerque, NM; April 1990.

Butler K. *Learning and Teaching Style in Theory and Practice.* Maynard, MA: Gabriel Systems; 1986.

Carkhuff R, Pierce R. *Training Delivery Skills II: Making the Training Delivery.* Amherst, MA: Human Resources Development Press; 1984.

Carliner S. *The six deadly sins of educational communication.* Performance and Instruction. 1991; November/December:29–32.

Caroline N. *Workbook in Emergency Medical Treatment: Review Problems for EMTs.* Boston: Little Brown and Company; 1982.

Carr C. *Is virtual reality virtually here?* Training and Development. 1992; October:37–41.

Cates W. *Fifteen principles for designing more effective instructional hypermedia/multimedia products.* Educational Technology. 1992; December:5–17.

Cherry R. *Keeping the spark alive.* JEMS. 1990; March: 62–65.

Conti G, Welborn R. *Teaching-learning styles and the adult learner.* Lifelong Learning. 1986; June:20–24.

Davenport J III, Davenport JA. *Andragogical-Pedagogical orientations of adult learners.* Lifelong Learning. 1986; September:58–59.

Davis L. *Planning, Conducting and Evaluating Workshops.* Austin, TX: Learning Concepts; 1974.

Dembo M. *Applying Educational Psychology in the Classroom.* White Plains, NY: Longman Publishing Group; 1991.

Dillon JT. *Research on questioning and discussion.* Educational Leadership. 1984; November:50–56.

Dunn R, Dunn K. *Practical Approaches to Individualizing Instruction.* West Nyack, NY: Parker;1972.

Edwards B. *Drawing on the Right Side of the Brain.* New York: St. Martin's Press; 1989.

Effective Training: A Guide for the Company Instructor. Intext, Inc; 1979.

EMT-Basic National Standard Curriculum; Department of Transportation;1994.

Eyres P. *Keeping the training department out of court.* Training. 1990; September:59–67.

Faulkner L. *Invincible Visual Job Aids.* Huntsville, AL: Faulkner Consulting Services; 1991.

Feuer D, Geber B. *Uh-oh. . . second thoughts about adult learning theory.* Training. 1988; December:31–39.

Friedman P, Yarbrough E. *Training Strategies from Start to Finish.* Englewood Cliffs, NJ: Prentice Hall; 1985.

Galbraith MW. *Adult Learning Methods*. Malaba, FL: Krieger Publishing; 1991.

Galbreath J. *The educational buzzword of the 1990's: multimedia, or is it hypermedia, or. . . ?* Educational Technology. 1992; April:15–19.

Gall M. *Synthesis of research on teacher's questioning*. Educational Leadership. 1984; November:40–46.

Garger S, Guild P. *Learning styles: the crucial differences*. Curriculum Review. 1984; 23:9–12.

Courseware GP. *Designing and Maintaining Instructional Programs*. Columbia, MD: General Physics Corporation; 1983.

Courseware GP. *Principles of Instructional Design*. Columbia, MD: General Physics Corporation; 1983.

Guild P, Garger S. *Marching to Different Drummers*. Alexandria, VA: Association for Supervision and Curriculum Development; 1985.

Gustafson C. *Increased stimulation with audiovisual aids in training*. JEMS. 1985; June:59–62.

Head J. *Instructor's Resource Manual: Emergency Care*. Englewood Cliffs: NJ; The Brady Company; 1990.

Helsel S. *Virtual reality and education*. Educational Technology. 1992; May:38–42.

Heron J. *The Facilitator's Handbook*. New York: Nichols Publishing; 1989.

Herrmann, N. *The Creative Brain*. Lake Lure, NC: Brain Books; 1988.

International Association of Fire Fighters (IAFF). *Hazardous Materials Instructor Training*. Washington, DC: IAFF; 1993.

James W, Galbraith M. *Perception learning styles: implications and techniques for the practitioner*. Lifelong Learning. 1985; January:20–23.

Kagen J, Rosman B, Day D, Albert J, Phillips W. *Information processing in the child: significance of analytic and reflective attitudes*. Psychological Monographs. 1964;78 (1, Whole No. 578).

Keirsey D, Bates M. *Please Understand Me*. Del Mar, CA: Prometheus Nemesis Book Company; 1984.

Kennedy Jr W. *Joggin' the noggin': developing memory aids for students*. JEMS 1990; October:85–88.

Knowles MS. *The Adult Learner: A Neglected Species*. Houston: Gulf Publishing Company; 1978.

Knowles M. *Andragogy in Action: Applying Modern Principles of Adult Learning*. San Francisco, CA: Jossey-Bass; 1984.

Krathwohl D, Bloom B, Masia B. *Taxonomy of Educational Strategies and Tactics*. Englewood Cliffs, NJ. Educational Technology Publications; 1964.

Laird D. *Approaches to Training and Development*, 2nd ed. Alexandria, VA: American Society for Training and Development; 1985.

Leshin C, Ploock J, Reigeluth C. *Instructional Design Objectives: Handbook II. Affective Domain*. New York: McKay; 1992.

Lierman B. *How to develop a training simulation*. Training and Development. 1994; February:50–52.

Mager R. *Developing Attitude Toward Learning*. Belmont, CA: Lake Publishing Company; 1984.

Mager R. *Preparing Instructional Objectives*, 2nd ed. Belmont, CA: Lake Publishing Company; 1984.

Magney J. *Game-based teaching*. The Education Digest, 1990; 55(5):54–57.

Malamed C. *Tapping into the mind: how to design graphics to be remembered*. AV Video. 1991; September:60–63.

Margolis F, Bell C. *Instructing for Results*. San Diego: University Assocaites, Inc. Pfeiffer & Co., and Minneapolis, MN: Lakewood Publications; 1986.

McAteer P. *Almost like on-the-job training*. Training and Development. 1991; October:19–24.

McCarthy B. *Using the 4MAT system to bring learning styles to schools*. Educational Leadership. 1990; 48(2):31–37.

McCarthy B. *What 4MAT training teaches us about staff development*. Educational Leadership. 1985; April:61–68.

McCarthy B. *The 4MAT System: Teaching to Learning Styles with Right/Left Mode Techniques*. Barrington, IL: Excel, Inc.; 1980.

McLagen P. *Helping Others Learn: Designing Programs for Adults*. Reading, MA: Addison-Wesley; 1978.

NEA Higher Education Advocate. *Newsletter for NEA Members in Higher Education*. May 9, 1988. Volume V, Number 11.

Newstrom JW, Lengnick-Hall ML. *One size does not fit all*. Training and Development. 1991; June:43–48.

Newstrom J, Scannel E. *Games Trainers Play*. New York: McGraw-Hill; 1980.

Newstrom J, Scannel E. *More Games Trainers Play*. New York: McGraw-Hill; 1984.

Newstrom J, Scannel E. *Still More Games Trainers Play*. New York: McGraw-Hill; 1986.

Pantilidis V. *Virtual reality in the classroom*. Educational Technology. 1993; April:23–27.

Pennsylvania Department of Health, Division of EMS *Emergency Medical Services Study Guide*. Harrisburg, PA: Pennsylvania Department of Health; 1990.

Porter R. *Learning it by living it: bring realism to EMS training*. JEMS. 1987; December:39–41.

Schlenger P. *Video visuals*. Training and Development. 1991; June:59–66.

Shaw M. *Group Dynamics: The Psychology of Small Group Behavior*. New York: McGraw-Hill; 1976.

Shea G. *Managing a Difficult or Hostile Audience*. Englewood Cliffs, NJ: Prentice-Hall; 1984.

Slack K. *Training for the real thing*. Training and Development. 1993; May:79–89.

Smith J. *Using models, mock-ups and simulators.* Training. 1978; December:97–98.

Strauss R. *Multimedia for the masses: designing for the TV screen.* AV Video. 1992; February:48–58.

Teaching Improvement Project Systems For Health Care Educators (TIPS). Lexington. KY: Center for Learning Resources, College of Allied Health Professionals, University of Kentucky.

Tubesing N, Tubesing D. *Structured Exercises in Health Management.* Duluth, MN: While Person Press; 1990.

United States Copyright Office. *Copyright Basics* (Document No. 1989–241–429 80.045.) Washington, DC: U.S. Government Printing Office; 1989.

Veilleux R. *Video production with fewer errors.* Training and Development. 1991; June:67–72.

Verduin J JR, Miller H, Greer C. *Adults Teaching Adults.* Austin, TX: Learning Concepts; 1977.

Weirsma W, Jurs S. *Educational Measurement and Testing.* Boston: Allyn and Bacon, Inc.; 1985.

Witkin H, Goodenough D. *Cognitive Styles: Essence and Origins.* New York: International Universities Press, Inc.; 1981.

Wlodowski R. *Enhancing Adult Motivation to Learn.* San Francisco, CA: Jossey-Bass; 1985.

Zemke R. *Learning to listen to trainees.* Training. 1977; July.

Zemke R, Zemke S. 30 *Things we know for sure about adult training.* Training. 1988; July:57–61.

Zimmerman G, Owen J, Seibert D. *Speech Communications,* 2nd ed. St. Paul, MN: West Publishing Company; 1980.

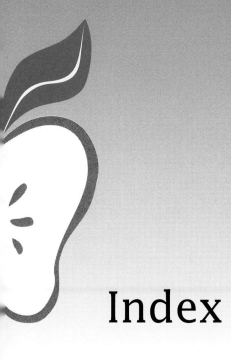

Index